D1727115

ATHEROSCLEROSIS REVIEWS
Volume 23

Atherosclerosis
Its Pathogenesis and the Role of Cholesterol

Atherosclerosis Reviews

Chief Editors: Antonio M. Gotto and Rodolfo Paoletti

Atherosclerosis Reviews
Volume 23

Atherosclerosis
Its Pathogenesis and the Role of Cholesterol

Editors

Peter C. Weber, M.D.
Universität München
Institut für Prophylaxe und
*   Epidemiologie der Kreislaufkrankheiten*
München, F.R.G.

Alexander Leaf, M.D.
Departments of Medicine and
*   Preventive Medicine*
Harvard Medical School
Massachusetts General Hospital
Boston, Massachusetts

Raven Press New York

Raven Press, 1185 Avenue of the Americas, New York, New York 10036

Made in the United States of America

Library of Congress Cataloging-in-Publication Data

Atherosclerosis: its pathogenesis and the role of cholesterol!
    editors, Peter C. Weber, Alexander Leaf.
        p.   cm.—(Atherosclerosis reviews; v. 23)
    "Contains the presentations at the Second Bayer AG "International Workshop on Atherosclerosis," held in Faro, Portugal, on November 27–December 2, 1990"—Pref.
    Includes bibliographical references and index.
    ISBN 0-88167-868-6
    1. Atherosclerosis—Pathogenesis—Congresses.   2. Cholesterol—
Pathophysiology—Congresses.   I. Weber, Peter C.   II. Leaf, Alexander, 1920–.
    III. Bayer AG "International Workshop on Atherosclerosis" (2nd: 1990: Faro, Portugal) IV. Series.
    [DNLM: 1. Atherosclerosis—etiology—congresses.
    2. Atherosclerosis—physiopathology—congresses.   3. Cholesterol—congresses.
    W1 AT385 v. 23/WG 550 A8684 1990]
    RC692.A729 vol. 23
    616.1'36 s—dc20
    [616.1'36]
    DNLM/DLC
    for Library of Congress   91-33779
                                                                               CIP

9 8 7 6 5 4 3 2 1

Contents

Atherosclerosis Reviews, Volume 23,
edited by P. C. Weber and A. Leaf.
Raven Press, Ltd., New York © 1991.

Preface

This book contains the proceedings of the second Bayer AG International Workshop on Atherosclerosis held in Faro, Portugal, November 27 through December 2, 1990. The contributions cover important aspects of the pathophysiology of atherosclerosis with a focus on the regulation of cholesterol and lipoproteins and their role in the pathogenesis of the disease. The summaries and reviews on plaque formation and progression; the cellular biology, genetics, and nutritional modification of lipoproteins, cholesterol, and fatty acids; as well as on lipid and peptide mediators of inflammation and cellular proliferation are presented by an expert panel of leading scientists in their field.

The paper of Dr. Weizel addresses practical problems in dealing with patients with hypercholesterolemia, but as organizers of the Workshop we would like to make a few comments in the interests of balancing Weizel's view. The clinical trials mentioned in his contribution had as their end points mortality figures. It is correct that differences in mortality were nonexistent or very small in these risk factor intervention trials, and this has led to calculations showing that the observed reductions of total cholesterol levels may increase life expectancy by a few weeks to a few months. It is also correct that the incidence of coronary events was very low (9.8% in the Lipids Research Clinics study and 4.1% in the Helsinki Heart study). However, in developed countries where life expectancy is already approaching the biologic limit of the human life span, no intervention to prevent disease will any longer importantly increase life expectancy.

Thus, the success of preventive interventions should be judged not on mortality figures but on morbidity. How we can be kept healthier, more vigorous, and active as long as the biologic limit of life permits, should be the measure of success of preventive measures. Diet is very important in this regard. The recommendations that we should eat a diet containing less saturated fats and cholesterol and reduce total fat intake deserves the support of all.

As to whom should, in addition, be treated by medications that is another matter. We believe that closer attention should be paid to the family history and targeting those for further investigations of cholesterol levels whose parents or siblings suffered coronary heart disease by age 55. This will extend the preventive net to a high-risk group without overextending expensive screening procedures. However, we do not agree that potent cholesterol-lowering medications can replace the need for the recommended dietary changes as they do not correct imbalances in dietary fats that are so prevalent in Western diets.

A better understanding of the key events initiating the atherogenic process and of the factors determining the natural course of atherosclerosis and its clinical manifestations will lead to the development of better strategies to prevent the disease and to the design of improved pharmacological modalities to intervene in a more causal way with the disease process.

At the Workshop, several presentations indicated that there may be other steps in the complex atherogenic processes at which interventions may be effectively targetted to prevent or regress the disease. Thus, preventing endothelial dysfunction, blocking oxidation of low-density lipoprotein (LDL) particles, interfering with release of growth factors and actions, and modulating the inflammatory response at the site of vessel injury and repair may all be effective new ways to cope with the disease process—in addition to current approaches such as lowering LDL cholesterol and triglyceride levels, inhibiting platelet function, lowering blood pressure, and normalizing glucose metabolism.

It is the aim of this and subsequent workshops to provide an overview of the progress in an important field of atherosclerosis research. Furthermore, it is our hope that this series of workshops will stimulate interaction among investigators studying atherosclerosis from either experimental or clinical approaches. We wish that this volume—as did the first one—also serves a useful function for a broader audience.

Peter C. Weber, M.D.
Alexander Leaf, M.D.

Acknowledgments

On behalf of all participants in the International Workshop on Atherosclerosis titled "Atherosclerosis—Its Pathogenesis and the Role of Cholesterol," held in Faro, Portugal, November 27–December 2, 1990, we thank Bayer AG for making the workshop possible. We are especially grateful to Dr. Jürgen Fritsch and Dr. Gunther Thomas for their invaluable contribution to the success of the workshop.

Atherosclerosis Reviews, Volume 23,
edited by P. C. Weber and A. Leaf.
Raven Press, Ltd., New York © 1991.

Cholesterol Transport in Lipoproteins

Richard J. Havel

Cardiovascular Research Institute, University of California,
San Francisco, California 94143-0130

Cholesterol transported in plasma lipoproteins is the precursor of cholesterol deposited in the arterial intima as an essential ingredient of the atherosclerotic plaque. In spite of much research and numerous recent observations, we do not yet have a comprehensive picture of the rates of cholesterol transport in plasma lipoproteins or a complete picture of the regulation of the processes by which cholesterol is transported in the blood. This is not to say that there are not some aspects of cholesterol transport that we understand reasonably well, but rather that we lack some crucial bits of information needed to develop a comprehensive understanding of how plasma cholesterol transport contributes to cholesterol homeostasis.

DIETARY CHOLESTEROL TRANSPORT

Dietary cholesterol is transported from the intestinal mucosa through the lymphatic system to the blood. This cholesterol is carried in chylomicrons (CYM) mainly as cholesteryl esters (CE) synthesized by acyl CoA acyl transferase (ACAT) in the mucosal cells; these are carried in the core of CYM particles together with dietary triglycerides (TG). After the bulk of the TG have been removed by the action of lipoprotein lipase in extrahepatic tissues (mainly adipose tissue and striated muscles), the CE—which remain with the resulting CYM "remnant"—are taken up chiefly by the liver via endocytosis into hepatocytes (12). The endocytic pathway for CYM, which resembles that for low-density lipoproteins (LDL) in the liver, is very efficient. The hepatic uptake system differs from that for LDL in a crucial respect: it does not appear to be down-regulated to any extent by accumulation of cholesterol in the hepatocyte (1)—an observation that suggests that the receptor for CYM remnants may be distinct from that for LDL. Although there is considerable evidence that CYM remnants bind to the LDL receptor (15,17), this view is supported by observations that show that the metabolism of chylomicron CE is little affected in rabbits (17) and humans (27) homozygous for mutations that greatly impair the function of the LDL receptor. The hypothesis that a receptor distinct from the LDL receptor is responsible for the endocytosis of CYM remnants has received considerable impetus from the discovery by Herz et al. of an LDL receptor-related protein (LRP) (14). LRP is an abundant protein on the surface of hepatocytes; like the LDL receptor, it is evidently a recycling receptor (13,24). Recently, LRP—a very large protein that spans the plasma membrane—has been shown to be the receptor for α_2 macroglobulin, a plasma protein that is thought to mediate the removal of proteases from the blood (22,29). The observation that CYM remnant removal is seriously impaired in humans with mutations of apolipoprotein (apo) E that impair its binding to the LDL receptor (28) is consistent with the notion that LRP (as well as the LDL receptor) recognize CYM remnants by binding to apoE. Chylomicron remnants and other lipoproteins rich in apoE do bind, albeit weakly, to LRP in ligand blots (24), but there is as yet no direct evidence that LRP has a major role in CYM remnant catabolism *in vivo.*

Our recent observations suggest that, as compared with LDL, the endocytosis of CYM remnants into hepatocytes of normal rats is delayed after initial removal of the particles from the blood (16). No such delay is observed in rats in which LDL receptors have been greatly increased by administration of 17-α-ethinyl estradiol for several days (15). We have postulated that endocytosis of CYM remnants in estradiol-treated rats is mediated chiefly by the LDL receptor, whereas a separate receptor contributes significantly to endocytosis of CYM remnants in normal rats.

Kowal et al. have observed that large β–very-low-density lipoproteins (β-VLDL) from cholesterol-fed rabbits, enriched in CE and apoE, interact poorly with LRP on fibroblasts from subjects with a null mutation of the LDL receptor; however, when the β-VLDL have been further enriched by addition of more apoE, the particles bind strongly to LRP in ligand blots and are readily endocytosed (20). They have suggested that LRP interacts specifically with particles containing a large number of apoE molecules.

Having observed that apoE is present on the microvillous plasma membrane surface of normal rat hepatocytes (10), from which it can be released by heparin or suramin, we have postulated that this apoE binds to CYM remnants, making them susceptible to strong interaction with LRP and leading to endocytosis. A number of years ago, we showed that C apoproteins can impair the hepatic uptake of CYM remnants or of CYM to which apoE had been added (30); a similar phenomenon has been observed by Kowal et al. for β-VLDL (21). Thus, C apoproteins can inhibit the endocytosis of apoE-enriched β-VLDL into fibroblasts from subjects with null mutations of the LDL receptor. These observations are consistent with, but do not establish, the role of LRP as a CYM remnant receptor. In addition, LRP in hepatocytes is not down-regulated by dietary cholesterol (23), as expected for a CYM remnant receptor.

Although the liver readily takes up dietary cholesterol, even in large amounts owing to apparent lack of down-regulation, the consequences of hepatic cholesterol uptake by this route vary widely among mammalian species. The rat liver readily excretes dietary cholesterol, mainly as bile acids, and the function of its LDL receptor remains unimpaired during cholesterol feeding, so that cholesterol does not accumulate in the blood (18). In the rabbit and several other species, including some nonhuman primates, excretion of dietary cholesterol by the liver is less efficient, so that CE (synthesized by ACAT and stored in oil droplets) accumulate, and hepatocytic LDL receptors are down-regulated (19). This has two effects. First, the lipoproteins (VLDL) synthesized and exported by the liver become enriched in CE. Second, the partially catabolized VLDL (VLDL remnants) accumulate in the blood because LDL receptors have been down-regulated. This phenomenon is most striking in rabbits, which have a very limited capacity to convert dietary cholesterol to bile acids. Interestingly, in a strain of rabbits that has a much lower tendency to develop hypercholesterolemia in response to dietary cholesterol, excretion of bile acids increases much more when cholesterol-rich diets are fed (26). Humans vary considerably in the extent to which dietary cholesterol increases plasma cholesterol levels, and there is some evidence that hyperresponsive individuals fail to reduce hepatic cholesterol synthesis appropriately (11). Whether they also have less capacity to increase bile acid synthesis is unclear.

ENDOGENOUS CHOLESTEROL TRANSPORT

In humans, most CE in the blood are in LDL, and it has been generally thought that these CE are produced by lecithin-cholesterol acyltransferase (LCAT) (7). This view may require some modification. LDL are derived chiefly from VLDL, and recent studies suggest that nascent VLDL may contain appreciable CE derived from hepatic ACAT (2,5). These esters are primarily cholesterol oleate, whereas LDL CE are predominantly cholesteryl linoleate, which is the main product of LCAT action in human blood plasma. LDL, however, circulate for days, during which their CE fatty acid composition can be modified by exchange of CE among lipoprotein species, leading to a predominance of cholesteryl linoleate, originally produced by LCAT. This exchange is made possible by the action of plasma cholesteryl ester transfer protein (CETP) acting upon species of high-density lipoproteins (HDL), as described below. There is no doubt that LCAT does contribute to LDL CE. In normal individuals, LDL contain more CE per particle than VLDL (5). Thus, during their lifetime, CE are acquired in a net sense from HDL, in addition to equilibration of CE species by CETP.

LCAT is thought to be the key enzyme of the pathway of reverse cholesterol transport, by which cholesterol in extrahepatic tissues is returned to the liver for excretion into the bile. LCAT, however, can utilize cholesterol preexisting in plasma lipoproteins as well as cholesterol transferred from cells to HDL, the site of LCAT action. We have no direct information on the fraction of the LCAT-substrate cholesterol derived from plasma lipoproteins or from cells—information required to estimate the magnitude of reverse cholesterol transport.

Recently, evidence has been obtained that cellular and plasma cholesterol used by LCAT to make plasma CE are channelled in distinct pathways. In model systems in which cultured cells are exposed to plasma, cellular cholesterol is transferred preferentially to a species of small HDL particles with pre-β mobility (6). These particles appear to fuse with each other to yield a larger form of pre-β HDL [which may resemble the discoidal HDL species that have been identified in rat liver perfusates as "nascent HDL" (9)]. These larger pre-β HDL associate with LCAT in a particle that also contains apoD, and these particles are the site of esterification of cell-derived CE. The newly formed esters are then transferred to other lipoproteins by CETP.

By contrast, cholesterol carried in LDL that is utilized by LCAT is first transferred to large α-migrating HDL and then to smaller α-HDL, where it is esterified (25). The extent to which cell-derived and lipoprotein-derived CE are transferred to VLDL and LDL also appears to differ. Whereas most cell-derived CE are transferred to HDL of α mobility, plasma-derived CE are transferred to a greater extent to VLDL and LDL. Thus, the latter would be available for uptake by the liver via the LDL receptor pathway, whereas the former would be taken up directly from HDL. The latter process is poorly understood. Most of the cell-derived cholesterol is transferred to particles that lack apoE and hence may not be taken up via the LDL receptor. In rats and some other mammals, HDL CE can be taken up by the liver and some other tissues by a pathway that does not involve removal of the protein component of HDL from the blood ("selective uptake" pathway) (7). The extent to which this pathway operates in humans *in vivo* is unclear; cell-derived CE may eventually be transferred to VLDL and LDL before they are removed from the blood. The fact that cell-derived CE tend to remain within α-migrating HDL is, however, consistent with the hypothesis that the concentration of cholesterol (mainly esters) in HDL is a function of the rate of reverse cholesterol transport. Nevertheless, there is no direct evidence of this relationship.

A number of mammals lack an active CETP in their blood. It seems likely that the pathways utilized by these species to carry out reverse cholesterol transport are quantitatively and perhaps qualitatively different from those in which this pathway is active, such as humans and rabbits. The rat represents a species that lacks an active CETP. It has been clear for many years that the CE in rat VLDL are produced by hepatocytic ACAT and delivered with the nascent VLDL particle into the blood (4,8). These CE (mainly cholesteryl oleate) are rapidly returned to the liver as a component of VLDL remnants, as few VLDL particles are normally converted to LDL in this species (4). The function of this liver-plasma-liver CE cycle is not known; in any event, VLDL CE do not appear to contribute to reverse cholesterol transport in the rat.

Recent studies have shown that nascent VLDL in hepatocytic Golgi compartments of the rat contain little unesterified cholesterol as compared with plasma VLDL, in which the content of unesterified cholesterol is considerably higher (8). Hepatic VLDL acquire cholesterol from erythrocytes during incubation *in vitro* (4). If this transfer occurs *in vivo,* the uptake of unesterified cholesterol into the liver during the endocytosis of VLDL remnants could make a significant contribution to reverse cholesterol transport because erythrocytic cholesterol may be enriched during exposure to endothelial cells, which in turn could acquire cholesterol by transfer from parenchymal cells in various tissues.

The extent to which cellular and plasma cholesterol used by LCAT are channeled in the rat is not known; but given the selective uptake pathway in the liver demonstrated in this species, HDL alone may mediate LCAT-dependent reverse cholesterol transport. It is unclear how the CE that enter cells, including the hepatocyte, via selective uptake are hydrolyzed and used by the cell. Recent studies in which rats have been transfected with the gene for human apoA-I, the major protein component of HDL, suggest that HDL containing the human protein are unable to mediate selective uptake of CE (3). If this intriguing observation is confirmed, differences in reverse cholesterol transport among species with and without an active CETP may be even greater than those that have been considered here.

SUMMARY

Cholesterol entering the blood from different sites is channeled through distinct pathways. Dietary cholesterol, transported in CYM chiefly as CE, is delivered efficiently to the liver and contributes little to the pool of circulating cholesterol. However, to the extent that it is retained in the liver, CYM cholesterol contributes to down-regulation of hepatic LDL receptors and thus has an important indirect effect in raising the concentration of cholesterol in VLDL and especially LDL. Hepatic cholesterol enters the blood chiefly as CE contained within VLDL; most of these esters are returned to the liver with VLDL remnants or LDL, and they do not contribute to the transport of extrahepatic cholesterol to the liver (reverse cholesterol transport). The pathway for reverse cholesterol transport appears to differ substantially among mammals that have or lack an active plasma cholesteryl ester transfer protein. In humans, with an active transfer protein, CE produced by plasma LCAT from cell-derived cholesterol are transferred from pre-β HDL, upon which they are produced, chiefly to α-migrating HDL species. By contrast, CE produced from lipoprotein cholesterol are synthesized on α-migrating HDL, but they are then transferred to a considerable extent to VLDL and LDL, and they can be taken up into the liver with these lipoproteins via the LDL receptor pathway. In the rat, HDL CE can be taken up by the liver selectively without uptake of the entire HDL particle. The extent to which this pathway is utilized in humans is unclear.

Increasing the uptake of plasma CE contained in VLDL and LDL via the LDL receptor pathway reduces the concentration of potentially atherogenic lipoprotein species in the blood, but the available data do not permit a conclusion that this reduction is accompanied by a more efficient reverse cholesterol transport. Although the concentration of CE in HDL could reflect the rate of esterification of cellular cholesterol by LCAT, this relationship has yet to be verified.

ACKNOWLEDGMENT

This work was supported in part by National Institutes of Health grant HL14237 Arteriosclerosis SCOR.

REFERENCES

1. Angelin, B., Raviola, C. A., Innerarity, T. I., and Mahley, R. W. (1983): *J. Clin. Invest.,* 71:816–831.
2. Bisgaier, C. L., Siebenkas, M. V., and Brown, M. L., et al. (1991): *J. Lipid Res.,* 32:21–33.
3. Chajek-Shaul, T., Hayek, T., Walsh, A. M., and Breslow, J. L. (1990): *Circulation,* 3:532.
4. Faergeman, O., and Havel, R. J. (1975): *J. Clin. Invest.,* 55:1210–1218.
5. Fielding, P. E., Ishikawa, Y., and Fielding, C. J. (1989): *J. Biol. Chem.,* 264:12462–12466.
6. Francone, O., Gurakar, A., and Fielding, C. J. (1989): *J. Biol. Chem.,* 264:7066–7072.
7. Gotto, A. M. J., Pownall, H. J., and Havel, R. J. (1986): *Methods Enzymol.,* 128:3–41.
8. Hamilton, R. L., Moorehouse, A., and Havel, R. J. (1991): *J. Lipid Res.,* 32:529–543.
9. Hamilton, R. L., Williams, M. C., Fielding, C. J., and Havel, R. J. (1976): *J. Clin. Invest.,* 58:667–680.
10. Hamilton, R. L., Wong, J. S., Guo, L. S. S., Krisans, S., and Havel, R. J. (1990): *J. Lipid Res.,* 31:1590–1603.
11. Havel, R. J. (1983): *Prog. Biochem. Pharmacol.,* 19:111–122.
12. Havel, R. J., and Hamilton, R. L. (1988): *Hepatology,* 8:1689–1704.
13. Herz, J., Kowal, R. C., Ho, Y. K., Brown, M. C., and Goldstein, J. L. (1990): *J. Biol. Chem.,* 265:21355–21362.
14. Herz, J. U. H., Rogne, S., Myklebost, O., Gausepohl, H., and Stanley, K. (1988): *EMBO J.,* 7:4119–4127.
15. Jäckle, S., Brady, S. E., and Havel, R. J. (1989): *Proc. Natl. Acad. Sci. USA,* 86:1880–1884.
16. Jäckle, S., Runquist, E., Brady, S., Hamilton, R. L., and Havel, R. J. (1991): *J. Lipid Res.,* 32:485–498.
17. Kita, T., Goldstein, J. L., Brown, M. S., Watanabe, Y., Hornick, C. A., and Havel, R. J. (1982): *Proc. Natl. Acad. Sci. USA,* 79:3623–3627.
18. Koelz, H. R., Sherrill, B. C., Turley, S. D., and Dietschy, J. M. (1982): *J. Biol. Chem.,* 257:8061–8072.
19. Kovanen, P. T., Brown, M. S., Basu, S. K., Bilheimer, D. W., and Goldstein, J. L. (1981): *Proc. Natl. Acad. Sci. USA,* 78:1396–1400.
20. Kowal, R. C., Herz, J., Goldstein, J. L., Esser, V., and Brown, M. S. (1989): *Proc. Natl. Acad. Sci. USA,* 86:5810–5814.
21. Kowal, R. C., Herz, J., Weisgraber, K. H., Mahley, R. W., Brown, M. S., and Goldstein, J. L. (1990): *J. Biol. Chem.,* 265:10771–10779.
22. Kristensen, T., Moestrup, S. K., Gliemann, J., Bendtsen, L., Sand, O., and Sottrup-Jensen, L. (1990): *FEBS Lett.,* 276:151–155.
23. Kütt, H., Herz, J., and Stanley, K. K. (1989): *Biochim. Biophys. Acta,* 1009:229–236.
24. Lund, H., Takahashi, K., Hamilton, R. L., and Havel, R. J. (1989): *Proc. Natl. Acad. Sci. USA,* 86:9318–9322.
25. Miida, T., Fielding, C. J., and Fielding, P. E. (1990): *Biochemistry,* 29:10469–10474.
26. Overturf, M. L., Smith, S. A., and Gotto, A. M., et al. (1990): *J. Lipid Res.,* 31:2019–2027.
27. Rubinsztein, D. C., Cohen, J. C., Berger, G. M., van der Westhuyzen, D. R., Coetzee, G. A., and Gevers, W. (1990): *J. Clin. Invest.,* 86:1306–1312.
28. Stalenhoef, A. F. H., Malloy, M. J., Kane, J. P., and Havel, R. J. (1986): *J. Clin. Invest.,* 78:722–728.
29. Strickland, D. K., Ashcom, J. D., Williams, S., Burgess, W. H., Migliorini, M., and Argraves, W. C. (1990): *J. Biol. Chem.,* 265:17401–17404.
30. Windler, E., Chao, Y.-S., and Havel, R. J. (1980): *J. Biol. Chem.,* 255:8303–8307.

Atherosclerosis Reviews, Volume 23,
edited by P. C. Weber and A. Leaf.
Raven Press, Ltd., New York © 1991.

Dietary Fatty Acids and the Regulation of Plasma Low-Density Lipoprotein Cholesterol Levels

John M. Dietschy, Laura A. Woollett, and David K. Spady

The University of Texas Southwestern Medical Center, Dallas, Texas 75235-8887

An evolving body of evidence shows that the intake of dietary lipids—both cholesterol and triacylglycerols—is largely responsible for the increased levels of plasma cholesterol carried in low-density lipoproteins (LDL cholesterol). In recent years, there have been major advances in our understanding of how the levels of this lipoprotein fraction are regulated and how specific lipids interact in this regulatory process. This chapter will briefly review how cholesterol and specific fatty acids interact to alter circulating levels of LDL cholesterol and explore a number of factors that may account for a variable response to these lipids in different individuals.

Figure 1 illustrates the important relationships between the regulation of cholesterol balance and the regulation of plasma LDL cholesterol levels. In every species, the liver is central to the maintenance of cholesterol homeostasis. Except for the small amounts of cholesterol that are lost from the body as steroid hormones or through the sloughing of skin and hair, any cholesterol that is synthesized in the extrahepatic tissues or absorbed from the intestine ultimately must reach the liver, where it is excreted from the body as either cholesterol or bile acids. Thus, the absolute rate of cholesterol synthesis in the liver must equal the absolute rate of sterol excretion in the feces minus the absolute quantity of cholesterol that is synthesized in the extrahepatic tissues and absorbed from the diet. In this manner, the concentration of cholesterol in virtually all of the tissues of the adult remains essentially constant throughout life.

This figure also emphasizes the central role of the liver in controlling the level of plasma LDL cholesterol. Very-low-density lipoproteins (VLDL) are secreted by the liver, and a portion of this lipoprotein fraction is converted to LDL. The rate at which this conversion occurs determines the LDL cholesterol production rate. The liver is also largely responsible for the uptake of circulating LDL cholesterol through the action of receptor-dependent LDL transport. It follows that the uptake of cholesterol and certain triacylglycerols into the liver may alter both the LDL cholesterol production rate and the level of receptor-dependent LDL cholesterol transport and thus alter the steady-state plasma level of LDL

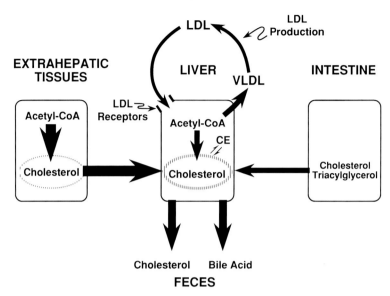

FIG. 1. Relationship between rates of cholesterol synthesis in the whole animal and the regulation of plasma LDL cholesterol levels. In the steady state, the excretion of sterol in the feces as either cholesterol or bile acid must equal the rate of cholesterol entry into the body through *de novo* synthesis or absorption from the gastrointestinal tract. The steady-state level of LDL cholesterol is largely determined by the rate of LDL cholesterol production and the activity of receptor-dependent LDL uptake by the liver. The flow of dietary cholesterol and triacylglycerol into the liver alters both the LDL production rate and receptor activity, and so alters the steady-state LDL cholesterol concentration.

cholesterol. The response of a given species or an individual within that species critically depends on the quantitative aspects of cholesterol synthesis and LDL cholesterol metabolism found in that species or individual (11).

IMPORTANCE OF DIFFERENT ORGANS
FOR CHOLESTEROL SYNTHESIS

The absolute rate of cholesterol synthesis in the whole animal generally varies with size. Small animals may have rates of cholesterol synthesis equal to approximately 100 mg/day per kg body weight, whereas larger animals like humans synthesize at rates of approximately 10 mg/day per kg body weight. Despite this large variation in the absolute rate of total body cholesterol synthesis, however, most extrahepatic tissues contribute a relatively constant percentage to total body synthesis. As illustrated in Fig. 2, for example, in most species the intestine accounts for approximately 10% to 20% of total body cholesterol synthesis (6,12). This is true for most of the other extrahepatic organs.

In contrast, the relative contribution of the liver to total body sterol synthesis varies significantly among species. As shown in Fig. 3, in the absence of dietary

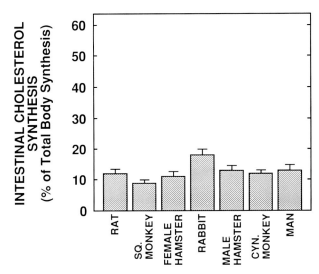

FIG. 2. The relative importance of cholesterol synthesis in the small intestine to total body sterol synthesis in animals maintained on a low-cholesterol, low-triacylglycerol diet. The absolute rates of cholesterol synthesis were measured *in vivo* in these animals using [³H]water (6,12, unpublished data from this laboratory).

cholesterol, the liver may account for as much as 40% to 50% of total body synthesis in species such as the rat and squirrel monkey but only 10% to 15% in other species such as the hamster, cynomolgus monkey, and humans (estimated) (6,12). Thus, not only does the absolute rate of cholesterol synthesis vary among species, the relative importance of the liver to total body synthesis also

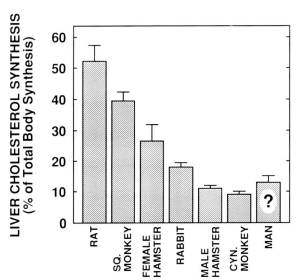

FIG. 3. The relative importance of cholesterol synthesis in the liver to total body sterol synthesis in animals maintained on a low-cholesterol, low-triacylglycerol diet (6,12, unpublished data from this laboratory).

varies. This observation is of considerable importance since it is those species with very low relative rates of hepatic cholesterol synthesis that respond most unfavorably to the addition of lipids to the diet. Furthermore, within a single species, the individual with the lowest rate of hepatic cholesterol synthesis responds with the most exaggerated elevation in LDL cholesterol to lipid feeding.

IMPORTANCE OF DIFFERENT ORGANS IN LDL-CHOLESTEROL DEGRADATION

Similar quantitative data on LDL metabolism are also available for many species. As shown in Fig. 4, in the hamster, rat, and rabbit, the absolute rate of LDL cholesterol uptake from the plasma also varies with the size of the animal. For example, a small animal, such as the hamster, will turn over the equivalent of 4 plasma pools of LDL cholesterol per day, whereas a larger animal, such as humans, will turn over approximately 0.4 pools per day. In all species for which data are now available, however, approximately three-fourths of this turnover is mediated by the receptor-dependent process whereas the remaining LDL uptake is accomplished through the receptor-independent transport mechanism (5,8,10). Furthermore, in all species, approximately 75% of LDL cholesterol clearance from the plasma occurs in the liver and—to a much lesser extent—the small bowel. The other organs are not important quantitatively in the uptake and degradation of LDL cholesterol. Furthermore, in these species, most of the

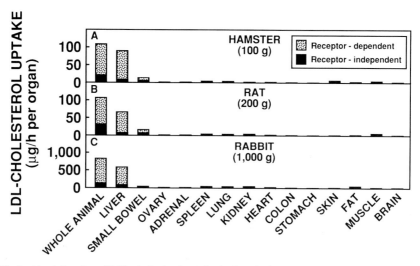

FIG. 4. Absolute rates of LDL cholesterol uptake in the whole animal and in the various tissues of these same animals. In the first column, the data show the absolute and relative importance of receptor-dependent and receptor-independent LDL transport in the uptake and degradation of LDL cholesterol in the whole animal. The other columns of data show the absolute and relative importance of each organ in the same animals.

receptor-dependent LDL transport that can be identified in the whole animal is accounted for by receptor activity found in the liver. Thus, like whole-body cholesterol synthesis, the absolute rate of LDL cholesterol uptake and degradation is inversely related to the size of the animal. Unlike its function in cholesterol synthesis, however, the liver plays a constant and central role in the degradation of LDL cholesterol. In every species for which data are available, the liver is the major organ for the removal of LDL cholesterol from the plasma and is essentially the only quantitatively significant site for receptor-dependent LDL transport.

QUANTITATIVE ASPECTS OF LDL-CHOLESTEROL METABOLISM

From these very brief considerations, it is apparent that the plasma LDL cholesterol concentration is essentially determined by two physiological processes: the rate at which VLDL is converted to LDL and the rate at which LDL is removed from the plasma by both receptor-dependent and receptor-independent transport processes. As illustrated in Fig. 5, the rate at which LDL cholesterol is formed is known as the LDL cholesterol production rate (J_t). This rate varies in circumstances where the rate of VLDL secretion changes, the percentage of the VLDL pool converted to LDL is altered, or the cholesterol/protein ratio of the particle is changed.

The LDL particle is removed from the plasma by both receptor-dependent and receptor-independent transport processes. Because the receptor-dependent process is saturable, it is characterized in terms of the maximal transport velocity (J^m) that could be achieved when all receptors are fully saturated and the functional affinity constant for this receptor-dependent process (K_m). J^m is a function of total body receptor number, whereas K_m is a function of the affinity of the LDL molecule for the LDL receptor mechanism *in vivo*. The velocity of the receptor-independent transport process varies as a linear function of the plasma

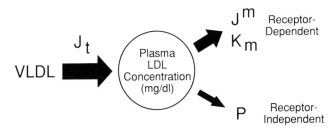

FIG. 5. Factors regulating the plasma LDL cholesterol concentration. Any change in the plasma LDL cholesterol concentration must be explained in terms of alteration in the LDL cholesterol production rate (J_t), the maximal transport velocity (J^m), and functional affinity constant (K_m) for the receptor-dependent transport process and the proportionality constant (P) for the receptor-independent process.

TABLE 1. *Values for the four major rate constants regulating LDL-cholesterol levels in four different species*

Species	Production rate J_t (mg/hr per kg)	Receptor-dependent J^m (mg/hr per kg)	Receptor-dependent K_m (mg/dl)	Receptor-independent P (mg/hr per kg per mg/dl)
Hamster	3.11	4.85	91	0.012
Rat	2.18	4.06	97	0.006
Rabbit	1.67	2.13	90	0.009
Humans	0.58	0.78	90	0.003

The values for the four rate constants in the hamster, rat, and rabbit were determined by direct measurements in animals that had been maintained on a diet essentially free of cholesterol and triacylglycerol (1). The values in humans have been estimated indirectly, as described elsewhere (2).

LDL cholesterol concentration and so can be described in terms of a simple proportionality constant (P). It should be emphasized that any change in the plasma LDL cholesterol concentration must be explained in terms of a change in one or more of these four rate constants.

Experimental means are now available for measuring these rate constants directly in the experimental animal (1,9) or indirectly in humans (2). These rate constants for four species are shown in Table 1. As is apparent, in the absence of dietary lipids (except in the case of humans), the rate of LDL cholesterol production varies from 3.11 mg/hr per kg in the hamster to only 0.58 mg/hr per kg in humans. The maximal rate of receptor-dependent LDL cholesterol uptake (J^m) is higher than these production rates, and the K_m values in all species are approximately 90–100 mg/dl. Thus, because the plasma LDL cholesterol concentration in essentially all species (on a low-cholesterol, low-triacylglycerol diet) is below these K_m values, the receptor-dependent LDL transport system is always operating well below maximum achievable velocities. The proportionality constant for the receptor-independent transport process also varies inversely with the size of the animal. Thus, in every species, the total rate of LDL cholesterol removal from the plasma equals the rate of LDL cholesterol production in the steady state; furthermore, the relative importance of these two transport processes is essentially the same in every species—at least under conditions where there is essentially no cholesterol or triacylglycerol in the diet.

DEPENDENCY OF THE LDL-CHOLESTEROL CONCENTRATION ON J_t AND J^m

With the availability of these four rate constants, it is possible to calculate how the LDL cholesterol concentration would change in any species under circumstances where one or more of these rate constants is altered. The expression that allows these calculations is as follows:

$$C_1 = \frac{J_t-J^m-PK_m + [(J_t-J^m-PK_m)^2 + 4PK_mJ_t]^{1/2}}{2P}$$

In this expression the concentration of LDL cholesterol (C_1) can be calculated at any value of the four transport parameters J_t, J^m, K_m, and P (3,4).

However, in the case of changes in LDL cholesterol levels brought about by most dietary or pharmaceutical manipulations, there is little or no change in the value of P and K_m. Rather, most alterations in the plasma cholesterol concentration are brought about by changes in the LDL cholesterol production rate (J_t) or total LDL receptor activity in the animal (J^m). The kinetic relationships between the steady-state plasma LDL cholesterol concentration and the relative values of J_t and J^m are shown in Fig. 6 in the case of the hamster. The solid data point represents the control hamster fed a standard laboratory chow diet containing little cholesterol or triacylglycerol. Such animals have a plasma LDL cholesterol concentration of about 25 mg/dl. The production rate and LDL receptor activity present in such animals have been set at 100% of activity. The lower curve illustrates how the plasma LDL cholesterol concentration would change under circumstances where J_t is kept constant while the relative receptor activity in the animal is systematically reduced from 100% to 0%. The upper curve shows the same relationship under circumstances where the production rate is increased to 200% of the control value.

Two points warrant emphasis. First, the relationship between the concentration

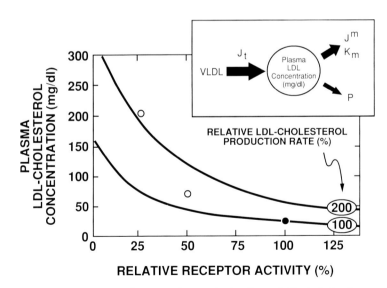

FIG. 6. The kinetic relationships between changes in the plasma LDL cholesterol concentration and alterations of either the LDL cholesterol production rate (J_t) or total body receptor activity (J^m). The solid data point represents the control animal fed a diet low in cholesterol and triacylglycerol where the values of J_t and J^m have been arbitrarily set at 100% activity.

of LDL cholesterol in the plasma and J^m is not linear. The concentration of LDL cholesterol increases markedly only after about 50% of the receptor activity has been lost. Second, the effect of an increase in the LDL cholesterol production rate is markedly dependent on the amount of receptor activity present in the animal. Thus, doubling the production rate increases the plasma LDL cholesterol concentration by only 30 mg/dl in the presence of 100% of receptor activity but by nearly 150 mg/dl in the presence of only 25% J^m. It is clear from these considerations that any manipulation that reduces the amount of receptor-dependent LDL transport in the animal at the same time there is also an increase in the LDL cholesterol production rate will be associated with significant increases in the plasma LDL cholesterol concentration.

EFFECT OF CHOLESTEROL ALONE ON THE KINETICS OF LDL-CHOLESTEROL

In experimental animals maintained on diets very low in cholesterol and triacylglycerol, LDL cholesterol production rates are low and receptor-dependent LDL uptake into the liver is occurring at maximal rates. When only cholesterol is added to the diet of such experimental animals, there is a modest increase in the plasma LDL cholesterol concentration, as is also true in humans (7). When the four parameters controlling LDL metabolism are measured in such animals, there is relatively little change in the parameters defining receptor-independent LDL uptake (P) and the affinity of the LDL particle for the receptor-dependent process (K_m). However, there is significant suppression of the maximal transport velocity (J^m) for the receptor-dependent process and relatively small increases in the LDL cholesterol production rate (J_t). Thus, in the hamster, for example, increasing amounts of cholesterol in the diet are associated with a progressive increase in the plasma LDL cholesterol concentration. This increase, in turn, is primarily the result of loss of hepatic LDL receptor activity (a decreasing value of J^m) accompanied by a progressive—but small—increase in LDL cholesterol production (J_t). The values for K_m and P remain essentially constant under these experimental circumstances (7).

THE EFFECT OF TRIACYLGLYCEROL FEEDING

The effects of different triacylglycerols are complex. Some lipids increase receptor activity whereas others decrease it, and the quantitative nature of these responses is very dependent on the relative concentration of cholesterol in the diet. The general principles involved in this situation are illustrated in Fig. 7. Feeding 0.12% cholesterol alone raises the plasma LDL cholesterol concentration in the experimental animal from approximately 25 mg/dl to 75 mg/dl. As is apparent, this is primarily due to loss of 50% of the receptor-dependent LDL transport process in the whole animal and to a small increase in the LDL cho-

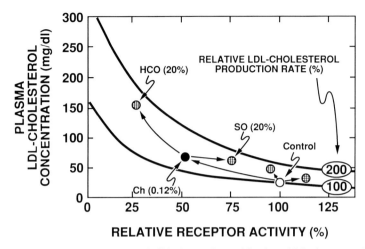

FIG. 7. The effect of feeding cholesterol (Ch) alone or in combination with hydrogenated coconut oil (HCO) or safflower oil (SO) on the plasma LDL cholesterol concentration.

lesterol production rate. When triacylglycerol-containing saturated fatty acids (hydrogenated coconut oil, HCO) are added to such a diet, there is further loss of receptor activity and a significant increase in the LDL cholesterol production rate. Hence, the plasma LDL cholesterol concentration increases to approximately 160 mg/dl.

In contrast, when an identical amount of triacylglycerol-containing unsaturated fatty acids is added to the diet, there is restoration of receptor activity. However, as is also apparent, this results in little change in the LDL cholesterol concentration, because the restoration of receptor activity is occurring on that horizontal portion of the curve where the plasma LDL cholesterol concentration is relatively unaffected by changes in receptor activity. Thus, one general principle that is seen in all species in which such experiments have been carried out is that saturated fatty acids routinely decrease receptor activity whereas unsaturated fatty acids increase receptor-dependent LDL transport. The effect of saturated fatty acids on the plasma LDL cholesterol concentration, however, are always much greater than changes associated with manipulation of the unsaturated fatty acid content of the diet.

A second general principle is also illustrated in Fig. 7. In general, the effects of either saturated or unsaturated fatty acids on plasma LDL cholesterol levels is critically dependent upon the concentration of cholesterol in the diet. Experimental results obtained in animals fed a diet free of cholesterol but containing the same quantities of HCO and safflower oil (SO) are shown in Fig. 7. The saturated fatty acids generally reduce receptor activity whereas the unsaturated fatty acids increase receptor activity, as was true in the presence of cholesterol. Nevertheless, the absolute magnitude of these changes is much smaller. Thus, for example, feeding 20% hydrogenated coconut oil in the absence of cholesterol

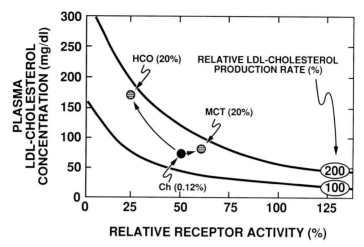

FIG. 8. The effect of saturated fatty acids of different chain lengths on the kinetic parameters controlling LDL cholesterol concentrations. The data show the effects of feeding either cholesterol (Ch) alone or in combination with hydrogenated coconut oil (HCO) or medium-chain-length triglycerides (MCT) (7,13).

increases the plasma LDL cholesterol concentration by approximately 25 mg/dl whereas feeding the same quantity of triacylglycerol in the presence of 0.12% cholesterol increases the LDL cholesterol concentration by over 125 mg/dl.

A third general principle of these lipid interactions is illustrated in Fig. 8. It is clear that not all saturated fatty acids behave in an identical manner. In this particular illustration, similar amounts of hydrogenated coconut oil and medium-chain-length triacylglycerols (MCT) were added to a diet containing a constant amount of cholesterol. It is clear that the MCT has relatively little effect on the plasma cholesterol level or on any of the parameters that regulate this level whereas HCO has a marked effect (13). In recent studies using synthesized triacylglycerols containing only a single fatty acid, it has been demonstrated that only one or two specific saturated fatty acids have the detrimental effects of decreasing receptor activity and increasing LDL cholesterol production rates. Similarly, if synthesized triacylglycerols that contain only one type of unsaturated fatty acid are used, the effects of restoration of receptor activity are characteristic of only a few specific types of fatty acid.

POTENTIAL SOURCES FOR VARIATION IN RESPONSE TO THESE DIETARY EFFECTS

The general effects produced by cholesterol and triacylglycerol have been demonstrated in several different animal species. Most of these studies have been carried out in inbred animals where the response to a specific dietary combination

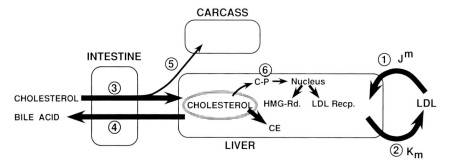

FIG. 9. Sites in the overall scheme of cholesterol metabolism that may account for a variable response of the plasma LDL cholesterol level to the dietary intake of cholesterol and triacylglycerols. Each of these specific steps is discussed in the text.

is uniform and reproducible. In genetically heterogenous populations, however, it is clear that the magnitude of these responses may vary significantly from individual to individual. This is clearly true in humans, various nonhuman primate species, and even experimental animals such as the hamster and rat. Furthermore, this hyper- or hyporesponsiveness often can be shown to be inheritable.

Figure 9 illustrates several circumstances in which genetic differences could account for variable responses of the plasma LDL cholesterol level to dietary challenge. First, there could be inherited abnormalities in the LDL receptor mechanism. Such abnormalities afflict approximately 0.2% of the human population. Second, there could be an abnormality of the apoB protein of LDL that is associated with a change in the effective K_m value for that particle. Such a defect has also been described in approximately 0.2% of the human population and accounts for some variability in plasma LDL levels. Other potential differences include variability in the percentage of cholesterol that is absorbed across the intestine (step 3), variability in the absolute rate of bile acid synthesis (step 4), shunting of significant amounts of cholesterol from the intestine to the extrahepatic organs (step 5), or changes in the sensitivity of the mechanisms responsible for "sensing" the size of the cholesterol pool in the hepatocyte (step 6). The nature of the defect responsible for such variability in the hyper- and hyporesponding animal is now being studied in detail in several laboratories.

Nevertheless, it now seems apparent that the significant increase in plasma LDL cholesterol levels found in most Western populations is, in a major way, dictated by the intake of a diet high in both cholesterol and triacylglycerols. The variable response of the plasma LDL cholesterol concentration to these dietary challenges must also be significantly influenced by genetic factors that alter one or more of the physiological responses to these dietary challenges.

ACKNOWLEDGMENT

The work outlined in this article is based on studies supported by U.S. Public Health Service grant HL-09610 and by a grant from the Moss Heart Fund.

REFERENCES

1. Dietschy, J. M., Spady, D. K., and Meddings, J. B. (1988): In: Suckling K. E., and Groot P. H. E., eds. *Hyperlipidaemia and atherosclerosis.* New York: Academic Press, pp. 17–32.
2. Meddings, J. B., and Dietschy, J. M. (1986): *Circulation,* 74:805–814.
3. Meddings, J. B., and Dietschy, J. M. (1987): In: Machleidt H., ed. *Contributions of chemistry to health.* Weinheim, F.R.G.: VCH, pp. 269–282.
4. Meddings, J. B., and Dietschy, J. M. (1987): In: *Progress in clinical biochemistry and medicine,* vol 5. Berlin: Springer-Verlag, pp. 1–24.
5. Spady, D. K., Bilheimer, D. W., and Dietschy, J. M. (1983): *Proc. Natl. Acad. Sci. USA,* 80: 3499–3503.
6. Spady, D. W., and Dietschy, J. M. (1983): *J. Lipid Res.,* 24:303–315.
7. Spady, D. K., and Dietschy, J. M. (1988): *J. Clin. Invest.,* 81:300–309.
8. Spady, D. K., Huettinger, M., Bilheimer, D. W., and Dietschy, J. M. (1987): *J. Lipid Res.,* 28: 32–41.
9. Spady, D. K., Meddings, J. B., and Dietschy, J. M. (1986): *J. Clin. Invest.,* 77:1474–1481.
10. Spady, D. K., Turley, S. D., and Dietschy, J. M. (1985): *J. Clin. Invest.,* 76:1113–1122.
11. Spady, D. K., Turley, S. D., and Dietschy, J. M. (1985): *J. Lipid Res.,* 26:465–472.
12. Turley, S. D., and Dietschy, J. M. (1988): In: Arias I. M., Jakoby W. B., Popper H., Schachter D., and Shafritz D. A., eds. *The liver: biology and pathobiology.* 2nd ed., New York: Raven, pp. 617–641.
13. Woollett, L. A., Spady, D. K., and Dietschy, J. M. (1989): *J. Clin. Invest.,* 84:119–128.

Atherosclerosis Reviews, Volume 23,
edited by P. C. Weber and A. Leaf.
Raven Press, Ltd., New York © 1991.

Roles for Cholesterol Biosynthetic Intermediates in the Covalent Modification of Proteins

Jasper Rine, William R. Schafer, Cynthia E. Trueblood,
and Matthew N. Ashby

*Department of Molecular and Cell Biology, University of California,
Berkeley, California 94720*

A decade ago, the covalent modification of proteins by intermediates of the cholesterol pathway had been observed in only a few exotic organisms that were far from the mainstream of biology. However, in the last 2 years, the number of examples has exploded to include some of the most interesting proteins in biology. Moreover, in contrast to N-linked glycosylation, for which it has been exceedingly difficult to establish a functional role, the importance of prenylation in the function of proteins has already been well established. In this chapter, we review briefly the discovery of prenylated proteins and the available information on the enzymes responsible for this modification. In addition, we speculate on the functional significance of this modification and what additional roles prenylation may play as suggested by studies in the yeast *Saccharomyces cerevisiae.*

DISCOVERY OF PRENYLATED PROTEINS

The discovery of covalent modification of proteins by intermediates of the cholesterol biosynthetic pathway came from two independent lines of investigation. The first examples came from studies of mating pheromones of the basidomycetous fungi *Rhodosporidium toruloides* and *Tremella brasiliensis,* which synthesize and secrete peptide pheromones containing carboxyl-terminal S-farnesyl cysteine (43,48). This same modification was later found as the carboxyl-terminal modification of the mating pheromone **a**-factor from the yeast *Saccharomyces cerevisiae,* an ascomycetous fungus (2). Because the divergence of fungi is as deeply rooted as the major branches of eukaryotic evolution, the existence of farnesylated peptides secreted from a wide variety of fungi suggests that farnesylated proteins and the secretion of farnesylated peptides are common to all eukaryotes.

A second route to the discovery of proteins modified by cholesterol intermediates came from experiments by Glomset and colleagues in which mammalian cells metabolically labeled with radiolabeled mevalonic acid were found to incorporate mevalonic acid into a number of cellular proteins, most of which are in the 20- to 30-kDa range (46). Although the identity of the labeled proteins remained elusive for a considerable time, recently some of these proteins have been identified, as has the nature of their modification. To date, the proteins radiolabeled by mevalonate have been shown to have either a farnesyl or a geranylgeranyl prenyl group attached in a thioether linkage to a carboxyl-terminal cysteine residue. We shall refer to all protein modifications of this type generically as "protein prenylation." Prenylated proteins include lamin B (15), and numerous G protein subunits (28,31,33,54). In addition, the lamin A precursor is apparently prenylated although the mature protein is not (5). Additional prenylated proteins are discussed in greater detail below.

PRENYLATION IS REQUIRED FOR Ras PROTEIN LOCALIZATION AND FUNCTION

The localization of Ras protein to the inner surface of the plasma membrane is essential for its transforming function. This membrane localization was long thought to be mediated by fatty acylation—in particular, palmitoylation of cysteine residues near the carboxyl terminus of the protein. This conclusion was based on the observation that mutation of the most C-terminal cysteine residue blocked palmitoylation and membrane localization (8,51). However, evidence from three different studies simultaneously led to the conclusion that prenylation and not fatty acylation was the functionally important modification. Perhaps the most unanticipated clue came from studies of yeast cells that were mevalonate auxotrophs due to mutations in HMG-CoA reductase, the enzyme that catalyzes the rate-limiting step in the cholesterol biosynthetic pathway. Surprisingly, when deprived of mevalonate, strains of the **a**-mating type, become unable to mate, whereas the mating ability of strains of the α-mating type is relatively unaffected by mevalonate limitation. This **a**-specific sterility is due to the inability of mevalonate-depleted strains to secrete active **a**-factor. We found that in mevalonate-starved cells, all the **a**-factor was retained within the cell in an unprocessed precursor form. Because mevalonate limitation would deplete cells of farnesyl diphosphate, farnesylation was apparently required for the other processing steps and for secretion (44). Previous studies had established that the posttranslational processing of **a**-factor and of the ras protein of yeast shared a common step(s) (17,40). Thus, because farnesylation of **a**-factor was required for its activity, posttranslational processing steps, and secretion, it was possible that ras protein was also modified by farnesylation. In genetic tests, mevalonate limitation suppressed the phenotypes associated with activated alleles of *RAS2* in yeast cells. Under these conditions, the RAS2 protein failed to associate with the plasma membrane and migrated with the mobility of the precursor form of RAS2, demonstrating a requirement for a mevalonate-derived molecule for the membrane localization and activity of ras protein (44).

These observations were extended to human ras by the discovery that lovastatin, an inhibitor of HMG-CoA reductase, could block the posttranslational processing and biological activity of oncogenic forms of human ras precursor upon injection into *Xenopus* oocytes (44). The carboxyl terminus of all ras proteins exhibits a sequence motif found in numerous other proteins, including a-factor precursor. This motif is referred to as CAAX, in which C denotes cysteine, X denotes any amino acid, and A denotes aliphatic amino acid. In a-factor, the C of the CAAX motif is the site of farnesylation. The corresponding cysteine in the RAS2 sequence and in the human ras sequence are residues known to be necessary for membrane localization (51) and, based upon the analogy to a-factor, are proposed as the site of farnesylation (44). Direct evidence for the farnesylation of Ras protein was provided by Casey et al., who, stimulated by the CAAX motif of a-factor and ras, found that Ras proteins were indeed farnesylated on a cysteine in a thioether linkage (10). Hancock et al. demonstrated that the prenyl group on ras proteins was indeed added to the cysteine of the CAAX sequence (22). They extended the similarity between ras and a-factor by demonstrating that the AAX of the CAAX motif was posttranslationally removed from ras and the resulting C-terminal cysteine was carboxymethylated (21), as is also true for a-factor (2).

IDENTIFICATION OF THE RAS PRENYLTRANSFERASE

Mutant yeast strains that were defective in the processing of ras and a-factor provided a logical starting point to identify the gene or genes encoding the enzyme responsible for the prenylation of the carboxyl terminus of Ras protein. The one gene known to affect both ras and a-factor function, referred to here as *RAM1/DPR1*, has been identified by several groups and given several names (17, 32,39,52). An *in vitro* assay was developed that measured the covalent modification of peptide substrates that mimic the carboxyl terminal sequence of both a-factor and ras. In this assay, it was possible for either radiolabeled isopentenyl diphosphate or farnesyl diphosphate to be covalently linked to the peptide substrate in an extract made from yeast cells. The assay revealed that modification of the peptide required both the cysteine of the CAAX sequence as well as the AAX in order to be labeled by the yeast extract and that human Ha-ras precursor was an effective substrate for prenylation. Extracts made from the *ram1/dpr1* mutants were deficient in this activity. One allele of the gene altered the buffer optimum of the reaction *in vitro*. In addition, extracts prepared from yeast strains that overproduce RAM1/DPR1 protein contain elevated protein prenyltransferase activity. Taken together, these results indicate that the polypeptide encoded by the *RAM1/DPR1* gene was a component of the protein prenyltransferase. The RAM1/DPR1 protein was purified following overexpression in *E. coli*. The purified product is inactive *in vitro* on the peptide substrates, yet when added to extracts made from *ram1/dpr1* mutants, the RAM1/DPR1 protein completely restores enzymatic activity. Thus, an additional component(s) is present in the extract that is required along with RAM1/DPR1 protein for activity (45). Similar conclusions have been reached by F. Tamanoi and colleagues (19).

A complementary biochemical study on mammalian prenyltransferase resulted in the purification to homogeneity of a rat brain prenyltransferase capable of linking a farnesyl moiety to a Ras substrate. This enzyme consists of two unrelated polypeptides, each of which is approximately 50 kDa in mass, both of which are necessary for activity (41). Thus, it is likely that the yeast *RAM1/DPR1* gene encodes one polypeptide of the corresponding yeast enzyme. At this point, the relative role of the two polypeptides is unknown, but it is possible that one subunit performs the catalytic function, whereas the other may provide recognition of the CAAX motif, the lipid donor, or both. We return to this issue in the following section.

OTHER PROTEIN PRENYLTRANSFERASES

The genetic properties of *ram1/dpr1* null alleles provide suggestive evidence for the existence of additional protein prenyltransferases in yeast cells. Specifically, since RAS function is essential for viability and the C-terminal cysteine is essential for Ras function, strains lacking the enzyme necessary to farnesylate this residue are expected to be inviable. Surprisingly, yeast strains containing a complete deletion of the *RAM1/DPR1* gene are fully viable when cultured at room temperature and are inviable only above 34°C. When this mutant is grown at the low temperature, there is still a small amount of ras protein in the membrane fraction. In contrast, mutant ras protein in which the C-terminal cysteine is mutated to serine is nonfunctional (12). These observations suggest the existence of at least one additional protein prenyltransferase capable of prenylating Ras at the lower temperature. The inability of mutant cells to grow at the high temperature could reflect intrinsic thermolability of the other protein prenyltransferase, or a demand for a higher level of prenylated Ras than can be provided by the other isozyme, or perhaps even that a different prenyl group has been added that is nonfunctional at the higher temperature.

If there is an additional protein prenyltransferase, which gene encodes it and what are its substrates *in vivo?* We can address this question indirectly by determining the identity of the essential substrates of RAM1/DPR1 protein. Overproduction of RAS2 protein can suppress the temperature sensitivity of *ram1/dpr1* mutants (Schafer and Rine, unpublished). Thus, it appears that ras is the only essential substrate for the RAM1/DPR1 enzyme. (As discussed below, there are likely to be other substrates for RAM1/DPR1 that are not essential.) Sequences related to *RAM1/DPR1* have been found in two other genes in yeast by Mark Goebl (personal communication). One of these genes, identified orig-

FIG. 1. Sequence similarity between the RAM1/DPR1 protein and two putative subunits of protein prenyltransferases. The references for the sequences are provided in the legend to Fig. 2.

inally as an open reading frame (*ORF2*) of unknown function at the 5' end of the *PRP4* gene (38), has since been shown to be essential for viability (37). The other homolog is *CDC43*, a gene that is required for establishment of cell polarity (23, D. I. Johnson, personal communication). The relationship of these three proteins is shown in Fig. 1. Although the proteins are clearly rather different, the degree of similarity is strong but not yet compelling evidence that *ORF2* and *CDC43* may be subunits of other protein prenyltransferases.

However, in addition to sequence similarity among themselves, there is some limited similarity between these proteins and the proposed allylic binding site of known prenyltransferases (Fig. 2). If this hypothesis is true, then we can use the phenotypes of mutations in these genes to gain insight into their presumptive substrates. A gene disruption of *ORF2* is lethal at all temperatures and is not suppressed by a mutation that bypasses the need for ras function. Thus ORF2, if a prenyltransferase, must have a different essential target than ras. However, it is possible that ORF2 encodes the residual protein prenyltransferase activity detected in the absence of *RAM1/DPR1*. *CDC43* was identified by alleles that cause isotropic growth without cell division at the high temperature. In the absence of a defined null allele, it is impossible to know whether *CDC43*, like *RAM1/DPR1*, is required only at high temperature or whether the existing alleles are in fact conditional. Interestingly, the hypothesis that this gene encodes a

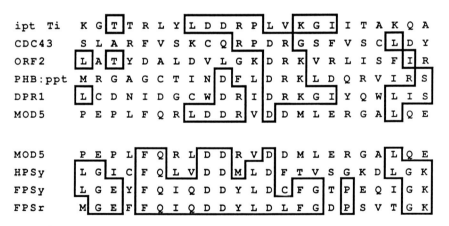

FIG. 2. Sequence identity between known prenyltransferases and DPR1/RAM1 homologues. The lower group of sequences represents the presumptive binding site for the allylic diphosphate in several prenyltransferases. With the exception of MOD5, these proteins are all polyprenyl synthetases. The upper group contains a number of protein sequences that bind allylic prenyl diphosphate substrates; they show slight identity to the sequences in the lower group and more significant identity to one another. The sequences are as follows: ipt Ti: cytokinin prenyltransferase from *Agrobacterium* plasmid Ti Bo542 (47); ORF2: yeast ORF2 protein (38); PHB:ppt: yeast p-hydroxybenzoate:polyprenyltransferase (4); CDC43, yeast CDC43 protein (23, D. Johnson, personal communication); DPR1: DPR1/RAM1 protein (20); MOD5: yeast tRNA: DMAPP transferase (34); HPSy: yeast hexaprenyl diphosphate synthetase (4); FPSy: yeast farnesyl diphosphate synthetase (3); FPSr: rat farnesyl diphosphate synthetase (11).

protein prenyltransferase is strengthened by the observation that two other genes involved in the establishment of polar growth, *RSR1* and *CDC42* (1,6) each encodes proteins with sequence similarity to small GTP binding proteins and with a CAAX sequence at their carboxyl termini (24). Thus, a reasonable hypothesis would be that CDC42 protein and RSR1 protein are substrates for prenylation by a *CDC43*-encoded prenyltransferase.

If protein prenyltransferases generally have two subunits, as found for the rat brain enzyme (41), then it is possible that yeast enzymes that have RAM1/DPR1, ORF2, or CDC43 as one subunit all share a common subunit. For example, if these three genes serve in providing target or lipid specificity, then in principle one catalytic subunit might service all three recognition subunits. We have been unable to find a mutation in the missing component of the RAM1/DPR1 prenyltransferase by the same screen that identified *ram1/dpr1* mutations. If the missing subunit were a shared subunit, it might be very difficult to recover alleles that would have specific effects.

It is worth noting that neither *RAM1/DPR1*, nor *CDC43*, nor *ORF2* was isolated in any systematic effort to identify protein prenyltransferases. Instead, each was found based either upon unrelated phenotypes or serendipitously by sequencing. Thus, there is no reason to believe that all protein prenyltransferases have been identified. Because the yeast genome is approximately 10% sequenced and three sequence homologs have been found, an upper estimate of 30 protein prenyltransferases in a yeast cell is conceivable. A large number of protein prenyltransferases would suggest that different enzymes prenylate different target proteins. Thus it may prove possible to develop inhibitors of different enzymes as a means of achieving selective effects such as blocking the localization and function of oncogenic forms of the ras proteins.

THE ROLE OF PRENYLATION IN G PROTEIN FUNCTION

Trimeric G proteins are a diverse group of structurally related proteins that participate in relaying information about events outside the cell, through receptors, to second messenger pathways inside the cell (7). The carboxyl-terminal CAAX sequence appears on several γ subunits of G proteins including the *STE18*-encoded γ subunit of the yeast Gm protein, a trimeric G protein that signals the response of cells to mating pheromones. In contrast to the Gs protein that couples adenylyl cyclase to the β-adrenergic receptor of mammalian cells, it is the $\beta\gamma$ subunit of Gm that stimulates the effector molecule in the yeast cell, resulting in the arrest of cell division upon treatment with pheromone. For this G protein, α is a negative regulator of $\beta\gamma$ such that α mutants are lethal because of the constitutive cell-cycle arrest provided by unregulated $\beta\gamma$ (14,50). The cysteine residue of the CAAX sequence is essential for the function of the G protein because mutations that affect this residue severely inhibit mating.

The importance of prenylation for the function of this trimeric G protein was demonstrated in two ways. First, strains starved for mevalonate and other iso-prenoids accumulate a precursor form of the γ subunit that fractionates in the soluble fraction of cell extracts. In wild-type cells, the γ subunit is exclusively of the mature size and in the membrane fraction. Thus, in this regard the pro-cessing and localization of the γ subunit are identical to the ras proteins. Fur-thermore, when added to a culture containing a lethal mutation in the gene for the α subunit of Gm, lovastatin, an inhibitor of the synthesis of mevalonate and all prenyl groups, is able to restore viability by reducing the level of functional γ subunit (16). A dramatic example of this assay is provided in Fig. 3. This simple Petri plate assay can be used to screen for inhibitors of the synthesis of prenyl groups as well as inhibitors of the prenyltransferase itself. Because it is likely that at least some protein prenyltransferases will exhibit some target spec-ificity, this screen may lead to the development of novel drugs that might, for example, block the processing of oncogenic forms of ras.

Direct evidence that G protein γ subunits are prenylated has recently been provided (31). Interestingly, the prenyl group on the transducin γ subunit is farnesyl, whereas the prenyl group on the γ subunit of a G protein from PC12 cells is geranylgeranyl (33). Indeed, geranylgeranyl prenyl groups may be the major class of prenyl modifications in mammalian cells (30). It is still unknown

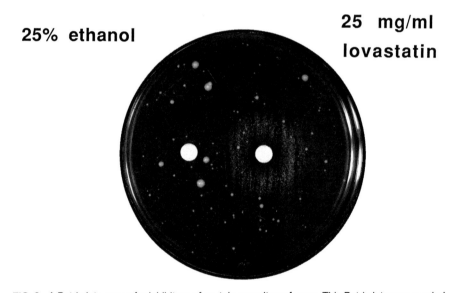

25% ethanol

25 mg/ml lovastatin

FIG. 3. A Petri plate assay for inhibitors of protein prenyltransferase. This Petri plate was seeded with yeast strains containing a temperature sensitive mutation in the gene encoding the α subunit of the trimeric G protein, Gm, which mediates response to yeast mating factors. The filter on the left was soaked in 25% ethanol and placed on the lawn, whereas the filter on the right was soaked in lovastatin (25 mg/ml) dissolved in 25% ethanol. The ring of growth around the lovastatin-soaked filter is due to inhibition of protein prenylation of the STE18-encoded γ subunit due to depletion of the prenyl donor pool (16).

whether the same protein prenyltransferase couples the farnesyl group and the geranylgeranyl group. Likewise, the factors that determine which lipid is attached to which protein are unknown. Because the RAM1/DPR1 prenyltransferase is responsible for the modification of both RAS2 and STE18 (γ subunit), the identification of the prenyl group on STE18 may shed some light on these issues.

SIGNIFICANCE OF STE6 HOMOLOGY WITH MDR

Because modifications of the fungal mating factors have been so instrumental in the development of the protein prenylation field, it is worth considering whether the mechanism by which these mating factors are secreted might offer insight into a novel and generally important route of secretion. STE6 is a polytopic integral membrane protein that is required for the export of a-factor. Mutations in the *STE6* gene specifically block the mating of cells of the a-mating type. The sequence of the *STE6* gene revealed extensive sequence identity to the mammalian *MDR* genes, which confer resistance to a number of drugs used as anticancer therapies (26,29). *MDR*, in turn, shares sequence identity with a class of bacterial membrane proteins whose role it is to transport molecules across cell membranes. These sequence similarities, which include ATP binding domains, suggest that the proteins act to pump their relevant substrates across membranes (as reviewed in 27). Thus the role of STE6 would be to bind and translocate a-factor across the membrane, providing an alternative route to the classic secretory pathway. Indeed, the STE6 protein has some sequence similarity to the a-factor receptor, which is found on α cells and is encoded by the *STE3* gene (26).

Mutants deficient in prenylation of a-factor accumulate a-factor precursor intracellularly, suggesting that prenylation might be required for recognition by the STE6 transporter. Because prenylation of the precursor precedes and is required for all subsequent posttranslational processing steps, it is difficult to establish a direct connection between prenylation and recognition by STE6. Nevertheless, the hypothesis that the prenyl group on mature a-factor may be required for its export remains attractive. Could prenylation play a role in the recognition or export of substrates by the MDR family of proteins? The natural substrate(s) of MDR is unknown. A clue that isoprenoids may be involved in the action of MDR proteins was provided by the discovery that two different synthetic isoprenoids could block the ability of MDR to confer resistance to vincristine and daunomycin in human KB cells (35). These observations lead to the possibility that the drugs may be prenylated *in vivo* and subsequently exported as prenylated mimics of the natural substrate of MDR. By this hypothesis, the synthetic isoprenoids would interfere with recognition of the modified drugs, blocking their export. As there is ample precedent for the prenylation of planar aromatic molecules such as heme a (49) and ubiquinone (36), it would be interesting to determine whether the drugs exported by the action of MDR are chemically altered, in particular by an isoprene group.

IS THERE A RECEPTOR FOR FARNESYLATED PROTEINS?

The role of a covalently linked lipid in localizing a protein to the plasma membrane may simply be to provide a hydrophobic anchor in the hydrophobic environment of the membrane. However, the available evidence suggests that this view is overly simplistic. The myristylated src protein is anchored in the membrane by means of a receptor that recognizes at least in part the myristate group. In the absence of the receptor or in the absence of the lipid, membrane attachment of src is blocked (42). Myristate is a 14-carbon fatty acid that, being completely saturated, would be more likely to spontaneously insert into a membrane than would a farnesyl group, which is of comparable length but unsaturated. Because myristate needs a receptor to mediate the association of linked proteins with a membrane, one would expect farnesyl also to require a receptor.

Another argument against farnesyl being completely responsible for the localization of farnesylated proteins is that one would then expect all farnesylated proteins to be localized in the same membranes, which they are not. For example, ras protein is in the plasma membrane whereas lamin B, is associated with the nuclear envelope (25). Although a receptor for lamin B has recently been identified (53), it is not yet known whether the farnesyl moiety of lamin B plays a role in recognition or binding by the receptor. The rho proteins, small GTP binding proteins that have sequence similarity to ras proteins, have recently been localized to the Golgi apparatus (M. Yamamoto, personal communication). The rho proteins end with a CAAX motif. Although there is no direct evidence that rho proteins are prenylated, there is a strong probability that they are. Therefore their Golgi localization argues against one single destination for all prenylated proteins. It will be interesting to learn whether the nature of the prenyl group on prenylated proteins (e.g., farnesyl versus geranylgeranyl) contributes to the localization of the protein.

Further evidence that the lipid attached to prenylated proteins may provide more than simply a hydrophobic domain comes from an imaginative experiment of Buss and colleagues on ras protein. The three-dimensional structure of ras is such that the amino terminus and carboxyl terminus of the protein are close together in space, and both are far from the site of GTP binding (13). To examine the relative importance of the particular lipid used to attach the protein to the plasma membrane, the carboxyl terminal CAAX sequence was removed and a consensus signal for protein myristylation was added to the amino terminus. Ras was localized by the myristate group to the plasma membrane in the absence of the CAAX motif. However, attachment of wild-type ras protein to the membrane by myristate created an activated form of the protein similar to that created by oncogenic mutations (9). Thus, the particular manner in which the protein is presented to the membrane can have profound effects on its activity.

SUMMARY

The most striking thread connecting prenylated proteins is a role in either cell division or the regulation of cell division. Mating pheromones arrest cells in cell-cycle specific manner in preparation for mating. Likewise, ras and related proteins control the decision to divide or remain quiescent. G proteins transmit the information about growth factors to second messengers. Nuclear lamins control the assembly and disassembly of the nucleus in mitosis. Is there a reason that membrane localization of these proteins is provided by a prenyl lipid and not, for example, by a fatty acid? As more examples of prenylated proteins accumulate, we will have a better understanding of whether the connection between prenylated proteins and cell division is a coincidence. One rationalization for a functional connection is that the mevalonate biosynthetic pathway is one of the most regulated pathways in the cell (18). Thus, prenyl groups, made from mevalonate, may be more accurate monitors of the physiological state of the cell. The prenyl linkage, however, is apparently very stable (22). Therefore if this linkage is to have a regulatory role, the role would likely involve either proper targeting of the protein, or controlling whether the protein becomes membrane associated or not. As there has been no report of significant levels of nonprenylated precursors in wild-type cells, it would seem that were membrane localization *per se* to be a point of regulation, nonprenylated precursors would have to be unstable. At this stage, a profound appreciation of unique properties providable only by prenylation remains elusive. If such properties exist, perhaps they will be recognized by examining more closely the mechanism by which prenylated proteins associate with membranes.

ACKNOWLEDGMENT

Work in the authors' lab has been supported by a grant from the National Institutes of Health (GM35827), the Lucille P. Markey Charitable Trust, the Tobacco-Related Disease Research Program of the State of California, a Damon Runyon–Walter Winchell Postdoctoral Fellowship (C.E.T.), and an NSF predoctoral fellowship (W.R.S.). We thank the members of our lab and Jeremy Thorner for many stimulating discussions of the ideas presented.

REFERENCES

1. Adams, A. E. M., Johnson, D. I., Longnecker, R. M., Sloat, B. J., and Pringle, J. R. (1990): *J. Cell Biol.,* 111:131–142.
2. Anderegg, R. J., Betz, R., Carr, S. A., Crabb, J. W., and Duntze, W. (1988): *J. Biol. Chem.,* 263: 18236–18240.
3. Anderson, M. S., Yarger, J. G., Burck, C. L., and Poulter, C. D. (1989): *J. Biol. Chem.,* 264: 19176–19184.
4. Ashby, M. N., and Edwards, P. A. (1990): *J. Biol. Chem.,* 265:13157–13164.
5. Beck, L. A., Hosick, T. J., and Sinensky, M. (1990): *J. Cell Biol.,* 110:1489–1499.
6. Bender, A., and Pringle, J. R. (1989): *Proc. Natl. Acad. Sci. USA,* 86:9976–9980.
7. Bourne, H. R., Sanders, D. A., and McCormick, F. (1990): *Nature,* 348:125–132.
8. Buss, J. E., and Sefton, B. W. (1986): *Molec. Cell Biol.,* 6:116–122.
9. Buss, J. E., Solski, P. A., Schaeffer, J. R., MacDonald, M. J., and Der, C. J. (1989): *Science,* 243: 1600–1603.
10. Casey, P. J., Solski, P. A., Der, C. J., and Buss, J. E. (1989): *Proc. Natl. Acad. Sci. USA,* 86: 8323–8327.
11. Clarke, C. F., Tanaka, R. D., Svenson, K., Wansley, M., Fogelman, A. M., and Edwards, P. A. (1987): *Mol. Cell Biol.,* 7:3138–3146.

12. Deschenes, R. J., and Broach, J. R. (1987): *Mol. Cell Biol.*, 7:2344–2351.
13. De Vos, A. M., Tong, L., and Milburn, M. V., et al. (1988): *Science*, 239:888–893.
14. Dietzel, C., and Kurjan, J. (1987): *Cell*, 50:1001–1010.
15. Farnsworth, C. C., Wolda, S. L., Gelb, M. H., and Glomset, J. A. (1989): *J. Biol. Chem.*, 264: 20422–20429.
16. Finegold, A. A., Schafer, W. R., Rine, J., Whiteway, M., and Tamanoi, F. (1990): *Science*, 249: 165–168.
17. Fujiyama, A., Matsumoto, K., and Tamanoi, F. (1987): *EMBO J.*, 6:223–228.
18. Goldstein, J. L., and Brown, M. S. (1990): *Nature*, 343:425–430.
19. Goodman, L. E., Judd, R. R., and Farnsworth, C. C., et al. (1990): *Proc. Natl. Acad. Sci. USA*, 87:9665–9669.
20. Goodman, L. E., Perou, C. M., Fujiyama, A., and Tamanoi, F. (1988): *Yeast*, 4:271–281.
21. Gutierrez, L., Magee, A. I., Marshall, C. J., and Hancock, J. F. (1989): *EMBO J.*, 8:1093–1098.
22. Hancock, J. F., Magee, A. I., Childs, J. E., and Marshall, C. J. (1989): *Cell*, 57:1167–1177.
23. Johnson, D. I., O'Brien, J. M., and Jacobs, C. W. (1990): *Gene*, 90:93–98.
24. Johnson, D. I., and Pringle, J. R. (1990): *J. Cell Biol.*, 111:143–152.
25. Krohne, G., Wolin, S. L., McKeon, F. D., Franke, W. W., and Kirschner, M. W. (1987): *EMBO J.*, 6:3801–3808.
26. Kuchler, K., Sterne, R. E., and Thorner, J. (1989): *EMBO J.*, 8:3973–3984.
27. Kuchler, K., and Thorner, J. (1990): *Curr. Opin. Cell Biol.*, 2:617–624.
28. Lai, R. K., Perez-Sala, D., Canada, F. J., and Rando, R. R. (1990): *Proc. Natl. Acad. Sci. USA*, 87:7673–7677.
29. McGrath, J. P., and Varshavsky, A. (1989): *Nature*, 340:400–404.
30. Maltese, W. A., and Erdman, R. A. (1989): *J. Biol. Chem.*, 264:18168–18172.
31. Maltese, W. A., and Robishaw, J. D. (1990): *J. Biol. Chem.*, 265:18071–18074.
32. Miyajima, I., Nakayama, N., Nakafuku, M., Kaziro, Y., Arai, K., and Matsumoto, K. (1988): *Genetics*, 119:797–804.
33. Mumby, S. M., Casey, P. J., Gilman, A. G., Gutowski, S., and Sternweiss, P. C. (1990): *Proc. Natl. Acad. Sci. USA*, 87:5873–5877.
34. Najarian, D., Dihanich, M. E., Martin, N. C., and Hopper, A. K. (1987): *Mol. Cell. Biol.*, 7: 185–198.
35. Nakagawa, N., Akiyama, S., Yamaguchi, T., Shiraishi, N., Ogata, J., and Kuwano, M. (1986): *Cancer Res.*, 46:4453–4457.
36. Olson, R. E., and Rudney, H. (1983): Biosynthesis of ubiquinone. *Vitam. Horm.*, 40:1–43.
37. Peterson-Bjorn, S., Harrington, T. R., and Friesen, J. D. (1990): *Yeast*, 6:345–352.
38. Peterson-Bjorn, S., Soltyk, A., Beggs, J. D., and Friesen, J. D. (1989): *Molec. Cell Biol.*, 9:3698–3709.
39. Powers, S., Kataoka, T., and Fasano, O., et al. (1984): *Cell*, 36:607–612.
40. Powers, S., Michaelis, S., Broek, D., et al. (1986): *Cell*, 47:413–422.
41. Reiss, Y., Goldstein, J. L., Seabra, M. C., Casey, P. J., and Brown, M. S. (1990): *Cell*, 62:81–90.
42. Resh, M. D. (1989): *Cell*, 58:281–286.
43. Sakagami, Y., Yoshida, M., Isogal, A., and Suzuki, A. (1981): *Science*, 212:1525–1527.
44. Schafer, W. R., Kim, R., Sterne, R., Thorner, J., Kim, S.-H., and Rine, J. (1989): *Science*, 245: 379–385.
45. Schafer, W. R., Trueblood, C. E., and Yang, C.-C., et al. (1990): *Science*, 249:1133–1139.
46. Schmidt, R. A., Schneider, C. J., and Glomset, J. A. (1984): *J. Biol. Chem.*, 259:10175–10180.
47. Strabala, T. J., Bednarek, S. Y., Bertani, G., and Amasino, R. M. (1989): *Mol. Gen. Genet.*, 216: 388–394.
48. Tsuchiya, E., Fukui, S., Kamiya, Y., Sakagami, Y., and Fujino, M. (1978): *Biochem. Biophys. Res. Commun.*, 85:459–463.
49. Weinstein, J. D., Branchaud, R., Beale, S. I., Bement, W. J., and Sinclair, P. R. (1986): *Arch. Biochem. Biophys.*, 245:44–50.
50. Whiteway, M., Hougan, L., and Dignard, D., et al. (1989): *Cell*, 56:467–477.
51. Willumsen, B. M., Norris, K., Papageorge, A. G., Hubbert, N. L., and Lowy, D. R. (1984): *EMBO J.*, 3:2581–2585.
52. Wilson, K. L., and Herskowitz, I. (1987): *Genetics*, 115:441–449.
53. Worman, H. J., Evans, C. D., and Blobel, G. (1990): *J. Cell Biol.*, 111:1535–1542.
54. Yamane, H. K., Farnsworth, C. C., and Xie, H., et al. (1990): *Proc. Natl. Acad. Sci. USA*, 87: 5868–5872.

Atherosclerosis Reviews, Volume 23,
edited by P. C. Weber and A. Leaf.
Raven Press, Ltd., New York © 1991.

Signal Transduction in the Arterial Wall

Role of Eicosanoids and the Cytokine Network in the Regulation of Cholesterol Metabolism

David P. Hajjar, Kenneth B. Pomerantz,
and Andrew C. Nicholson

*Departments of Biochemistry and Pathology, Cornell University
Medical College, New York, New York 10021*

Cholesteryl ester (CE)–laden foam cells of monocytic or smooth muscle cell (SMC) origin underlying intact endothelium are a characteristic feature of the human atherosclerotic lesion. However, the mechanisms that promote lipid accumulation in cells comprising the atheroma have not been fully elucidated. Owing to potential autocrine and paracrine interactions of these cells, the regulation of cholesterol metabolism in macrophages and SMC is complex. In response to injury or activation, endothelial cells (EC) release eicosanoids, chemoattractants, and growth factors; develop pro-coagulant properties; and express surface glycoproteins that promote the adhesion of inflammatory cells (30). Studies in nonhuman primates indicate that an inflammatory infiltrate consisting of monocyte/macrophages and T lymphocytes precedes SMC migration, proliferation, and lipid accumulation (10). These observations imply that soluble mediators derived from activated EC and inflammatory cells recruited into the lesion could influence cholesterol deposition in intimal SMC and macrophages. Recently, our laboratory has focused on the contribution of endothelial and monocyte-derived soluble mediators on cholesterol metabolism in arterial SMC and macrophages in order to define the pathogenesis of foam cell development. This brief review will highlight the recent progress made by our laboratory and others on the regulation of intracellular cholesterol metabolism in the vessel wall.

THE ENDOTHELIAL CELL

The endothelial cell (EC) has a pivotal role in maintaining normal hemostatic and hemodynamic function and may mediate the initial events in the development of atherosclerosis. Under physiological conditions, EC serve as a selectively permeable barrier to circulating macromolecules (including plasma lipoproteins) and elaborate substances that maintain thromboresistance and vascular tone. In response to injury or activation, EC release soluble mediators that promote the adhesion of neutrophils, monocytes, and platelets. In this respect, the histologic features of the atherosclerotic lesion (consisting of monocyte/macrophages and T lymphocytes) are similar to other chronic inflammatory lesions. The presence of this inflammatory infiltrate precedes or coincides with SMC migration, proliferation, and cholesterol accumulation, implying that cellular interactions contribute to these processes (19).

In an attempt to define the role of the endothelium in lipid accretion processes in the underlying smooth muscle cells, we de-endothelialized rabbit thoracic aortae and allowed for re-endothelialization; we found that CE accumulated to a greater extent under re-endothelialized (rather than de-endothelialized) areas of denuded rabbit aorta *in vivo* (12). We concluded that the endothelium could modulate lipid accretion in the blood vessel wall (12). Through subsequent experiments, we found that the lipid was trapped in the re-endothelialized areas by proteoglycan (24). Subsequently, we demonstrated that EC can also modulate normal SMC cholesterol metabolism *in vivo* (21) and *in vitro* (22,23).

Endothelial cells modulate numerous aspects of SMC function, including their phenotype, proliferative capacity, and lipoprotein catabolism. However, the factors that contribute to dysregulation of cholesterol metabolism in cells of the atheroma is still obscure. We propose that the normal EC and its constitutively expressed repertoire of soluble mediators are important in the maintenance of low vascular cholesterol content and that dysregulation of endogenous mediator production by EC following activation or trauma may promote net cholesterol and CE accumulation within SMC and macrophages.

ENDOTHELIAL CELL–DERIVED MEDIATORS

Two important mechanisms should be considered in examining the means by which normal EC regulate cellular cholesterol content in underlying SMC and macrophages. First, EC regulate cholesterol flux between the intra- and extravascular compartments. This may be ultimately dependent on the plasma concentrations of low-density lipoproteins (LDL) and high-density lipoproteins (HDL). Normally, EC effectively restrict plasma lipoprotein flux; only after injury is LDL permeability increased (29). Second, the normal EC may constitutively express or secrete a repertoire of agents, including eicosanoids (PGI_2, PGE_2, and 12-HETE) or EC-derived growth factors (PDGF) that promote CE hydrolysis and subsequent efflux in underlying SMC (Fig. 1). Upon stimulation or injury, EC may elaborate substances that not only increase EC permeability to LDL but also may inhibit net cholesterol efflux. Our laboratory and others have direct experimental evidence to demonstrate that EC modulate CE metabolism in SMC

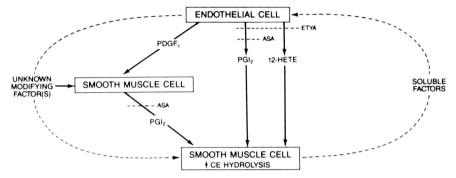

FIG. 1. Transcellular signalling and regulation of cholesteryl ester catabolism in smooth muscle cells by eicosanoids. Endothelial cells secrete humoral factors such as eicosanoids (e.g., PGI$_2$ and 12-HETE) and growth factors (e.g., PDGF) that increase cholesteryl ester (CE) hydrolysis in smooth muscle cells. Enhancement by eicosanoids and growth factors is abolished by pre-incubating endothelial cells with cyclooxygenase/lipoxygenase inhibitors and antibodies to PDGF, respectively. In addition, smooth muscle cells secrete soluble factors such as cytokines (TNF, IL-1), which activate endothelial cells to produce more PDGF (see Fig. 2) or other soluble mediators that can enhance CE catabolism. (From ref. 23 with permission.)

via soluble factors (Fig. 1) (23). Some investigators have shown that PDGF stimulates eicosanoid production by activating phospholipase A$_2$ and by stimulation of the transcription and translation of cyclooxygenase and PGI$_2$ synthase genes. In our laboratory, we have shown that EC-derived PDGF can also stimulate lysosomal (acid) CE hydrolase (ACEH) activities in arterial SMC (23). Eicosanoid dependency of these observations was established when aspirin or ETYA treatment of EC abolished EC stimulation of CE hydrolysis in SMC (23). Exogenously added PDGF stimulated CE hydrolytic activity almost twofold in SMC cultured alone or co-cultured with EC, but not in the presence of aspirin-treated EC (23). PGI$_2$ synthesis and ACEH activity in SMC were also stimulated by HDL in an eicosanoid-dependent manner (36). Apo A-1, the principal apoprotein in HDL, is synthesized by vascular EC and is identical to PGI$_2$ stabilizing factor, which prolongs the chemical half-life of PGI$_2$, increasing its ability to stimulate NCEH activity. In summary, these observations indicate that EC can modulate cholesterol content in underlying SMC and macrophages through growth factor/eicosanoid/lipoprotein type interactions.

CHOLESTEROL, VASCULAR WALL, AND GROWTH FACTORS

Cellular cholesterol content is ultimately dependent on the activity of the processes of (a) cholesterol influx [by cholesterol donors such as LDL and β-VLDL via the LDL receptor, and modified LDL, via the scavenger receptor(s)], (b) metabolism (lysosomal and cytoplasmic CE hydrolysis, cholesterol esterification, and trafficking to the cell membrane), and (c) efflux (by plasma cholesterol acceptors, including HDL, via its receptor). Clearly, the regulation of these processes will determine the cholesterol and CE content of SMC and macrophages, whereas dysregulation of these processes would result in lipid accumulation. Low-density lipoprotein (LDL) receptor-mediated cholesterol metabolism is regulated by cellular cholesterol levels, acting via sterol-mediated down-regulation of genes whose products control the processing of LDL-CE and *de novo* cholesterol synthesis via HMG-CoA reductase and the LDL receptor (4). Because LDL receptor activity varies inversely with levels of cellular cholesterol, LDL receptor-independent pathways of cholesterol uptake are important in cholesterol accumulation and eventual foam cell development. Macrophages and EC accumulate CE via receptors distinct from the LDL receptor, termed "scavenger receptors" (3), whose gene has recently been cloned (39) and whose expression is not down-regulated by cholesterol (4). Scavenger receptor uptake of modified forms of LDL—including oxidized LDL (41), LDL–heparin–fibronectin aggregates (13,14), and LDL complexes (42)—may be an important mechanism that circumvents the tight control of cellular cholesterol content and leads to foam cell development. Conversely, cholesterol efflux from SMC and macrophages is affected by plasma cholesteryl acceptor proteins, the most efficacious of which is high-density lipoprotein (HDL). HDL is known to be a negative risk factor for atherosclerosis, as documented by epidemiological studies. The mechanism by which HDL promotes net cholesterol efflux is complex. Bierman and his colleagues have demonstrated specific receptors for HDL, which, in association with the plasma enzyme LCAT, esterify cellular-free cholesterol to form HDL core lipid (5,32).

There is accumulating evidence that soluble mediators derived from EC, including growth factors, cytokines, and eicosanoids, modulate cholesterol metabolism in underlying vascular tissue. Growth factors, including platelet-derived growth factor (PDGF) (31), acidic and basic fibroblast growth factor (aFGF and bFGF) (46), and transforming growth factor-β (TGF-β) (38) are locally synthesized by vascular cells under physiological and pathophysiological conditions. PDGF secretion by EC is inducible by endotoxin, thrombin, and TGF-β; it is inhibited by bFGF. FGF is not secreted but is either intracellular or bound to extracellular matrix. Its release follows cell injury or exposure to heparin or heparinases. TGF-β is secreted into the extracellular milieu in a latent form and may be activated by plasmin and cathepsin D. EC and SMC in co-culture produce activated TGF-β, whereas EC and SMC cultured alone produce only the latent form.

These growth factors have been implicated in the regulation of cholesterol metabolism through their effect on the LDL and scavenger receptors. For example, PDGF (5) and FGF (8) promote the binding and uptake of LDL in SMC. PDGF also increases LDL receptor gene transcription in fibroblasts (28). PDGF increases fluid phase endocytosis in the absence of a storage pool of cellular cholesterol and renders the cell dependent on cholesterol synthesis to affect the proliferative response to PDGF. In addition, TGF-β activates LDL receptor activity and the CE cycle in arterial SMC (unpublished observations). The stimulation of LDL receptor activity by growth factors may stem from the need for cholesterol to provide for membrane biogenesis accompanying the proliferative response to these agents. However, growth factors may also modulate scavenger receptor activity, whose role in proliferation is unclear, but whose role in the accumulation of intracellular CE by the macrophage is considered to be of major importance. Macrophages produce a factor (not PDGF) that stimulates acetyl-LDL–induced cholesterol esterification (40), whereas bacterial endotoxin downregulates the scavenger receptor on human monocytes (43). Moreover, exposure of vascular cells to modified LDL modulates growth factor expression. Modified LDL suppresses PDGF production from EC by a free radical-dependent mechanism (18). Acetylated LDL also impairs the ability of EC to release erythroid growth factors (7) but stimulates granulocyte-macrophage colony-stimulating factor (GM-CSF) release (37). CE-enrichment stimulates macrophage release of plasminogen activator (11). In addition, oxidized LDL suppresses the expression of TNF-α mRNA in stimulated murine peritoneal macrophages (26). These data suggest that lipoproteins and EC- and macrophage-derived growth factors interact to regulate SMC and macrophage cholesterol metabolism.

CYTOKINES, EICOSANOIDS, AND CHOLESTEROL

Although cytokines are believed to mediate inflammatory events, including recruitment and adhesion of inflammatory cells, the role of cytokines in the regulation of cholesterol metabolism is only beginning to be appreciated. Cytokines, including IL-1, TNF, and GM-CSF, are synthesized by inflammatory cells and activated arterial cells. Cytokines also stimulate growth factor production (25) (Fig. 2). In addition, cytokines may also modulate macrophage and SMC cholesterol metabolism. Fogelman et al. have shown that products of activated lymphocytes decrease the activity of the LDL and scavenger receptors (17). Oppenheimer et al. have recently demonstrated that γ-interferon up-regulates HDL receptor expression in human skin fibroblasts (32), which may be an important mechanism by which γ-interferon inhibits the development of atherosclerosis in rabbits (45). TNF and GM-CSF lower serum cholesterol in humans, but the mechanism by which this occurs is still unclear.

A general consequence of growth factor and cytokine activation of cells is increased eicosanoid generation. PGI_2, PGE_2, and 12-HETE are the major eicosanoids synthesized by arterial EC and SMC. Macrophages and neutrophils also secrete leukotrienes and HETE in response to agonists, including growth factors. In addition to its properties as a vasodilator and inhibitor of platelet aggregation, PGI_2, its metabolites, and 12-HETE display anti-atherosclerotic properties *in vitro*. Exogenously added PGI_2 and 12-HETE stimulate acidic (lysosomal) and neutral (cytoplasmic) CE hydrolytic activities in SMC with no

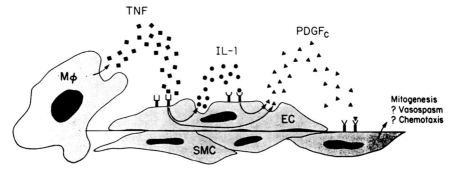

FIG. 2. Model depicting the cytokine-induced activation of growth factor production by the endothelium. Tumor necrosis factor (TNF) or interleukin (IL-1) can stimulate platelet-derived growth factor (PDGF) production and secretion from endothelial cells. The released PDGF can, in turn, stimulate arterial smooth muscle proliferation or enhance eicosanoid production by these cells (see Fig. 1).

change in ACAT activities, thereby increasing net CE hydrolysis. PGI_2 and 12-HETE were shown to enhance cytoplasmic CE hydrolase by increasing the cyclic AMP-dependent protein kinase (20,22), whereas PGE_2 inhibited ACAT activity (Fig. 3). PGI_2 is antiproliferative for SMC (1) and fibroblasts, and it antagonizes the mitogenic effects of growth factors and cytokines (27).

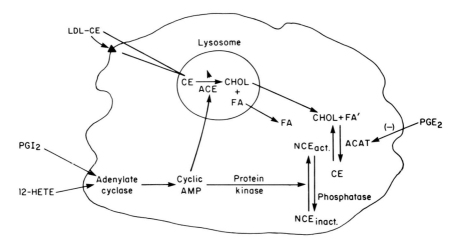

FIG. 3. Eicosanoids alter intracellular cholesterol metabolism. Hypothetical model describing the influence of eicosanoids on cellular cholesterol metabolism. PGI_2 and 12-HETE stimulate cyclic AMP production, which directly increases acid cholesteryl ester (CE) hydrolase (ACEH) activity and lysosomal CE hydrolysis. Increased cyclic AMP activates neutral CE hydrolase (NCEH) activity via phosphorylation by protein kinase, stimulating cytoplasmic CE hydrolysis. Increases in these CE hydrolases result in the degradation of CE derived from low-density lipoproteins as well as CE in cytoplasmic droplets. Cellular synthesis of PGE_2 inhibits cholesterol esterification via acyl CoA:cholesterol acyltransferase (ACAT). (From ref. 47 with permission.)

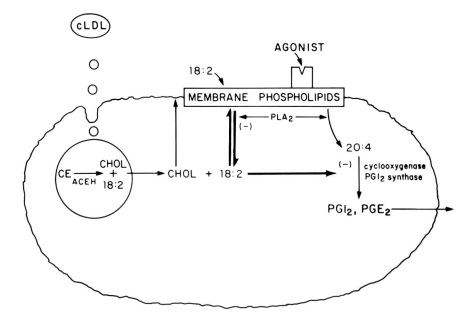

ARTERIAL SMOOTH MUSCLE CELL

FIG. 4. Effect of cholesterol enrichment on smooth muscle cell eicosanoid metabolism. Cholesterol esters enter the cell via derivitized LDL. These lipids are hydrolyzed in the lysosomes by ACEH. Linoleate from LDL-derived cholesteryl esters (CE) are incorporated into membrane phospholipids that compete for arachidonate release by phospholipase A_2 and conversion to PGI_2 and PGE_2. Linoleate can, in turn, also inhibit the eicosanoid synthetic machinery in the cell, affecting overall metabolism if the cell becomes substantially engorged with lipid.

These observations are of significance because most studies have demonstrated that reduced PGI_2-synthetic capacity accompanies atherosclerosis (33,44). The effects of CE accumulation on macrophage eicosanoid production is controversial, since both increased and decreased eicosanoid synthetic capacity by CE-enriched macrophages have been reported. This laboratory has demonstrated that CE-enriched SMC are deficient in their ability to synthesize eicosanoids, due principally to coordinate inhibition of phospholipase A_2, cyclooxygenase, and PGI_2 synthase (35) (Fig. 4). Decreased capacity to produce PGI_2 may have significance because a decrease in the formation of this eicosanoid may result in decreased CE hydrolysis and subsequent CE accumulation.

CELLULAR INTERACTIONS

Finally, the interaction of inflammatory cells (neutrophils and macrophages) with activated EC provides additional mechanisms by which soluble mediators could alter SMC and macrophage cholesterol metabolism. Platelets are abundant

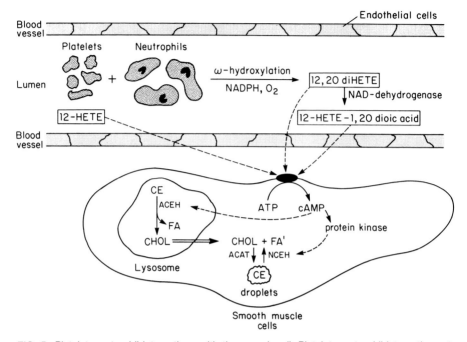

FIG. 5. Platelet–neutrophil interactions with the vessel wall. Platelet–neutrophil interactions at the surface of the blood vessel wall produce metabolic products of 12-HETE, 12,20, diHETE, and 12-HETE-1,20 dioic acid by ω-hydroxylation/reduction processes. These three hydroxy acids stimulate the cyclic AMP–dependent protein kinase in smooth muscle cells to activate cytoplasmic CE hydrolysis via the neutral CE hydrolase. This NCEH enzyme can subsequently hydrolyze CE-enriched droplets in the atherosclerotic foam cell. (From ref. 22 with permission.)

in fatty streaks in hypercholesterolemic nonhuman primates and can serve as cholesterol donors for both SMC and macrophages (6). Platelet products (ADP, serotonin, fibrinogen, and fibronectin) enhance LDL-receptor activity and inhibit scavenger receptor activity in human macrophages (2). Transcellular metabolism of eicosanoids, cholesterol, and cytokines may be altered during close interaction of these cells. Co-culture of neutrophils with either endothelial or smooth muscle cells permitted transcellular metabolism of LTA_4 to LTC_4 (15,16), 12-HETE to 12,20-di-HETE (22). 12,20-di-HETE stimulated CE-hydrolytic activity (Fig. 5), as was the case with PGI_2 and 12-HETE (Fig. 3) by the protein kinase A cascade (22). These data support the concept that interactions of inflammatory cells may be important in the generation of mediators capable of altering SMC and macrophage cholesterol metabolism.

Thus, the results of our experiments and those of others (17) have supported the hypothesis that soluble mediators derived from endothelial/inflammatory cell interactions are central to major signal transducing pathways involved in the regulation of SMC and macrophage cholesterol metabolism (Fig. 6). These findings on the mechanisms responsible for lipid accumulation in the vessel wall

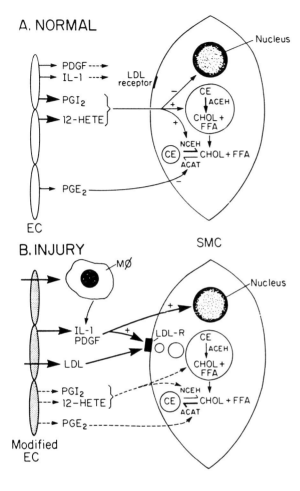

FIG. 6. Alterations in SMC function as a result of injury and hyperlipidemia. **(A)** Under normal conditions, endothelial cell (EC)- and SMC-derived eicosanoids maintain SMC in a quiescent state and maintain low CE content by stimulating lysosomal (ACEH) and cytoplasmic (NCEH) CE hydrolases. **(B)** Under conditions of injury, EC and monocyte release of interleukin-I (IL-1) and platelet-derived growth factor (PDGF) causes SMC proliferation as well as an increase in the activity of the low-density lipoprotein receptor (LDL-R). In the absence of hyperlipidemia, endogenously synthesized eicosanoids may modulate these effects. However, in the presence of hyperlipidemia, eicosanoid production is attenuated, leading to unrestricted cell growth and accumulation of CE. PGI$_2$ = prostacyclin, 12-HETE = 12-hydroxy-eicosatetraenoic acid, CHOL = cholesterol, FFA = free fatty acid, ACAT = acyl-CoA:cholesterol acyltransferase, MO = macrophage. (From ref. 47 with permission.)

following EC activation or injury will undoubtedly have an impact on our understanding of the pathogenesis of foam cell development during atherogenesis.

REFERENCES

1. Akopov, S., Orekhov, A., Tertov, V., Khashimov, K., Gabrielyan, E., and Smirnov, V. (1988): *Atherosclerosis,* 72:245–248.
2. Aviram, M. (1989): *Metabolism,* 38:425–430.
3. Brown, M., and Goldstein, J. (1983): *Ann. Rev. Biochem.,* 52:223–261.
4. Brown, M., and Goldstein, J. (1986): *Science,* 232:34–47.
5. Chait, A., Ross, R., Albers, J., and Bierman, E. (1980): *Proc. Natl. Acad. Sci. USA,* 77:4084–4088.
6. Chao, F., Blanchette-Machie, E., and Chen, Y., et al. (1990): *Am. J. Pathol.,* 136:169–179.
7. Dainiak, N., Warren, H., and Kreczko, S., et al. (1988): *J. Clin. Invest.,* 81:834–843.
8. Davies, P., and Kerr, C. (1982): *Biochim. Biophys. Acta,* 712:26–32.

9. Eldor, A., Falcone, D., Hajjar, D., Minick, C., and Weksler, B. (1981): *J. Clin. Invest.,* 67:735–741.
10. Faggiotto, A., Ross, R., and Harker, L. (1984): *Arteriosclerosis,* 4:323–330.
11. Falcone, D., and Ferenc, M. (1988): *J. Cell. Physiol.,* 135:387–396.
12. Falcone, D., Hajjar, D., and Minick, C. (1980): *Am. J. Pathol.,* 99:81–104.
13. Falcone, D., Mateo, N., Shio, H., Minick, C., and Fowler, S. (1984): *J. Cell Biol.,* 99:1266–1274.
14. Falcone, D., and Salisbury, B. (1988): *Arteriosclerosis,* 8:263–273.
15. Feinmark, S., and Cannon, P. (1986): *J. Biol. Chem.,* 261:16466–16472.
16. Feinmark, S., and Cannon, P. (1987): *Biochim. Biophys. Acta,* 922:125–135.
17. Fogelman, A., Seager, J., Haberland, M., Hokom, M., Tanaka, R., and Edwards, P. (1982): *Proc. Natl. Acad. Sci. USA,* 79:922–926.
18. Fox, P., Chisolm, G., and DeCorleto, P. (1987): *J. Biol. Chem.,* 262:6046–6054.
19. Gown, A., Tsukada, T., and Ross, R. (1986): *Am. J. Pathol.,* 125:191.
20. Hajjar, D. (1986): *Arch. Biochem. Biophys.,* 247:49–56.
21. Hajjar, D., Falcone, D., Fowler S., and Minick C. (1981): *Am. J. Pathol.,* 102:28–39.
22. Hajjar, D., Marcus, A., and Etingin, O. (1989): *Biochemistry,* 28:8885–8891.
23. Hajjar, D., Marcus, A., and Hajjar, K. (1987): *J. Biol. Chem.,* 262:6976–6981.
24. Hajjar, D., and Salisbury, B. (1986): *Pathol. Immunopathol. Res.,* 5:437–454.
25. Hajjar, K., Hajjar, D., Silverstein, R., and Nachman, R. (1987): *J. Exp. Med.,* 166:235–245.
26. Hamilton, T., Ma, G., and Chisolm, G. (1990): *J. Immunol.,* 144:2343–2350.
27. Hori, T., Kashiyama, S., and Hayakawa, M., et al. (1989): *J. Cell. Physiol.,* 141:275–280.
28. Mazzone, T., Basheerruddin, K., Ping, L., Frazer, S., and Getz, G. (1989): *J. Biol. Chem.,* 264:1787–1792.
29. Munick, C., Stemerman, M., and Insull, W. (1979): *Am. J. Pathol.,* 95:131–158.
30. Munro, J., and Cotran, R. (1988): *Lab. Invest.,* 58:249–261.
31. Nilsson, J., Sjolund, M., Palmberg, L., Thyberg, J., and Heldin, C. (1985): *Proc. Natl. Acad. Sci. USA,* 82:4418–4422.
32. Oppenheimer, M., Oram, J., and Bierman, E. (1988): *J. Biol. Chem.,* 2630:19318–19323.
33. Pfitster, S., Schmitz, J., Willerson, J., and Campbell, W. (1988): *Prostaglandins,* 36:515–532.
34. Piomelli, D., Feinmark, S., and Cannon, P. (1987): *J. Pharm. Exp. Ther.,* 241:763–770.
35. Pomerantz, K., and Hajjar, D. (1989): *J. Lipid Res.,* 30:1219–1231.
36. Pomerantz, K., and Hajjar, D. (1990): *Biochemistry,* 29:1892–1899.
37. Rajavashisth, T., Andalibi, A., and Territo, M., et al. (1990): *Nature,* 344:254–256.
38. Rappolee, D., Mark, D., Banda, M., and Werb, Z. (1988): *Science,* 241:708–712.
39. Rohrer, L., Freeman, M., Kodama, T., Penman, M., and Krieger, M. (1990): *Nature,* 343:570–572.
40. Shimokado, K., and Numano, F. (1989): *Arteriosclerosis,* 7:501A.
41. Steinbrecher, U., Lougheed, M., Kwan, W., and Dirks, M. (1989): *J. Biol. Chem.,* 264:15216–15223.
42. Tertov, V., Sobenin, I., Gabbasov, Z., Popov, E., and Orkehov, A. (1989): *Biochem. Biophys. Res. Commun.,* 163:489–494.
43. Van Lentin, B., Fogelman, A., Seager, J., Ribi, E., Haberland, M., and Edwards, P. (1985): *J. Immunol.,* 134:3718–3721.
44. Wang, J., Lu, Y., Guo, Z., Zhen, E., and Shi, F. (1989): *Atherosclerosis,* 75:219–225.
45. Wilson, A., Schaub, R., Goldstein, R., and Kuo, P. (1990): *Arteriosclerosis,* 10:208–214.
46. Winkles, J., Friesel, R., and Burgess, W. (1987): *Proc. Natl. Acad. Sci. USA,* 84:7124–7128.
47. Pomerantz, K., and Hajjar, D. (1989): *Atherosclerosis,* 9:413–429.

Atherosclerosis Reviews, Volume 23,
edited by P. C. Weber and A. Leaf.
Raven Press, Ltd., New York © 1991.

Dietary Fat, Lipoprotein Structure, and Atherosclerosis in Primates

Lawrence L. Rudel, Janet K. Sawyer, and John S. Parks

Departments of Biochemistry and Comparative Medicine, Bowman Gray School of Medicine of Wake Forest University, Winston-Salem, North Carolina 27103

Epidemiologic studies have shown that plasma lipoprotein cholesterol concentrations vary among individuals and that certain patterns can predispose individuals to premature coronary heart disease (CHD). The pattern that places people at highest risk is the one in which high-density lipoprotein (HDL) cholesterol is low whereas low-density lipoprotein (LDL) cholesterol is high. In addition to the differences in lipoprotein cholesterol concentration, numerous studies in both experimental animals and humans have indicated that factors affecting plasma lipoprotein composition also may lead to premature coronary artery atherosclerosis. Among the more well-studied of these predisposing factors are dietary cholesterol and fat, which we have examined in nonhuman primate models of atherosclerosis. The use of experimental animals facilitates the study of the effects of dietary fat on coronary artery atherosclerosis because complete modification of diet is assured. Further, plasma lipoproteins and atherosclerosis in primate models are similar to those in humans.

We studied numerous characteristics of plasma lipoproteins in four groups of primates during a period of atherosclerosis induction. The diets contained 40% of calories as fat. The effects of saturated fat were compared to those of polyunsaturated fat enriched with n-6 fatty acids (study I) and with n-3 fatty acids (study II). Enough cholesterol was added to the diets to induce plasma cholesterol concentrations in the 300 mg/dl to 400 mg/dl range to predispose the animals to develop atherosclerosis. At the end of the diet induction period, the animals were killed, and the extent of atherosclerosis was quantitated morphometrically. The characteristics most highly correlated with atherosclerosis were the compositional modifications of LDL, such as the enrichment of LDL with higher melting cholesteryl esters in the saturated fat diet group. Other factors as yet undefined that are associated with increased size of the LDL particle may also be important, but the presence of increased numbers of more easily oxidized lipids in LDL was associated with less atherosclerosis. HDL cholesterol and apoA-I concentrations generally correlated negatively to atherosclerosis in these animals, and HDL cholesterol concentrations were generally reduced by the polyunsaturated fat diets. The effects of HDL appear to assume more importance in individuals in which LDL have become atherogenic.

MATERIALS AND METHODS

The experimental primates used in these two studies were feral male *Cercopithecus aethiops* or African green monkeys. In study I, the animals were of the vervet subspecies (*C. aethiops pygerythrus*); in study II, the animals were of the grivet subspecies (*C. aethiops aethiops*).

Atherosclerosis was induced by feeding, for a period of 5 and 2.5 years for studies I and II, respectively, a diet containing 40% of calories as fat and cholesterol (0.8 mg/kcal) to induce mild-to-moderate hypercholesterolemia. The effects of diets enriched in saturated fat (principally lard) have been compared with those of diets containing isocaloric substitutions of about half of the saturated fat with polyunsaturated fat (either safflower oil in the n-6 fatty acid–enriched diet of study I or fish oil in the n-3 fatty acid–enriched diet of study II) (1,7). Plasma lipoproteins were isolated and characterized and apolipoprotein concentrations measured by methods that have been previously described (3,4,9). Atherosclerosis quantitations were done using morphometric procedures on aortae that were removed at necropsy and fixed and stained as previously described (6).

For purposes of this communication, the data were analyzed as two separate studies. Statistical comparisons were made using two-tailed, unpaired *t* tests between the saturated and polyunsaturated fat group of each study. The atherosclerosis data were transformed to natural log data to normalize the distributions within groups before the statistical analyses were performed.

RESULTS AND DISCUSSION

We have published two studies on the effects of dietary fat on plasma lipoproteins and apolipoproteins (1,7); the data are summarized in Table 1. Both of these studies contained a group of animals fed a similar saturated fat diet. In the vervet monkey study (study I), the polyunsaturated fat diet contained half of the fat calories as safflower oil; in the grivet monkey study (study II), the polyunsaturated fat diet contained half of the fat calories as menhaden oil. It is apparent that the values for the two saturated fat groups are similar. Compared to animals fed saturated fat, animals given diets enriched in polyunsaturated fat (both n-6 and n-3) had generally lower total plasma LDL and HDL cholesterol concentrations; however, for these data, only the differences in HDL cholesterol concentration were statistically significant. Other larger data sets—particularly for the safflower oil comparison—have shown that the difference in total plasma cholesterol concentration is of the same order of magnitude and statistically significant (1). Plasma triglyceride (TG) concentrations were generally lower in the n-6 polyunsaturated fat group, but they were significantly higher in the n-3

TABLE 1. *Dietary fat effects on plasma lipids, lipoproteins, and apolipoproteins*

Group	Sub-species	N	TPC	TG	VLDL + ILDL (mg/dl)	LDL	HDL	ApoB	ApoA-I
						Cholesterol		Apolipoprotein	
Study I									
SAT	VER	13	355 ± 41	31 ± 5	15 ± 1	224 ± 47	103 ± 9[b]	129 ± 7[a]	244 ± 16
POLY (n-6)	VER	11	280 ± 24	20 ± 2	22 ± 6	161 ± 25	81 ± 5	108 ± 9	232 ± 15
Study II									
SAT	GR	12	371 ± 60	15 ± 1[c]	18 ± 2	249 ± 63	105 ± 8[c]	134 ± 12	223 ± 20[b]
POLY (n-3)	GR	11	251 ± 35	24 ± 1	12 ± 3	167 ± 37	72 ± 8	141 ± 14	161 ± 18

All values are mean ± SEM.

SAT, saturated; POLY, polyunsaturated; VER, vervet; GR, grivet: TPC, total plasma cholesterol concentration; TG, triglyceride; VLDL + ILDL, very-low-density lipoproteins plus intermediate-sized low-density lipoproteins; LDL, low-density lipoproteins; HDL, high-density lipoproteins; ApoB, apolipoprotein B; ApoA-I, apolipoprotein A-I.

[a] $p = 0.06$
[b] $p \leq 0.05$.
[c] $p \leq 0.01$.

polyunsaturated fat animals. In all cases, the TG concentrations were low, as is typical for monkeys. The differences were not primarily associated with altered VLDL concentrations but rather reflect LDL and HDL triglyceride concentrations. ApoA-I concentrations were significantly lower in the polyunsaturated (n-3) group. ApoB concentrations were generally comparable among groups, although the apoB of the n-6 polyunsaturated fat group was marginally lower. Thus, both types of polyunsaturated fat appeared to lower the concentration of the "good" cholesterol (HDL and apoA-I), while the effect to lower the "bad" cholesterol (LDL and apoB) was also present (although more modest in degree). The effects on LDL and apoA-I were less than previously reported for polyunsaturated (n-6) fat (10), but this is apparently due to the fact that the dietary fat for the present study is not as rich in polyunsaturated fatty acids (P/S = 2 versus P/S = 7).

The dietary effects on plasma LDL size and composition in studies I and II are shown in Table 2. The average LDL particle size which was estimated using gel filtration chromatography (9), was smaller in the n-3 polyunsaturated fat group than in the other groups. In general, the numbers of molecules of phospholipid and free cholesterol per particle were present in proportion to particle size, as was the number of cholesteryl ester molecules. The largest and most statistically significant difference for this data set on LDL composition was for the cholesterol ester fatty acid (CEFA) ratio between the polyunsaturated (n-6) and saturated groups of study I. The difference in cholesteryl ester composition led to the differences in transition temperature.

The relationship between cholesteryl ester content and particle size is shown in Fig. 1. The content of cholesteryl linoleate was not proportional to particle size in the saturated fat groups (the line shown did not have a slope significantly

TABLE 2. *Dietary fat effects on plasma LDL composition*

Group	N	Sub-species	LDLMW (g/μmole)	PL	FC	TG	CE	CEFA ratio	TM (°C)
				LDL					
				(molecules/particle)					
Study I									
SAT	13	VER	3.20	805	621	180	2166	1.18^c	36.1^a
			± 0.11	± 37	± 43	± 89	± 148	± 0.07	± 1.1
POLY (n-6)	11	VER	3.19	781	621	61	2234	0.59	33.6
			± 0.10	± 40	± 34	± 20	± 94	± 0.03	± 0.5
Study II									
SAT	12	GR	3.43^b	1006^a	802^b	26^c	2431^a	1.69	37.9^c
			± 0.12	± 31	± 47	± 3	± 138	± 0.16	± 0.8
POLY (n-3)	11	GR	2.91	869	636	65	1965	1.43	26.3
			± 0.13	± 59	± 39	± 5	± 135	± 0.11	± 1.1

All values are mean ± SEM.

LDLMW, low-density lipoprotein molecular weight; PL, phospholipid; FC, free cholesterol; TG, triglyceride; CE, cholesteryl ester; CEFA ratio, saturated + monounsaturated fatty acids/polyunsaturated fatty acids in cholesteryl esters; Tm, peak melting temperature of LDL representing a liquid crystalline to liquid transition. Others as in Table 1.

^{a} $p \le 0.05$.
^{b} $p \le 0.01$.
^{c} $p \le 0.0001$.

different from 0), but the relationship was diet group–specific. The animals fed linoleate rich diets had the highest numbers of cholesteryl linoleate molecules per particle; the animals fed the fish oil–enriched diet had the lowest. For the numbers of cholesteryl oleate per particle, LDL particles from all diet groups fit on the same line. The extent of increase in numbers of cholesteryl ester molecules per particle (proportional to size) was the greatest for this cholesteryl ester, suggesting that increased availability of this ester is the primary reason for the increase in LDL size. Fewer numbers of cholesteryl palmitate molecules were present in the LDL particles, but the numbers of molecules of this ester also increased with size. The data for all diet groups except the n-3 polyunsaturated fat group fit on the same line. The numbers of cholesteryl palmitate molecules per LDL particle were generally higher in the n-3 polyunsaturated fat group. Another study (4) has shown that the LDL particles from the animals fed fish oil had n-3 fatty acid–containing cholesteryl esters that increased in number as LDL particle size increased, with numbers in the 200–400 molecules/particle range. The LDL of the other diet groups had no detectable n-3 fatty acid–containing cholesteryl esters.

The increase in the content of cholesteryl oleate in the LDL particles indicates that a significant portion of the increased numbers of cholesteryl esters in LDL are derived in the liver from the acyl CoA:cholesterol acyltransferase enzyme (ACAT). ACAT activities are high in the livers of each of these high-fat diet groups, although the livers of animals fed fish oil have lower activities (Carr and Rudel, unpublished data). In liver perfusion studies, we showed that at least some of the increased numbers of cholesteryl esters of the plasma LDL were

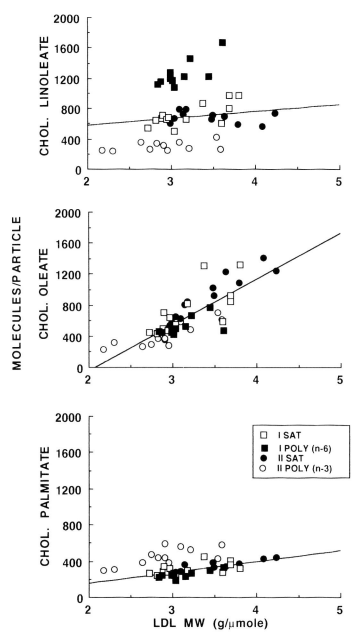

FIG. 1. Relationships between LDL particle size (MW) and individual cholesteryl ester content in molecules per LDL particle. LDL samples from individual animals in the study were analyzed and a point for each was plotted. Diet groups are indicated in the inset. Together, the three esters in this figure make up >80% of the cholesteryl esters in the LDL particles. The lines shown are the least-squares, best-fit regression lines. The slope for the line for cholesterol linoleate was not significantly different from zero, and the line shown is only for the animals in the saturated groups. For cholesteryl oleate, $R^2 = 0.66$ ($p < 0.0001$) and all groups are included. For cholesteryl palmitate, $R^2 = 0.52$ ($p < 0.0001$); the line represents three groups, excluding the n-3 polyunsaturated fat group.

likely derived from cholesteryl ester secreted by the liver. The amount of cholesterol secreted *in vitro* by the liver during perfusion was highly correlated ($r = 0.9$) to the size of the LDL *in vivo* (2). Overall, the result of such diet-induced alterations in cholesteryl ester metabolism is to increase the content of higher-melting cholesteryl esters, particularly in the saturated fat group, resulting in larger LDL particles with higher average liquid crystalline to liquid transition temperatures (Table 2). This modification in physical properties may reflect changes in the characteristics of the LDL particle, both in the core and in core-surface interactions; however, the exact nature of such modifications presently is only a matter of speculation. The varying cholesteryl ester compositions in LDL particles may be of importance in determining the relative atherogenicity of different LDL populations.

The change in dietary fatty acid composition also results in modification of LDL phospholipid fatty acid composition, but this has not been as well documented as the change in cholesteryl ester composition. Table 3 summarizes available data on total plasma lipoprotein phospholipid fatty acid composition in the three diet groups (5; Parks and Rudel, unpublished observations) and should reflect similar alterations in LDL phospholipids. Compared to the saturated fat group, the percentage of linoleic acid in the sn-2 position was nearly doubled in the n-6 fat group; however, the total number of paired double bonds in the phospholipid fatty acids of these two diet groups is almost the same. In the fish oil group, the percentage of fatty acids with five and six double bonds is greatly increased compared to either of the other diet groups, and the total number of double bonds in the phospholipid fatty acids of this group is almost 50% higher than in either of the two other groups. These alterations in phos-

TABLE 3. *Fatty acid distribution of isolated plasma phospholipids from monkeys fed three dietary fats*

	Saturated			Polyunsaturated (n-6)			Polyunsaturated (n-3)		
	% Comp. total	% in sn-1	% in sn-2	% Comp. total	% in sn-1	% in sn-2	% Comp. total	% in sn-1	% in sn-2
16:0	21.8 ± 0.5[a]	92	8	21.1 ± 0.4	88	12	22.6 ± 0.7	86	14
18:0	18.5 ± 1.0	97	3	19.0 ± 0.7	91	9	18.5 ± 0.4	91	9
18:1	8.2 ± 0.1	37	63	5.0 ± 0.1	58	42	4.9 ± 0.1	44	56
18:2	15.3 ± 0.1	7	93	27.4 ± 0.1	8	92	4.1 ± 0.1	10	90
20:4	19.9 ± 0.2	11	89	14.2 ± 0.4	3	97	10.9 ± 0.7	9	91
20:5 (n-3)	N.D.	—	—	N.D.	—	—	13.9 ± 0.2	11	89
22:5 (n-3)	3.6 ± 0.0	14	86	2.7 ± 0.1	0	100	4.5 ± 0.1	12	88
22:6 (n-3)	4.8 ± 0.0	11	89	4.2 ± 0.1	0	100	14.6 ± 0.3	10	90
Other	7.9			6.4			6.0		

N.D., not detectable.
[a] Mean $\pm$ SEM ($n = 3$) for two separate plasma pools for each diet group.

pholipid fatty acids are believed to have consequences for the plasma LCAT reaction (5). Other effects may also be present. Certainly, the increase in the numbers of double bonds that occurs in the lipoprotein phospholipids (together with those in the other lipids) of the polyunsaturated fat groups would be expected to predispose the lipids to peroxidation. However, the antioxidant status of these particles has not been measured; *in vivo,* no difference in peroxidation may actually be realized.

Given the extensive and growing *in vitro* evidence that oxidation of LDL may be a factor in atherogenesis as well as the marked modifications in plasma lipoproteins induced by dietary fat, it was important to determine the actual extent of atherosclerosis. Dietary polyunsaturated fats lowered the plasma LDL cholesterol concentrations somewhat, although the effect was not statistically significant in these groups. The plasma HDL cholesterol concentrations were significantly lowered by polyunsaturated fats, which could predispose these groups to more atherosclerosis. The most remarkable alterations appeared in the composition of the LDL particles. If the oxidation of LDL lipids was a major factor in the initiation or exacerbation of atherosclerosis, the increased number of double bonds in the LDL in the polyunsaturated fat groups might well result in more atherosclerosis.

Table 4 shows several measures of the extent of aortic atherosclerosis in the experimental animals of these studies. The abdominal aorta intimal area, percentage of surface area covered with atherosclerotic lesions, and the percent of stenosis was significantly less in the n-6 polyunsaturated fat group than in the saturated fat group. The percent of surface covered with fatty streaks was significantly less in the n-3 polyunsaturated group, and the percent covered with all types of lesions was marginally less ($p = 0.07$) in this group than in the

TABLE 4. *Dietary fat effects on abdominal aorta atherosclerosis*

				Abdominal aorta		
Group	N	Sub-species	% Fatty str.	% Athero.	Intimal A (mm^2)	% Stenosis
Study I						
SAT	13	VER	25.49 ± 8.80	50.61 ± 9.77[a]	2.54 ± 1.05[b]	19.57 ± 6.65[c]
POLY (n-6)	11	VER	13.80 ± 5.20	26.40 ± 8.02	0.40 ± 0.09	4.66 ± 0.86
Study II						
SAT	12	GR	52.96 ± 6.65[a]	66.86 ± 8.57[d]	1.21 ± 0.31	11.38 ± 2.95
POLY (n-3)	9	GR	33.17 ± 7.97	43.62 ± 10.23	1.14 ± 0.48	11.69 ± 4.56

All values are mean ± SEM.

% Fatty str., % of surface with fatty streak; % Athero., % of surface with atherosclerotic lesions; Intimal A, average intimal area of five selected sections of abdominal aorta; % Stenosis, percent of aortic lumen occupied by intimal lesion. Others as in Table 1.

[a] $p \le 0.05$.
[b] $p \le 0.01$.
[c] $p \le 0.005$.
[d] $p \le 0.07$.

saturated fat group. Thus, the changes in lipoproteins that occurred in the poly-unsaturated fat groups actually resulted in less rather than more atherosclerosis.

The relationships between plasma LDL and atherosclerosis were determined using correlation analysis, as shown in Fig. 2, since all of the plasma lipoprotein measurements as well as the atherosclerosis measurements were made in each animal of both studies. Even though atherosclerosis was induced in the animals in study II for a shorter time, the extent of disease was similar (Table 4), probably because the grivet subspecies is more susceptible to atherosclerosis induction. In any case, this outcome made it possible to combine the data from all four groups. For all animal groups, LDL particle size is plotted against the percent of surface area covered with an atherosclerotic lesion. The best fit regression line shows that a significant relationship exists, with the $R^2 = 0.34$ ($p < 0.0001$) for these data. These data strongly suggest that the compositional alterations in LDL we have described are important in the development of atherosclerosis in these animals. LDL size is a measure of the change in LDL composition that has been noted before to correlate to the extent of atherosclerosis (8). Clearly, the changes in LDL particles associated with LDL cholesteryl ester enrichment that are exaggerated when saturated fat is fed are also associated with increased atherosclerosis in these monkeys.

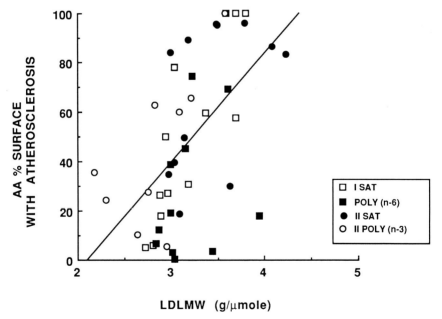

FIG. 2. Relationship between LDL particle size (MW) and the percent of the abdominal aorta surface containing an atherosclerotic lesion. Each point represents data from a single animal. The diet groups are indicated in the inset. The line shown is the least squares, best fit regression line, for which $R^2 = 0.34$ ($p < 0.0001$).

The implications of these findings are significant. The result of feeding polyunsaturated fat instead of saturated fat to nonhuman primates was to ameliorate the development of dietary cholesterol-induced atherosclerosis. Although it is clear that polyunsaturated fat diets increase the potential for oxidation of LDL lipids by increasing the number of paired double bonds per LDL particle, the oxidation of LDL during atherosclerosis development is apparently quite well buffered by the antioxidant status in the animal, so that atherosclerosis is less extensive in animals fed polyunsaturated fat. Instead, other factors that might predispose to atherosclerosis, such as the physical state of the LDL core lipid, appear to be more important.

Clearly, these studies support the hypothesis that the enlargement of LDL particle size and enrichment of LDL particles with cholesteryl oleate represent atherogenic alterations in LDL particle composition. On the other hand, our studies in no way have established mechanisms of LDL-induced atherosclerosis. Only when we understand the effects on the artery wall of the various physical and chemical properties of LDL will we be able to define how polyunsaturated fats protect against atherosclerosis. In animals fed polyunsaturated fat, we assume that the changes in LDL composition account for the relative degree of atherogenicity, since atherosclerosis was less extensive in spite of decreased HDL cholesterol concentrations. It would appear that HDL are needed to protect against atherosclerosis only when LDL are atherogenic, as defined by particle concentration or composition. Regardless of the mechanisms, however, polyunsaturated fats in the diet are likely to have a beneficial rather than detrimental effect on the development of atherosclerosis.

ACKNOWLEDGMENT

This work has been supported by grants HL-14164 (SCOR in Arteriosclerosis), HL-30342, and HL-24736 from the National Institutes of Health.

REFERENCES

1. Babiak, J., Lindgren, F., and Rudel, L. L. (1988): Effects of saturated and polyunsaturated dietary fat on the concentrations of HDL subpopulations in African green monkeys. *Arteriosclerosis,* 8: 22–32.
2. Johnson, F. L., St. Clair, R. W., and Rudel, L. L. (1983): Studies of the production of low density lipoproteins by perfused livers from nonhuman primates: effect of dietary cholesterol. *J. Clin. Invest.,* 72:221–236.
3. Koritnik, D. L., and Rudel, L. L. (1983): Measurement of apolipoprotein A-I concentration in nonhuman primate serum by enzyme-linked immunosorbent assay (ELISA). *J. Lipid Res.,* 24: 1639–1645.
4. Parks, J. S., and Bullock, B. C. (1987): Effect of fish oil versus lard diets on the chemical and physical properties of low density lipoproteins of nonhuman primates. *J. Lipid Res.,* 28:173–182.
5. Parks, J. S., Bullock, B. C., and Rudel, L. L. (1983): The reactivity of plasma phospholipids with lecithin: cholesterol acyltransferase is decreased in fish oil-fed monkeys. *J. Biol. Chem.,* 264: 2545–2551.

6. Parks, J. S., Kaduck-Sawyer, J., Bullock, B. C., and Rudel, L. L. (1990): Effect of dietary fish oil on coronary artery and aortic atherosclerosis in African green monkeys. *Arteriosclerosis,* 10: 1102–1112.
7. Parks, J. S., Martin, J. A., Sonbert, B. L., and Bullock, B. C. (1987): Alteration of high density lipoprotein subfractions of nonhuman primates fed fish-oil diets. Selective lowering of HDL subfractions of intermediate size and density. *Arteriosclerosis,* 7:71–79.
8. Rudel, L. L., Bond, M. G., and Bullock, B. C. (1985): LDL heterogeneity and atherosclerosis in nonhuman primates. *Ann. N.Y. Acad. Sci. U.S.A.,* 454:248–253.
9. Rudel, L. L., Marzetta, C. A., and Johnson, F. L. (1986): Separation and analysis of lipoproteins by gel filtration. *Methods Enzymol.,* 129:45–57.
10. Rudel, L. L., Parks, J. S., and Bond, M. G. (1986): Dietary polyunsaturated fat effects on atherosclerosis and plasma lipoproteins in African green monkeys. In: Scarpelli, D. G., and Migake, G., eds. *Current topics in nutrition and disease. Nutritional diseases: research directions in comparative pathobiology,* Vol. 15. New York: Alan R. Liss, pp. 501–523.

Atherosclerosis Reviews, Volume 23,
edited by P. C. Weber and A. Leaf.
Raven Press, Ltd., New York © 1991.

Genetic Defects in the Human Plasma Apolipoproteins

H. Bryan Brewer Jr., Silvia Santamarina-Fojo, and Jeffrey M. Hoeg

Molecular Disease Branch, National Heart, Lung, and Blood Institute, National Institutes of Health, Bethesda, Maryland 20892

Apolipoproteins play a pivotal role in the biosynthesis, transport, intravascular remodeling, and catabolism of plasma lipoproteins. To date, 10 major human plasma apolipoproteins have been isolated, and their covalent structures elucidated. Molecular defects that result in characteristic dyslipoproteinemias have been identified in several of the apolipoprotein genes. This report summarizes the structural mutations that lead to the major clinical dyslipoproteinemias.

HUMAN APOLIPOPROTEINS

The major human plasma apolipoproteins are listed in Table 1 (2,34,58). ApoA-I and apoA-II are the two major proteins of high-density lipoproteins (HDL), and apoB-100 is the principal apolipoprotein in low-density lipoproteins (LDL). Apolipoproteins A-IV, C-I, C-II, C-III, D, and E are present in several different density classes of lipoproteins. Apo(a) is a unique protein present on Lp(a). The genes for apoA-I, apoC-II, and apoA-IV are clustered on chromosome 11 and those for apoE, apoC-II, and apoC-I are tandemly organized on chromosome 19.

Human apoB exists as two isoproteins designated apoB-48 and apoB-100 (29). The structural basis for the two apoB isoproteins has been elucidated and involves apoB mRNA editing (4,21,25,41). A single copy of the apoB gene is located on chromosome 2. ApoB-100 contains 4,536 amino acids and is translated from the full length apoB mRNA; apoB-48 contains 2,152 amino acids and is the amino-terminal half of apoB-100. Two different species of apoB mRNA can be synthesized from the single apoB gene. One mRNA codes for apoB-100, whereas the other apoB mRNA contains a premature in-frame stop codon in which a single base substitution of a U for C occurs at nucleotide 6,666, converting the CAA codon for glutamine residue 2,153 in apoB-100 to a UAA in-frame stop codon. The 2,152 amino acid apoB-48 is translated from the edited apoB mRNA. In humans, the two major sites of synthesis of the apoB isoproteins (21), are the

TABLE 1. *Major human plasma apolipoproteins*

Apolipoprotein	Chromsome	Approximate molecular weight (kDa)	Major density class	Major site of synthesis
A-I	11	28	HDL	Liver, intestine
A-II	1	18	HDL	Liver
A-IV	11	45	Chylomicrons, VLDL, HDL	Intestine
B-48	2	500	Chylomicrons, VLDL, IDL, LDL	Intestine
B-100	2	250	Chylomicrons, VLDL, IDL	Liver, intestine
C-I	19	7	Chylomicrons, VLDL, HDL	Liver
C-II	19	10	Chylomicrons, VLDL, HDL	Liver
C-III$_{0-2}$	11	10	Chylomicrons, VLDL, HDL	Liver
E$_{2-4}$	19	34	VLDL, IDL, HDL	Liver
Apo(a)	6	500	LDL, HDL	Liver

intestine, which synthesizes approximately 85% apoB-48 and 15% apoB-100 (24), and the liver, which secretes virtually only apoB-100 (9).

The major functions of the plasma apolipoproteins in lipoprotein metabolism are summarized in Table 2 and include the following: (a) Apolipoproteins function as structural proteins that are required for the biosynthesis, assembly, and secretion of lipoprotein particles. ApoA-I is necessary for the formation of HDL; apoB-100 and apoB-48 are required for the secretion of triglyceride-rich lipoproteins from the liver and intestine, respectively (20,30,40). (b) Apolipoproteins also function as cofactors or activators of enzymes involved in lipid and lipoprotein metabolism. ApoC-II activates lipoprotein lipase, the enzyme that is responsible for the hydrolysis of plasma lipoprotein triglycerides to free fatty acids and monoglycerides (19,32). ApoA-I modulates the activity of lecithin–

TABLE 2. *Functions of the plasma apolipoproteins in lipoprotein metabolism*

Function	Apolipoprotein
Structural protein on lipoprotein particles	
Intestinal chylomicron	B-48, B-100
Hepatic VLDL	B-100
HDL	A-I
Cofactor for enzymes	
Lipoprotein lipase	C-II
Lecithin–cholesterol acyltransferase	A-I
Ligand on lipoprotein particles for interaction with receptor sites on cells	
Remnant receptor	E
LDL receptor	B-100, E
HDL receptor	A-I, A-II

cholesterol acyltransferase (LCAT), which catalyzes the esterification of plasma cholesterol to cholesteryl esters (11). (c) Apolipoproteins play a critical role in the metabolism of lipoproteins as ligands on lipoprotein particles that interact with high-affinity cellular receptors for specific lipoproteins. ApoB-100 and apoE interact with the LDL receptor and initiate absorptive endocytosis and the cellular uptake of LDL and small remnant lipoproteins (3,49). ApoE has also been proposed to interact with the putative remnant receptor, which facilitates the hepatic removal of lipoprotein remnants secreted by the intestine and liver (7,11,36). ApoA-I, apoA-II, and apoA-IV have been reported to interact with a putative 110 kDa HDL receptor (1,10,22,39). The interaction of apoA-I-containing lipoproteins with cells has been shown to facilitate the removal of cholesterol from peripheral cells for transport to the liver, where cholesterol is excreted from the body (1).

During the last decade, specific genetic defects in the plasma apolipoproteins that lead to characteristic disorders of lipoprotein metabolism have been identified. The major dyslipoproteinemias are reviewed in the following sections.

CHYLOMICRON–VLDL METABOLISM

ApoC-II

The physiological importance of apoC-II as an activator of lipoprotein lipase (LPL) has been established by the discovery of patients with a deficiency of apoC-II and severe hypertriglyceridemia (6). Patients who are homozygotes for apoC-II deficiency present at an early age with eruptive xanthomas, hepatosplenomegaly, lipemia retinales, and frequent episodes of abdominal pain or pancreatitis.

The molecular defects that lead to a deficiency of apoC-II have been identified in several kindreds (for review, see ref. 12). The defects are summarized in Table 3, and include an absolute deficiency of apoC-II, mutant variants of the apolipoprotein resulting from single base substitutions in the gene, and single base

TABLE 3. *Genetic defect in apolipoproteins C-II associated with the hyperchylomicronemia syndrome*

Kindred	Mutation	Amino acid	RFLP
Padova	C → A	tyr_{37} → stop codon	Rsal
Hamburg	G → C	Donor splice site mutation in the first base of intron 2	Ddel, Hphl
Nijmegen	G deletion	Val_{18} → stop	Hphl
Bari	C → G	tyr_{37} → stop codon	Rsal
Paris₁	A → G	met_{22} → Val	—
Paris₂	C → T	arg_{19} → stop codon	Nlall
Toronto	T deletion	leu_{75} → stop codon	NR

NR, not reported.

changes that introduce premature stop codons and the synthesis of truncated C-II apolipoproteins. In several kindreds, the genetic defect has altered the normal endonuclease restriction pattern of the apoC-II gene, thus allowing rapid screening and identification of affected members of the kindred.

ApoE

ApoE serves as an important ligand for the LDL receptor and has also been proposed to be an important ligand for the putative remnant receptor, which is genetically distinct from the LDL receptor (11,23,36,50). Structure–function analysis of human apoE has revealed that basic amino acids within residues 140–160 are critical in the binding of apoE-containing lipoprotein particles to the LDL receptor.

ApoE is a polymorphic apolipoprotein in human plasma, and the major isoproteins apoE-2, apoE-3, and apoE-4 are products of the three major alleles (ϵ-2, ϵ-3, ϵ-4) at a single genetic locus (8,54,65). Three common homozygous phenotypes (apoE-2/2, apoE-3/3, and apoE-4/4) and three heterozygous phenotypes including apoE-3/2, apoE-3/4, and apoE-2/4 have been identified. Charge differences in the apoE isoproteins permit the identification of the apoE phenotypes by isoelectrofocusing of plasma or delipidated very-low-density lipoproteins (VLDL).

The structural basis for the major apoE isoproteins has been established. ApoE-3 is considered to be the parent isoprotein, and apoE-2 and apoE-4 are common structural variants. The most frequent form of apoE-2 differs from apoE-3 at amino acid 158, where a cysteine residue is replaced by arginine (7,15,43,53,57). ApoE-4 differs from apoE-3 by the replacement of the cysteine at residue 112 by arginine (7,15,43,53,57). A deficiency or structural mutation in apoE is associated with dysbetalipoproteinemia or type III hyperlipoproteinemia. Type III hyperlipoproteinemia is characterized by elevated plasma cholesterol and triglycerides, and by the accumulation of cholesterol-rich remnants of chylomicrons and VLDL that have been designated β-VLDL. The clinical manifestations of type III hyperlipoproteinemia include planar as well as tuboeruptive xanthomas and an increased risk of premature cardiovascular disease.

Recently, the molecular defects in apoE associated with type III have been classified as apoE deficiency, recessive type III hyperlipoproteinemia, and dominant type III hyperlipoproteinemia (Table 4). The kindred with apoE deficiency is of particular interest as the only apparent clinical manifestation of apoE deficiency is the dyslipoproteinemia whereas the immunological, neurological, and endocrine functions in the homozygotes are normal (13,46).

The majority of individuals with type III hyperlipoproteinemia have the autosomal-recessive form of dysbetalipoproteinemia. These patients usually have the apoE-2/2 phenotype with the arginine 158 → cysteine substitution; most subjects with the apoE-2/2 phenotype are normocholesterolemic or hypocho-

TABLE 4. *Classification of mode of inheritance of the genetic defects in apoE associated with type III hyperlipoproteinemia*

Mutation	ApoE phenotype
Dominant inheritance	
apoE-1$_{Harrisburg}$ (lys$_{146}$ → glu)	E-1
lys$_{146}$ → gln	E-2
arg$_{142}$ → cys	E-2
seven amino acid insertion at amino acid 121	E-3
Recessive Inheritance	
arg$_{158}$ → cys	E-2

lesterolemic (7,16,28,35). The development of hyperlipidemia requires the presence of additional dyslipoproteinemias or other genetic and environmental factors such as obesity or hypothyroidism.

Patients with the dominant form of inheritance of type III hyperlipoproteinemia develop hyperlipidemia as heterozygotes. The apoE variants associated with the dominant form include mutations at residues 142 and 146, and a seven amino acid insertion at residue 121 (Table 4) (37,42,51,56).

Individuals with the apoE-4 variant have elevated plasma levels of total as well as LDL cholesterol when compared to subjects with the apoE-3/3 phenotype. Kinetic studies utilizing radiolabeled apoE isoproteins have established that apoE-4 is catabolized more rapidly than apoE-3 (15,17). Based on these results, it has been proposed that patients with the apoE-4 phenotype have a more rapid clearance of plasma chylomicron and VLDL remnants by the liver than apoE-3 subjects. The increased rate of clearance of these particles into the liver leads to a downregulation of the LDL receptor, which results in higher plasma cholesterol and LDL levels as well as an increased level of remnant particles. An increased level of plasma LDL would be expected to increase the risk of premature cardiovascular disease in patients with the apoE-4 phenotype.

LDL METABOLISM

ApoB

Familial Defective ApoB-100

Recently, a new genetic disease, familial defective apoB-100, that is characterized by elevated plasma levels of cholesterol and LDL has been identified (27,52). These patients may have an increased risk of premature cardiovascular disease. The molecular defect in this dyslipoproteinemia is a defective apoB-100 due to a G to A mutation in the apoB gene that results in the substitution of a glutamine for arginine at amino acid 3,500. This mutation in apoB-100 is associated with reduced binding of the mutant LDL to the LDL receptor and delayed clearance of plasma LDL. Thus, LDL containing the arginine for glutamine substitution is a poor ligand for the LDL receptor and results in hypercholesterolemia as well as the potential for premature heart disease. The clinical effects of this mutation in apoB are comparable to familial hypercholesterolemia, where the structural defect is in the LDL receptor. Thus, a defect has now been identified in both the ligand as well as the receptor in the LDL receptor system. A patient presenting with type II hyperlipoproteinemia may have a defect in either the ligand apoB-100, resulting in the dyslipoproteinemia being designated as familial defective apoB-100, or the LDL receptor, resulting in familial hypercholesterolemia.

Familial Hypobetalipoproteinemia

Patients with the homozygous form of familial hypobetalipoproteinemia are characterized clinically by malabsorption, mild spinocerebellar ataxia, atypical retinitis pigmentosa, and acanthocytosis. Plasma chylomicrons, VLDL, intermediate-density lipoproteins (IDL), and LDL are absent, and the only lipoprotein circulating is HDL (20). The disease has an autosomal-dominant mode of inheritance, with heterozygotes having LDL levels that are 50% of normal.

The genetic defect in homozygous hypobetalipoproteinemia is due to a mutation in the apoB gene (33,45). The genetic defects in two kindreds with homozygous hypobetalipoproteinemia have been identified. In the first kindred, a defect in exon 21 is present resulting in a complete absence of secretion of apoB-containing lipoproteins (45). In the second kindred, the plasma apoB levels are <2% of normal and a G deletion at the splice junction of intron–exon 28 resulted in a frame-shift mutation with the introduction of a premature stop codon and the synthesis of a truncated B-87 apolipoprotein (31).

Several kindreds in which the patients are heterozygotes or compound heterozygotes for hypobetalipoproteinemia have been identified with truncated forms of apoB. These patients have decreased plasma apoB and LDL levels; however, there are no clinical symptoms of malabsorption or ataxia. The size of the truncated apoB variants ranges from apoB-25 to apoB-89 (5,18,26,31,60–64). Based on an analysis of the plasma level of the truncated apoB isoprotein and the hydrated density of the lipoprotein particles containing the apoB variants, it has been concluded that a minimal length of approximately 30% of apoB-100 is required for the secretion of an apoB-containing plasma lipoprotein. Furthermore, apoB mutants ranging in size from apoB-31 to apoB-40 were isolated in the HDL density range, whereas apoB mutants apoB-46 or larger have the hydrated density of VLDL. Thus, it appears that approximately 45% of the structure of apoB-100 is required for assembly of a lipoprotein particle that has the density of VLDL.

It is interesting to note that there is no significant clinical sequelae in the heterozygotes of familial hypobetalipoproteinemia due to a truncated apoB, despite the relatively low plasma levels of LDL cholesterol.

HDL METABOLISM

ApoA-I

ApoA-I is the major structural apolipoprotein of HDL. As a major ligand for interaction with the putative HDL receptor, apoA-I has been proposed to be an important apolipoprotein in reverse cholesterol transport.

ApoA-I is of clinical interest due to its inverse association with the development of premature cardiovascular disease (14,44,59). Screening for potential apoA-I mutations that would affect HDL levels has been the focus of several laboratories, and several point mutations in apoA-I have been identified; however, the majority of these mutations have not been associated with significant changes in plasma apoA-I and HDL cholesterol levels. Two mutations (the deletion of apoA-I lysine 107 and the substitution of apoA-I proline 165 → arginine) are associated with reduced levels of HDL cholesterol (55).

Mutations in the apoA-I gene that lead to a virtual absence of plasma apoA-I and HDL cholesterol are associated with severe premature heart disease. Three kindreds have been reported with a selective deficiency of apoA-I, markedly reduced levels of HDL, and premature vascular disease. The proband in the first kindred with apoA-I deficiency is a 5-year-old Turkish female with planar xanthomas and a markedly reduced level of plasma HDL (48). Clinical features included mild hepatomegaly, but no splenomegaly, neuropathy, or tonsillar hypertrophy. Plasma apoA-I was absent, apoA-II was reduced to 10% of normal, and apoC-III as well as apoA-IV levels were similar to controls. The molecular defect in this kindred was shown to be a deletion of a base resulting in a frame shift introducing a premature stop codon at residue 27 in apoA-I.

The proband in the second kindred was a 45-year-old female with mild corneal opacities and premature heart disease (40,47). There were no xanthomas, organomegaly, or orange tonsils. Plasma triglycerides and VLDL were reduced, LDL and apoB were normal, and HDL was markedly deficient. Plasma apolipoproteins A-I, C-III, and A-IV were not detectable, and apoA-II was decreased to <10% of normal. The genetic defect in this kindred was a 7.5 kb deletion resulting in the failure of transcription of the apoproteins A-I, C-III, and A-IV genes.

Probands in the third kindred were two females aged 31 and 32 years with mild corneal opacities and planar xanthomas on the trunk, neck, and eyelids, and severe coronary artery disease (30,38). Plasma levels of VLDL were reduced, LDL was normal, and HDL was severely decreased. ApoA-I and apoC-III were absent and apoA-II was reduced to <5% of normal. The molecular defect was shown to be a rearrangement in the apoA-I and apoC-III gene complex (30,38).

These three kindreds illustrate two important points. First, the close proximity of the genes for apolipoproteins A-I, C-III, and A-IV on chromosome 11 permits the loss of the expression of up to three apolipoproteins by a single mutation; second, the absence of plasma apoA-I alone or in combination with reduced levels of apoC-III or apoC-III and apoA-IV results in the virtual absence of HDL and an increased risk of premature heart disease.

SUMMARY

The determination of the molecular structure of the plasma apolipoproteins has permitted the elucidation of the physiological functions of the apolipoproteins in lipoprotein metabolism. This information has facilitated the characterization of the molecular defects in patients with dyslipoproteinemias and the development of new techniques to identify these patients, particularly those at risk for the development of early heart disease. The ability to recognize selectively those individuals at risk for cardiovascular disease will enable the physician to initiate therapy at an early stage of the disease and reduce the potential for development of premature vascular disease.

REFERENCES

1. Barbaras, R., Puchois, P., Grimaldi, P., Barkia, A., Fruchart, J. C., and Ailhaud, G. (1987): Relationship in adipose cells between the presence of receptor sites for high density lipoproteins and the promotion of reverse cholesterol transport. *Biochem. Biophys. Res. Commun.,* 149:545–554.
2. Breslow, J. L. (1988): Apolipoprotein genetic variation and human disease. *Physiol. Rev.,* 68: 85–132.
3. Brown, M. S., and Goldstein, J. L. (1986): A receptor-mediated pathway for cholesterol homeostasis. *Science,* 232:34–47.
4. Chen, S. H., Habib, G., Yang, C. Y., Gu, Z. W., Lee, B. R., Weng, S. A., Silberman, S. R., Cai, S. J., Deslypere, J. P., Rosseneu, M., Gotto, A. M. Jr., Li, W. H., and Chan, L. (1987): Apolipoprotein B-48 is the product of a messenger RNA with an organ-specific in-frame stop codon. *Science,* 238:363–366.
5. Collins, D. R., Knott, T. J., Pease, R. J., et al. (1988): Truncated variants of apolipoprotein B cause hypobetalipoproteinaemia. *Nucleic. Acids. Res.,* 16:8361–8375.
6. Cox, D. W., Breckenridge, W. C., and Little, J. A. (1978): Inheritance of apolipoprotein C-II deficiency with hypertriglyceridemia and pancreatitis. *N. Engl. J. Med.,* 299:1421–1424.
7. Davignon, J., Gregg, R. E., and Sing, C. F. (1988): Apolipoprotein E polymorphism and atherosclerosis. *Arteriosclerosis,* 8:1–21.
8. Dousset, J. C., Fourcade, A., Lamy, J. N., and Soula, G. (1980): Changing relative proportions of apolipoproteins of VLDL in chronic male alcoholics. *Pathol. Biol. (Paris),* 28:453–456.
9. Edge, S. B., Hoeg, J. M., Schneider, P. D., and Brewer, H. B. Jr. (1985): Apolipoprotein B synthesis in humans: liver synthesizes only apolipoprotein B-100, *Metabolism,* 34:726–730.
10. Fidge, N. H. (1986): Partial purification of a high density lipoprotein-binding protein from rat liver and kidney membranes. *FEBS Lett.,* 199:265–268.
11. Fielding, C. J., Shore, V. G., and Fielding, P. E. (1972): Lecithin:cholesterol acyltransferase: effects of substrate composition upon enzyme activity. *Biochim. Biophys. Acta,* 270:513–518.
12. Fojo, S. S., and Brewer, H. B. Jr. (1991): The familial hyperchylomicronemia syndrome. *JAMA,* 265:904–908.
13. Ghiselli, G., Schaefer, E. J., Gascon, P., and Brewer, H. B. Jr. (1981): Type III hyperlipoproteinemia associated with apolipoprotein E deficiency. *Science,* 214:1239–1241.
14. Gordon, T., Castelli, W. P., Hjortland, M. C., Kannel, W. B., and Dawber, T. R. (1977): High density lipoprotein as a protective factor against coronary heart disease. The Framingham study. *Am. J. Med.,* 63:707–714.
15. Gregg, R. E., and Brewer, H. B. Jr. (1988): The role of apolipoprotein E and lipoprotein receptors

in modulating the in vivo metabolism of apolipoprotein B-containing lipoproteins in humans. *Clin. Chem.,* 34:B28–B32.

16. Gregg, R. E., Zech, L. A., Schaefer, E. J., and Brewer, H. B. Jr. (1981): Type III hyperlipoproteinemia: defective metabolism of an abnormal apolipoprotein E. *Science,* 211:584–586.
17. Gregg, R. E., Zech, L. A., Schaefer, E. J., Stark, D., Wilson, D., and Brewer, H. B. Jr. (1986): Abnormal in vivo metabolism of apolipoprotein E-4 in humans. *J. Clin. Invest.,* 78:815–821.
18. Hardman, D. A., Pallinger, C. R., Kane, J. P., and Malloy, M. J. (1989): Molecular defect in normotriglyceridemic abetalipoproteinemia. *Circulation,* 80:1853a.
19. Havel, R. J., Shore, V. G., Shore, B., and Bier, D. M. (1970): Role of specific glycopeptides of human serum lipoproteins in the activation of lipoprotein lipase. *Circ. Res.,* 27:595–600.
20. Herbert, P. N., Gotto, A. M. Jr., and Frederickson, D. S. (1978): Familial lipoprotein deficiency (abetalipoproteinemia, hypobetalipoproteinemia, and Tangier disease). In: Stanbury, J. B., Wyngaarden, J. B., and Frederickson, D. S., eds. *Metabolic basis of inherited disease.* New York: McGraw-Hill, pp. 544–588.
21. Higuchi, K., Hospattankar, A. V., Law, S. W., Megalin, N., Cortright, J., and Brewer, H. B. Jr. (1988): Identification of two distinct apoB mRNAs, an mRNA with the apoB-100 sequence and an apoB mRNA containing a premature in-frame translational stop codon, in both liver and small intestine. *Proc. Natl. Acad. Sci. U.S.A.,* 85:1772–1776.
22. Hoeg, J. M., Demosky, S. J. Jr., Edge, S. B., Gregg, R. E., Osborne, J. C. Jr., and Brewer, H. B. Jr. (1985): Characterization of a human hepatic receptor for high density lipoproteins. *Arteriosclerosis,* 5:228–237.
23. Hoeg, J. M., Demosky, S. J. Jr., Gregg, R. E., Schaefer, E. J., and Brewer, H. B. Jr. (1985): Distinct hepatic receptors for low density lipoprotein and apolipoprotein E in humans. *Science,* 227:759–761.
24. Hoeg, J. M., Sviridov, D. D., Tennyson, G. E., et al. (1990): Both apolipoproteins apoB-100 and apoB-48 are synthesized by the human intestine. *J. Lipid Res.,* 31:1761–1769.
25. Hospattankar, A. V., Higuchi, K., Law, S. W., Meglin, N., and Brewer, H. B. Jr. (1987): Identification of a novel in-frame translational stop codon in human intestine apoB mRNA. *Biochem. Biophys. Res. Commun.,* 148:279–285.
26. Huang, L. S., Ripps, M. E., Korman, S. H., Deckelbaum, R. J., and Breslow, J. L. (1989): Hypobetalipoproteinemia due to an apolipoprotein B gene exon 21 deletion derived by Alu-Alu recombination. *J. Biol. Chem.,* 264:11394–11400.
27. Innerarity, T. L., Weisgraber, K. H., Arnold, K. S., Mahley, R. W., Krauss, R. M., Vega, G. L., and Grundy, S. M. (1987): Familial defective apolipoprotein B-100: low density lipoproteins with abnormal receptor binding. *Proc. Natl. Acad. Sci. U.S.A.,* 84:6919–6923.
28. Innerarity, T. L., Weisgraber, K. H., Arnold, K. S., Rall, S. C. Jr., and Mahley, R. W. (1984): Normalization of receptor binding of apolipoprotein E2. Evidence for modulation of the binding site conformation. *J. Biol. Chem.,* 259:7261–7267.
29. Kane, J. P., Hardman, D. A., and Paulus, H. E. (1980): Heterogeneity of apolipoprotein B: isolation of a new species from human chylomicrons. *Proc. Natl. Acad. Sci. U.S.A.,* 77:2465–2469.
30. Karathanasis, S. K., Zannis, V. I., and Breslow, J. L. (1983): A DNA insertion in the apolipoprotein A-I gene of patients with premature atherosclerosis. *Nature (Lond),* 305:823–825.
31. Krul, E. S., Kinoshita, M., Talmud, P., et al. (1989): Two distinct truncated apolipoprotein B species in a kindred with hypobetalipoproteinemia. *Arteriosclerosis,* 9:856–868.
32. LaRosa, J. C., Levy, R. I., Herbert, P., Lux, S. E., and Fredrickson, D. S. (1970): A specific apoprotein activator for lipoprotein lipase. *Biochem. Biophys. Res. Commun.,* 41:57–62.
33. Leppert, M., Breslow, J. L., Wu, L., et al. (1988): Inference of a molecular defect of apolipoprotein B in hypobetalipoproteinemia by linkage analysis in a large kindred. *J. Clin. Invest.,* 82:847–851.
34. Li, W. H., Tanimura, M., Luo, C. C., Datta, S., and Chan, L. (1988): The apolipoprotein multigene family: biosynthesis, structure, structure-function relationships, and evolution. *J. Lipid Res.,* 29:245–271.
35. Mahley, R. W. (1988): Apolipoprotein E: cholesterol transport protein with expanding role in cell biology. *Science,* 240:622–630.
36. Mahley, R. W., Hui, D. Y., Innerarity, T. L., and Weisgraber, K. H. (1981): Two independent lipoprotein receptors on hepatic membranes of dog, swine, and man. Apo-B,E and apo-E receptors. *J. Clin. Invest.,* 68:1197–1206.

37. Mann, W. A., Gregg, R. E., Sprecher, D. L., and Brewer, H. B. Jr. (1989): Apolipoprotein E-1 Harrisburg: a new variant of apolipoprotein E dominantly associated with type III hyperlipoproteinemia. *Biochim. Biophys. Acta.,* 1005:239–244.

38. Norum, R. A., Lakier, J. B., Goldstein, S., Angel, A., Goldberg, R. B., Block, W. D., Noffze, D. K., Dolphin, P. J., Edelglass, J., Bogorad, D. D., and Alaupovic, P. (1982): Familial deficiency of apolipoproteins A-I and C-III and precocious coronary-artery disease. *New Engl. J. Med.,* 306: 1513–1519.

39. Oram, J. F., Brinton, E. A., and Bierman, E. L. (1983): Regulation of high density lipoprotein receptor activity in cultured human skin fibroblasts and human arterial smooth muscle cells. *J. Clin. Invest.,* 72:1611–1621.

40. Ordovas, J. M., Cassidy, D. K., Civeira, F., Bisgaier, C. L., and Schaefer, E. J. (1989): Familial apolipoprotein A-I, C-III, and A-IV deficiency and premature atherosclerosis due to deletion of a gene complex on chromosome 11. *J. Biol. Chem.,* 264:16339–16342.

41. Powell, L. M., Wallis, S. C., Pease, R. J., Edwards, Y. H., Knott, T. J., and Scott, J. (1987): A novel form of tissue-specific RNA processing produces apolipoprotein-B48 in intestine. *Cell,* 50: 831–840.

42. Rall, S. C. Jr., Newhouse, Y. M., Clarke, H. R., Weisgraber, K. H., McCarthy, B. J., Mahley, R. W., and Bersot, T. P. (1989): Type III hyperlipoproteinemia associated with apolipoprotein E phenotype E3/3. Structure and genetics of an apolipoprotein E3 variant. *J. Clin. Invest.,* 83: 1095–1101.

43. Rall, S. C. Jr., Weisgraber, K. H., and Mahley, R. W. (1982): Human apolipoprotein E. The complete amino acid sequence. *J. Biol. Chem.,* 257:4171–4178.

44. Rhoads, G. G., Gulbrandsen, C. L., and Kagan, A. (1976): Serum lipoproteins and coronary heart disease in a population study of Hawaii Japanese men. *New Engl. J. Med.,* 294:293–298.

45. Ross, R. S., Gregg, R. E., Law, S. W., et al. (1988): Homozygous hypobetalipoproteinemia: a disease distinct from abetalipoproteinemia at the molecular level. *J. Clin. Invest.,* 81:590–595.

46. Schaefer, E. J., Gregg, R. E., Ghiselli, G., Forte, T. M., Ordovas, J. M., Zech, L. A., and Brewer, H. B. Jr. (1986): Familial apolipoprotein E deficiency. *J. Clin. Invest.,* 78:1206–1219.

47. Schaefer, E. J., Ordovas, J. M., Law, S. W., et al. (1985): Familial apolipoprotein A-I and C-III deficiency, variant II. *J. Lipid Res.,* 26:1089–1101.

48. Schmitz, G., and Lackner, K. (1989): High density lipoprotein deficiency with xanthomas: a defect in apoA-I synthesis. In: Crepaldi, G., and Baggio, G., eds. *Atherosclerosis VIII.* Rome: Tekno Press, pp. 399–403.

49. Schmitz, G., Robenek, H., Lohmann, U., and Assmann, G. (1985): Interaction of high density lipoproteins with cholesteryl ester-laden macrophages: biochemical and morphological characterization of cell surface receptor binding, endocytosis, and resecretion of high density lipoproteins by macrophages. *EMBO J.,* 4:613–622.

50. Shepherd, J., and Packard, C. J. (1987): Apolipoprotein B metabolism in man. *Acta Med. Scand. Suppl.,* 715:61–66.

51. Sing, C. F., and Davignon, J. (1985): Role of the apolipoprotein E polymorphism in determining normal plasma lipid and lipoprotein variation. *Am. J. Hum. Genet.,* 37:268–285.

52. Soria, L. F., Ludwig, E. H., Clarke, H. R., Vega, G. L., Grundy, S. M., and McCarthy, B. J. (1989): Association between a specific apolipoprotein B mutation and familial defective apolipoprotein B-100. *Proc. Natl. Acad. Sci. U.S.A.,* 86:587–591.

53. Utermann, G., Langenbeck, U., Beisiegel, U., and Weber, W. (1980): Genetics of the apolipoprotein E system in man. *Am. J. Hum. Genet.,* 32:339–347.

54. Utermann, G., Steinmetz, A., and Weber, W. (1982): Genetic control of human apolipoprotein E polymorphism: comparison of one- and two-dimensional techniques of isoprotein analysis. *Hum. Genet.,* 60:344–351.

55. von Eckardstein, A., Funke, H., Henke, A., Altland, K., Benninghoven, A., and Assmann, G. (1989): Apolipoprotein A-I variants. Naturally occurring substitutions of proline residues affect plasma concentration of apolipoprotein A-I. *J. Clin. Invest.,* 84:1722–1730.

56. Wardell, M. R., Weisgraber, K. H., Havekes, L. M., and Rall, S. C. Jr. (1989): Apolipoprotein E3-Leiden contains a seven-amino acid insertion that is a tandem repeat of residues 121–127. *J. Biol. Chem.,* 264:21205–21210.

57. Weisgraber, K. H., Innerarity, T. L., and Mahley, R. W. (1982): Abnormal lipoprotein receptor-binding activity of the human E apoprotein due to cysteine–arginine interchange at a single site. *J. Biol. Chem.,* 257:2518–2521.

58. Williams, D. L. (1985): Molecular biology in arteriosclerosis research. *Arteriosclerosis,* 5:213–227.
59. Wilson, P. W., Garrison, R. J., Castelli, W. P., Feinleib, M., McNamara, P. M., and Kannel, W. B. (1980): Prevalence of coronary heart disease in the Framingham Offspring Study: role of lipoprotein cholesterols. *Am. J. Cardiol.,* 46:649–654.
60. Young, S. G., Bertics, S. J., Curtiss, L. K., and Witztum, J. L. (1987): Characterization of an abnormal species of apolipoprotein B, apolipoprotein B-37, associated with familial hypobetalipoproteinemia. *J. Clin. Invest.,* 79:1831–1841.
61. Young, S. G., Bertics, S. J., Curtiss, L. K., Dubois, B. W., and Witztum, J. L. (1987): Genetic analysis of a kindred with familial hypobetalipoproteinemia. Evidence for two separate gene defects: one associated with an abnormal apolipoprotein B species, apolipoprotein B-37; and a second associated with low plasma concentrations of apolipoprotein B-100. *J. Clin. Invest.,* 79: 1842–1851.
62. Young, S. G., Hubl, S. T., Smith, R. S., Snyder, S. M., and Terdiman, J. F. (1990): Familial hypobetalipoproteinemia caused by a mutation in the apolipoprotein B gene that results in a truncated species of apolipoprotein B (B-31). A unique mutation that helps to define the portion of the apolipoprotein B molecule required for the formation of buoyant, triglyceride-rich lipoproteins. *J. Clin. Invest.,* 85:933–942.
63. Young, S. G., Northey, S. T., and McCarthy, B. J. (1988): Low plasma cholesterol levels caused by a short deletion in the apolipoprotein B gene. *Science,* 241:591–593.
64. Young, S. G., Peralta, F. P., Dubois, B. W., Curtiss, L. K., Boyles, J. K., and Witztum, J. L. (1987): Lipoprotein B37, a naturally occurring lipoprotein containing the amino-terminal portion of apolipoprotein B100, does not bind to the apolipoprotein B,E (low density lipoprotein) receptor. *J. Biol. Chem.,* 262:16604–16611.
65. Zannis, V. I., and Breslow, J. L. (1981): Human very low density lipoprotein apolipoprotein E isoprotein polymorphism is explained by genetic variation and posttranslational modification. *Biochemistry,* 20:1033–1041.

Atherosclerosis Reviews, Volume 23,
edited by P. C. Weber and A. Leaf.
Raven Press, Ltd., New York © 1991.

Genetics and Clinical Importance of Lp(a) Lipoprotein

Kåre Berg

Institute of Medical Genetics, University of Oslo, and Department of Medical Genetics, Ullevål University Hospital, Oslo, Norway

The Lp(a) lipoprotein (4) was detected by the use of antisera produced in animals. The immune sera was submitted to an absorption procedure aimed at identifying differences in individual human sera. Adequately absorbed rabbit immune sera distinguished between categories of human sera. One category gave a definite precipitin reaction with absorbed antiserum in agar gel double immunodiffusion experiments and one did not (4). In addition, a small number of human sera gave a weak or doubtful precipitin reaction in tests with absorbed antiserum. Early genetic studies indicated that the capacity of human serum to produce distinct precipitin bands with absorbed immune serum segregated as an autosomal dominant trait in families, and single locus control was proposed (4). The terms Lp(a+) and Lp(a−), respectively, were introduced for human sera which had the capacity to react with absorbed anti-Lp(a) serum and those that lacked this capacity. It was found that the Lp(a) antigen(s) resides on lipoprotein particles that are different from all other lipoproteins in serum. The Lp(a) lipoprotein particles share antigens (residing in apolipoprotein B (apoB)) with low-density lipoprotein (LDL), the presence of the Lp(a) antigen(s) being their unique characteristic. The antigenic properties of Lp(a) lipoprotein still form the basis for Lp(a) lipoprotein determination. The Ag system (2) of allotypes in LDL was known when the Lp(a) lipoprotein was detected. Formal genetic analysis as well as studies at the molecular level showed that Lp(a) lipoprotein was independent of the homospecific LDL antigens constituting the Ag polymorphism (2) [for review of early studies of Lp(a) lipoprotein, see (5)].

EARLY GENETIC STUDIES ON Lp(a) LIPOPROTEIN PHENOTYPES

The first genetic studies of Lp(a) lipoprotein phenotypes were soon significantly expanded. By 1968, we had examined 175 Norwegian nuclear families and 30 nuclear families from Easter Island with respect to capacity of human serum to react with specific anti-Lp(a) serum (5). We found one Lp(a+) child among 273 children of parents who both typed as Lp(a−) in double immunodiffusion. With this exception, the data strongly supported single locus control and dominant inheritance of the Lp(a+) phenotype.

Studies were also conducted in several other European laboratories. By 1971, more than 500 families with almost 1,500 offspring had been examined. The findings strongly supported the concept of autosomal dominant determination of the Lp(a+) phenotype (4). The early genetic studies (4,6,13) also included a search for genetic linkage (29), but no linkage to any marker known at the time was discovered.

QUANTITATIVE MEASUREMENT OF Lp(a) LIPOPROTEIN

In addition to the problem posed by occasional exceptions to the proposed autosomal dominant mode of inheritance, a small number of very weak or doubtful precipitin reactions were observed (6,7) in the early double immuno-diffusion analyses. Some of these reactions may have been caused by antisera that cross-reacted with serum components other than Lp(a) lipoprotein particles (especially LDL or plasminogen) or by other technical problems. However, the possibility had to be considered that small amounts of Lp(a) lipoprotein could be present in serum that did not exhibit a distinct precipitin band in agar gel double immunodiffusion experiments. This hypothesis was substantiated when more sensitive and quantitative immunological techniques were applied. Today there is broad agreement that small amounts of Lp(a) lipoprotein are present in most or all sera that type as Lp(a−) in double immunodiffusion experiments.

In the 1970s, several laboratories introduced quantitative immunoelectro-phoresis to determine Lp(a) lipoprotein levels. Although some laboratories have successfully worked with other and more sensitive techniques such as radioim-munoassays (1,35), quantitative immunoelectrophoresis remains the method of choice for determination of Lp(a) lipoprotein concentration. With this technique, the immunological reaction can actually be observed as a precipitin "rocket" (Fig. 1). Any problem of cross-reactivity with serum components other than Lp(a) lipoprotein would be identified as an additional precipitin "rocket" (or "rockets"). The homology between the polypeptide chain carrying the Lp(a) antigen(s) and plasminogen (18,27) makes the issue of cross-reactivity of anti-Lp(a) sera with plasminogen a very important one. In quantitative immuno-electrophoresis, it is possible to confirm the lipoprotein nature of the reacting antigen by staining the precipitin "rocket" for lipid.

The use of monoclonal antibodies for quantitative Lp(a) lipoprotein deter-mination (by techniques other than quantitative immunoelectrophoresis) is questionable, because it cannot be taken for granted that a given monoclonal antibody reacts equally well with the different isoforms (19,41) of the polypeptide chain carrying the Lp(a) antigen(s) (see below). Furthermore, the isoform problem makes it difficult to make a valid reference preparation for radioimmunoassay or ELISA tests.

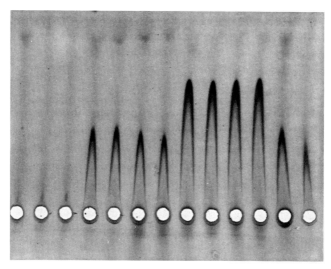

FIG. 1. Determination of Lp(a) lipoprotein concentration in serum by quantitative immunoelectrophoresis in antiserum-containing agarose gel. Individual human sera were introduced into the circular wells and submitted to electrophoresis. The area under the precipitin "rocket" reflects the concentration of Lp(a) lipoprotein in any given sample. Note very wide variation between sera with respect to Lp(a) lipoprotein concentration.

At least some of the commercially offered kits are open to criticism because of cross-reactivity with plasminogen, the use of monoclonal rather than polyvalent antisera, or because of inadequate standardization when compared with the reference technique of quantitative immunoelectrophoresis. There are very few sources of high-quality antisera to Lp(a) lipoprotein, but only reagents from such sources should be used.

The level of Lp(a) lipoprotein is remarkably stable in the serum of a given individual, at least over a great many years. Numerous determinations over the course of a lifetime are therefore not necessary. This should make even a somewhat laborious method of analysis acceptable.

We have shown (8,9) that there is a plausible relationship between the results of Lp(a) phenotyping by double immunodiffusion and quantitative measurements of Lp(a) lipoprotein level. The phenotyping by double immunodiffusion detects all samples in the top quartile of Lp(a) lipoprotein concentrations as Lp(a+) individuals as well as some samples below the top quartile.

Lp(a) LIPOPROTEIN AS A QUANTITATIVE GENETIC TRAIT

Important studies of Lp(a) lipoprotein as a quantitative genetic trait were conducted by Schultz et al. (35) and Sing et al. (37); single locus control was again confirmed. A particularly extensive quantitative study was conducted by

Morton et al. (30), who analyzed 227 families with a total of 557 children. They found strong indications of a major locus with a dominant gene and no evidence against Mendelian transmission. Several twin studies have resulted in heritability estimates of unity or very close to unity for Lp(a) lipoprotein concentration. Thus, the genetic determination of Lp(a) lipoprotein level appears to be adequately documented.

Lp(a) POLYPEPTIDE CHAIN ISOFORMS

Antigenic heterogeneity was observed in the early studies of Lp(a) lipoprotein (5). At an early stage, Rittner (34) noted a strong association between Lp(a) lipoprotein phenotypes and electrophoretic variants of lipoproteins in the density area of Lp(a) lipoprotein. Fless et al. (19) detected heterogeneity between individuals of the polypeptide chain carrying the Lp(a) antigen(s) based on variation in size of this polypeptide chain. Further studies of this phenomenon were carried out by Utermann et al. (41), who demonstrated several isoforms. The familial nature of these isoforms was also confirmed by Utermann et al. (39).

Only a limited number of genetic studies have been carried out on the isoforms. The frequency of a "null" allele has been changing, presumably as techniques have been improved. Nevertheless, the early studies of the isoforms did not uncover any genetic irregularity. However, Gaubatz et al. (20) observed lack of Hardy-Weinberg equilibrium of the isoforms and also noted that isoforms did not always behave as Mendelian traits in families. Technical problems may underlie the apparent departures from Hardy-Weinberg equilibrium and Mendelian inheritance.

Although there is an association between isoforms of the polypeptide chain carrying the Lp(a) antigen(s) and serum Lp(a) lipoprotein level, the range of concentrations within any isoform pattern is wide. On this basis, Utermann et al. (40) calculated that only about 40% of the population variation in Lp(a) lipoprotein level reflects the isoform polymorphism. This has led some workers to suggest that at least one additional locus is involved in determining Lp(a) lipoprotein level. This position is strongly contradicted by genetic linkage data.

LPA-PLASMINOGEN LINKAGE

Eaton et al. (18) demonstrated extensive homology at the protein level between the polypeptide chain carrying the Lp(a) antigen(s) and plasminogen. McLean et al. (27) cloned and sequenced cDNA representing the total LPA gene. They found extensive homology, indicating an evolutionary relationship between the LPA and plasminogen genes. Plasminogen has one copy of each of five different "kringle" structures. The polypeptide chain carrying the Lp(a) antigen(s), which is much larger than plasminogen, has no region homologous to "kringles" I–III of plasminogen but a high number of structures homologous to "kringle" IV. The sample examined by McLean et al. had 37 copies (27).

TABLE 1. Lod scores for the LPA-plasminogen
linkage relationship (Oslo series)

	Recombination fraction			
Segregation from	0.00	0.10	0.20	0.30
Males	2.71	1.97	1.25	0.62
Females	4.82	3.73	2.58	1.42
All	7.53	5.70	3.83	2.04

Adapted from ref. 9.

The evidence for an evolutionary relationship between the Lp(a) polypeptide chain and plasminogen led several workers to conduct genetic linkage analyses. Weitkamp et al. (43) examined a plasminogen protein polymorphism in a series of families who had been scored with respect to Lp(a) phenotype by double immunodiffusion. They found very strong evidence of close linkage. Phenotyping by double immunodiffusion detects high levels of Lp(a) lipoprotein (8), and it may be assumed that the study of Weitkamp et al. was in fact an analysis of segregating high Lp(a) lipoprotein levels in families.

Drayna et al. (16) found close linkage between isoforms of the polypeptide chain carrying the Lp(a) antigen(s) and DNA polymorphism at the plasminogen locus. The results would have been the same if segregating high Lp(a) lipoprotein levels had been used to score for linkage, instead of isoforms. Berg, studying segregation in families of high Lp(a) lipoprotein levels and DNA polymorphisms at the plasminogen locus, found strong evidence for close genetic linkage (8,9). The lod score from the last study alone exceeds 7 for recombination fraction zero (Table 1). Taken together, the lod scores from these three studies where segregating high level of Lp(a) lipoprotein was analyzed, exceed 20. Studies analyzing protein isoforms of the Lp(a) polypeptide chain and DNA variants at the plasminogen locus have produced similar results.

It must be concluded that Lp(a) lipoprotein level, isoforms, and Lp(a) phenotypes scored by double immunodiffusion are determined by one and the same locus—the LPA locus, which is very close to the plasminogen locus on chromosome 6 (6q25–6q27).

SIGNIFICANCE OF THE LPA-PLASMINOGEN LINKAGE IN RELATION TO Lp(a) LIPOPROTEIN LEVEL

The linkage demonstrated definitely proves a single-locus determination of high Lp(a) lipoprotein concentration, whether this is determined by double immunodiffusion that detects only people with the highest values or measured by quantitative immunoelectrophoresis. If other relatively frequent genes contribute to a high Lp(a) lipoprotein concentration, recombination should have been observed in families where segregation of high Lp(a) lipoprotein levels were analyzed with respect to the plasminogen linkage. The absence of recombination makes the speculation (38) that genes at other loci also contribute to the serum level of Lp(a) lipoprotein implausible, at least with respect to the concentrations that are of clinical interest—those in the top quartile or near the top quartile of the population distribution. Thus, the linkage data prove single-locus control of Lp(a) lipoprotein level and make it highly unlikely that other genes with a major effect will be found.

DNA VARIATION AT THE LPA LOCUS

Thanks to the cloning and sequencing of cDNA representing the LPA gene (27), the gene is accessible for direct study. We have reported a quantitative DNA polymorphism at the LPA locus (25). A 2.0-kilobase (kb) fragment produced following digestion with the restriction enzyme MspI exhibited wide quantitative variation between individuals (Fig. 2). This variation could also be detected following digestion with other restriction enzymes. Under optimal conditions, the 2.0-kb fragment did not hybridize with plasminogen probes. This quantitative variation was also detected with an Lp(a) probe that detects only "kringle" IV structures, as well as with a synthetic oligonucleotide constructed on the basis of the reported cDNA sequence of copy 2 of "kringle" IV in the LPA gene, where 20 of 79 bases differ between the Lp(a) and plasminogen genes. This quantitative DNA variation is likely to reflect variation between individuals in numbers of a structure homologous to "kringle" IV of plasminogen. It seems likely that this is the basis for the variation observed at the protein level as the isoform polymorphism. The size variation is also probably caused by varying numbers of "kringle" IV structures. If the isoform variation reflects this quan-

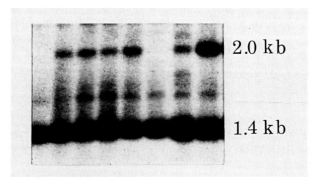

FIG. 2. Section of Southern blot showing quantitative DNA variation at the Lp(a) locus. The vertical lanes show individual DNA samples following digestion with the restriction enzyme MspI. The DNA fragments have been visualized by use of a radioactive cDNA probe that detects "kringle" IV structures in the LPA gene. Note wide variation in amount of a 2.0-kilobase (kb) fragment between individuals. Quantitative estimates may be obtained by relating the variable 2.0-kb fragment to the constant 1.4-kb fragment. It is likely that the quantitative variation in the 2.0-kb fragment reflects variation between individuals in number of "kringle" IV structures.

titative variation in DNA, DNA analysis may well turn out to be the method of choice to study this genetic variation.

We have also detected an MpsI restriction site polymorphism using a probe covering several copies of "kringle" IV and extending into the 3' area beyond the LPA gene (11). This polymorphism is not convincingly detectable with probes that only detect "kringle" IV structures and cannot be visualized using plasminogen probes under suitable conditions. It appears that this restriction site polymorphism may be 3' to the last "kringle" IV in the LPA gene.

In limited family studies, both DNA polymorphisms have behaved as Mendelian traits, and both have co-segregated with Lp(a) lipoprotein level in informative families. Neither polymorphism has exhibited an impressive correlation with Lp(a) lipoprotein level in unrelated people. However, there was an almost significant shortage of homozygotes for presence of the MspI restriction site in people belonging to the top quartile of Lp(a) lipoprotein levels. It seems plausible that more extensive studies will indeed detect a significant correlation between each of the two polymorphisms and Lp(a) lipoprotein concentration.

Lp(a) LIPOPROTEIN AS A GENETIC RISK FACTOR FOR CORONARY HEART DISEASE

In 1974, Berg et al. (10) reported an association between Lp(a) lipoprotein and coronary heart disease (CHD). This discovery has since been confirmed in a long series of studies. Lp(a) lipoprotein determination was a feature of four of the studies performed in our laboratory at the Institute of Medical Genetics, University of Oslo. The result of the four studies are summarized in Table 2. These case control studies, which all yielded significant results, comprised a total of 702 patients.

A particularly informative study was conducted by Rhoads et al. (33), who found a risk of 28% for contracting myocardial infarction (MI) prior to age 60 in men with an Lp(a) lipoprotein concentration in the top quartile of the population distribution (Table 3). Significantly, the risk was as high as 13% even for the age group 60 through 69 years and 14% when all cases of MI (n = 303) were

TABLE 2. *Case-control studies showing higher frequency of phenotype Lp(a+) (studies 1–3) or higher measured level of Lp(a) lipoprotein (study 4) in coronary heart disease (CHD) patients than in controls*

Study	Population	No. of patients	p value[a]
1	Finnish	153	0.002–0.005
2	Swedish	58	0.036
3	Norwegian	188	<0.0001
4	Japanese	303	<0.005
	Total	702	

[a] For differences between patients and controls.

TABLE 3. Odds ratio for history of myocardial infarction at different ages and population attributable risk for men with an Lp(a) lipoprotein concentration in the top quartile of the population distribution (33)

Age at study	Odds ratio	Population attributable risk (%)
<60	2.54	28
60–69	1.57	13
70+	1.22	5
All	1.65	14

considered. In England, Durrington et al. (17) found that the source of practically all familial aggregation of cases of premature CHD (in the absence of Mendelian hyperlipidemias) was a high level of Lp(a) lipoprotein.

There are now more than 20 published studies confirming the association between a high Lp(a) lipoprotein level and CHD. A high Lp(a) lipoprotein concentration is well established as a genetic risk factor (14). No consistent correlation has been observed between Lp(a) lipoprotein level and other risk factors. Correlation coefficients between Lp(a) lipoprotein level and various established or potential risk factors or protective factors with respect to CHD from one of our studies are given in Table 4. However, an apparent association between Lp(a) lipoprotein concentration and cholesterol disappeared when cholesterol was adjusted for cholesterol present in Lp(a) lipoprotein particles. Thus, a high Lp(a) lipoprotein level is a genetic risk factor in its own right that is not detected by any of the traditional methods for risk factor analysis.

TABLE 4. Correlation coefficients (Pearson) between Lp(a) lipoprotein level and various established or potential risk factors or protective factors with respect to CHD in a study of healthy, unrelated Norwegians (the number of subjects varied between 147 and 160)

Parameter	r
Total serum cholesterol	0.26
LDL cholesterol	0.20
HDL cholesterol	0.02
Fasting triglycerides	−0.04
Apolipoprotein AI	0.05
Apolipoprotein B	0.11
Homocysteine	−0.04
Fibrinogen	0.17
Plasminogen	0.08
Serum cholesterol adjusted for cholesterol in Lp(a) lipoprotein	0.04

POSSIBLE MECHANISMS UNDERLYING THE ASSOCIATION BETWEEN A HIGH Lp(a) LIPOPROTEIN LEVEL AND ATHEROSCLEROTIC DISEASE

It was established by the earliest studies that Lp(a) lipoprotein particles aggregate very easily. Several years ago, we compared the aggregation of Lp(a) lipoprotein and LDL particles, respectively, under conditions mimicking those in arterial walls. We found that Lp(a) lipoprotein forms aggregates at near physiological concentrations of calcium ions and massive aggregates in the presence of both glycosaminoglycans and calcium (15). These results were in excellent agreement with studies reported by Walton (42), who detected apparently intact Lp(a) lipoprotein particles in atherosclerotic lesions. This finding has recently been confirmed; the amount of Lp(a) lipoprotein deposited in the arterial wall has been shown to correlate with Lp(a) lipoprotein concentration in serum (32).

The characteristics of Lp(a) lipoprotein particles and their "dose-dependent" deposition in arterial walls could explain the association between Lp(a) lipoprotein and CHD. The finding of extensive homology between the polypeptide chain carrying the Lp(a) antigen(s) and plasminogen (18,27) suggests alternative mechanisms that may explain the association between a high Lp(a) lipoprotein level and CHD. There are already several *in vitro* studies indicating that Lp(a) lipoprotein may interfere with fibrinolytic/thrombolytic processes. Thus, Harpel et al. (23) demonstrated an affinity between Lp(a) lipoprotein and protease-modified fibrinogen or fibrin; Hajjar et al. (22) demonstrated Lp(a) lipoprotein modulation of endothelial cell surface fibrinolysis; and Miles et al. (28) detected Lp(a) lipoprotein competition for plasminogen receptors by molecular mimickry. We have observed an apparent (but relatively weak) association between Lp(a) lipoprotein and fibrinogen levels.

The presence of Lp(a) lipoprotein in atherosclerotic lesions makes it reasonable to regard this lipoprotein as atherogenic. If the *in vitro* studies suggesting an inhibitory capacity on fibrinolysis/thrombolysis are confirmed, it would seem that a high Lp(a) lipoprotein level contributes to CHD risk by two different mechanisms. This may explain why Lp(a) lipoprotein make people susceptible to CHD at much lower serum concentrations than LDL.

Lp(a) LIPOPROTEIN AND THE LOW DENSITY LIPOPROTEIN RECEPTOR

The question of whether the LDL receptor plays a role in the regulation of Lp(a) lipoprotein concentration has been a subject of considerable interest. In our own studies using radiolabeled Lp(a) lipoprotein, we failed to find saturation characteristics or differences in receptor function parameters between cultured cells from healthy people and homozygotes for LDL receptor deficiency (26). Furthermore, we did not observe competition between unlabeled Lp(a) lipoprotein and labeled LDL in cell culture studies. A restriction fragment length polymorphism (RFLP) in the LDL receptor gene that exhibits association with cholesterol level (31) was not associated with Lp(a) lipoprotein concentration.

With the exception of nicotinic acid (21), all tested drugs have failed to reduce Lp(a) lipoprotein concentration. This has been the case even when a dramatic reduction in LDL concentration has been achieved with HMGCoA reductase inhibitors (12). This finding, which illustrates the metabolic independence of LDL from Lp(a) lipoprotein, makes it implausible that the LDL receptor plays a major role in the regulation of Lp(a) lipoprotein level under physiological or near physiological circumstances. However, transgenic mice expressing a very high level of activity of human LDL receptor clear injected Lp(a) lipoprotein faster than normal mice (24). Thus, the LDL receptor is important in clearing Lp(a) lipoprotein in this exceptional situation.

The reported observation of a higher mean level of Lp(a) lipoprotein in a series of British patients with familial hypercholesterolemia (40) than in healthy people in Austria does not necessarily mean that the LDL receptor is of importance in the regulation of Lp(a) lipoprotein level. Even if the comparison between British patients and Austrian controls were valid, there would be problems. Plausibly, having both a high cholesterol level and a high Lp(a) lipoprotein level would increase an individual's chance of appearing as a patient in a clinical setting. This notion is supported by the observations of Armstrong et al. (3), who found that in the absence of classical hypercholesterolemia, having a high level of Lp(a) lipoprotein may be particularly unfortunate when the LDL level is also increased. In a study of patients with familial hypercholesterolemia, Seed et al. (36) in fact observed a higher Lp(a) lipoprotein level in patients who had manifest CHD than in those who did not.

Only future studies can resolve the extent to which the LDL receptor is involved in Lp(a) lipoprotein clearing. By nature of the laborious *in vitro* analyses involved, Lp(a) lipoprotein from only a small number of people has been included in any single LDL receptor study on cultured cells. It is crucial to consider whether differences between individuals may have caused apparently conflicting results. Perhaps the polypeptide chain carrying the Lp(a) antigen(s) is not attached to the same cysteine residue in apoB in all people. If this were the case, some Lp(a) polypeptide chains could interfere with LDL receptor binding of apoB and others not. This possibility warrants further study.

CLINICAL USE OF Lp(a) LIPOPROTEIN DETERMINATION

Determination of Lp(a) lipoprotein level should be part of the diagnostic workup of patients with premature CHD (before 55–60 years in men or 60–65 years in women). In patients with early MI, a high Lp(a) lipoprotein level should be suspected when traditional risk factors are absent.

Therapeutic and preventative goals in people with a high Lp(a) lipoprotein level must be to alter in a favorable direction all risk factors that can be manipulated—including cigarette smoking, unhealthy diet, other lifestyle factors, blood pressure, and blood lipids. The possibility that a high Lp(a) lipoprotein level interferes with thrombolysis/fibrinolysis makes it reasonable to reduce the propensity to thrombus formation as much as possible.

These observations suggest that particularly aggressive efforts to reduce total and LDL cholesterol should be made in people with a high Lp(a) lipoprotein concentration. If cholesterol is not reduced to a satisfactory level by dietary and lifestyle changes alone, the physician should not be reluctant to try drug treatment at lower cholesterol values.

Even in the presence of monogenic hypercholesterolemia there may be some reluctance to institute aggressive lipid lowering regimens in women because of their lower CHD risk. It seems rational to be more aggressive in treating increased lipid levels in women if they have a high Lp(a) lipoprotein concentration than if they do not.

Finally, aggressive lipid-lowering regimens may be contemplated in people with a high Lp(a) lipoprotein level who have just had cardiac bypass operations. The purpose would be to reduce the propensity to develop atherosclerosis in the grafts for patients who are at special risk.

Lp(a) ANALYSES IN PREVENTATIVE MEDICINE

A particularly strong reason for examining Lp(a) lipoprotein concentration in individuals with premature CHD is to be able to examine close relatives, particularly children. The aim is to offer preventative advice to close relatives who are found to be at risk but are still healthy at the time of examination. The advice would make it possible for motivated people to make use of every preventative measure available. It is a plausible expectation that such measures would be more effective if they were started early in life, when the coronary arteries are free from severe atherosclerosis. Compliance with preventative advice would undoubtedly be better if the motivation were stronger, and presumably increased risk in one's family and oneself would be a strong motivating factor. Disease prevention and health promotion should become an important project for the whole family in a setting of family-oriented preventative medicine.

With our present knowledge that a high Lp(a) lipoprotein level is a strong genetic risk factor for premature CHD, Lp(a) lipoprotein determination should not be limited to situations where serious CHD has already occurred. Provided that screening is offered on a voluntary basis and the test results are treated in the strictest confidence, such analyses should be available to persons who want it for the purpose of disease prevention.

SUMMARY

Single-locus control of Lp(a) lipoprotein level has been firmly established. The locus controlling quantitative Lp(a) variation (the LPA locus) has been assigned to chromosome 6. Size isoforms of the polypeptide chain carrying the Lp(a) antigen(s) are controlled from the same chromosomal area, because isoforms as well as segregating high Lp(a) lipoprotein levels exhibit strong genetic linkage (no recombination observed) with normal genetic variation at the plasminogen locus. A DNA polymorphism at the LPA locus that probably reflects varying numbers of "kringle" IV structures and a restriction site polymorphism have been detected. Neither the DNA polymorphisms nor the isoforms of the polypeptide chain carrying the Lp(a) antigen(s) have shown a striking correlation with Lp(a) lipoprotein level. This suggests that the amount of Lp(a) lipoprotein is determined by an area of the gene that is not close to these polymorphisms.

A high Lp(a) lipoprotein level is by itself a significant risk factor for CHD, but there is evidence that the risk increases significantly if serum cholesterol level is also increased. Once a high Lp(a) lipoprotein level is detected, the goal of physician and patient should be to reduce all CHD risk factors that can be manipulated. Lp(a) lipoprotein analysis should be used in any diagnostic workup of people with premature CHD and their families as well as in other attempts to prevent CHD.

At present, there is no evidence that examination of isoforms of the polypeptide chain carrying the Lp(a) antigen(s) or of DNA variation at the LPA locus will improve the prediction of CHD risk any more than simply making quantitative Lp(a) lipoprotein measurements.

ACKNOWLEDGMENT

Work in the author's laboratory is supported by the Norwegian Council on Cardiovascular Diseases, the Norwegian Research Council for Science and the Humanities, and Anders Jahres Foundation for the Promotion of Science, as well as by grant EDC-1 1 RO1 HD26746-01 GT from the National Institute of Child Health and Human Development, National Institutes of Health, Bethesda, Maryland. Part of this article was written while the author was a scholar in residence at the Fogarty International Center for Advanced Studies in the Biomedical Sciences, National Institutes of Health, Bethesda, Maryland. I am indebted to Dr. Richard Lawn of Stanford University and Dr. Dennis Drayna of Genentech, Inc., San Francisco, for cDNA probes used to examine the LPA gene.

REFERENCES

1. Albers, J. J., Adolphson, J. L., and Hazzard, W. R. (1977): *J. Lipid Res.,* 18:331–338.
2. Allison, A. C., and Blumberg, B. S. (1961): *Lancet,* 1:634–637.
3. Armstrong, V. W., Cremer, P., and Eberle, E., et al. (1986): *Atherosclerosis,* 62:249–257.
4. Berg, K. (1963): *Acta Pathol. Microbiol. Scand.,* 59:369–382.
5. Berg, K. (1968): *Ser. Haematol.,* 1:111–136.
6. Berg, K. (1971): In: de Grouchy, J., Ebling, F. J. G., Henderson, I., and François, J., eds. *Human genetics: proceedings of the IVth International Congress of Human Genetics Paris 1971,* Amsterdam: Excerpta Medica, pp. 352–362.

7. Berg, K. (1979): In: Scanu, A. M., Wissler, R. M., and Getz, G. S., eds. *The biochemistry of atherosclerosis.* New York: Marcel Dekker, pp. 419–490.
8. Berg, K. (1990): In: Scanu, A. M., ed. *Lipoprotein (a).* New York: Academic Press, pp. 1–23.
9. Berg, K. (1990): In: Berg, K., Retterstøl, N., and Refsum, S., eds. *From phenotype to gene in common disorders.* Copenhagen: Munksgaard, pp. 138–162.
10. Berg, K., Dahlén, G., and Frick, M. H. (1974): *Clin. Genet.,* 6:230–235.
11. Berg, K., Kondo, I., Drayna, D., and Lawn, R. (1990): *Clin. Genet.,* 37:473–480.
12. Berg, K., and Leren, T. (1989): *Lancet,* 2:812.
13. Berg, K., and Mohr, J. (1963): *Acta Genet.,* 13:349–360.
14. Brown, M. S., and Goldstein, J. L. (1987): *Nature,* 330:113–114.
15. Dahlén, G., Ericson, C., and Berg, K. (1978): *Clin. Genet.,* 14:36–42.
16. Drayna, D. T., Hegele, R. A., Hass, P. E., et al. (1988): *Genomics,* 3:230–236.
17. Durrington, P. N., Hunt, L., Ishola, M., Arrol, S., and Bhatnagar, D. (1988): *Lancet,* 1:1070–1073.
18. Eaton, D. L., Fless, G. M., Kohr, W. J., et al. (1987): *Proc. Natl. Acad. Sci. USA,* 84:3224–3228.
19. Fless, G. M., Rolih, C. A., and Scanu, A. M. (1984): *J. Biol. Chem.,* 259:11470–11478.
20. Gaubatz, J. W., Ghanem, K. I., Guevara, J., Nava, M. L., Patsch, W., and Morrisett, J. D. (1990): *J. Lipid Res.,* 31:603–613.
21. Gurakar, A., Hoeg, J. M., Kostner, G., Papadopoulos, N. M., and Brewer, H. B. (1985): *Atherosclerosis,* 57:293–301.
22. Hajjar, K. A., Gavish, D., Breslow, J. L., and Nachman, R. L. (1989): *Nature,* 339:303–305.
23. Harpel, P. C., Gordon, B. R., and Parker, T. S. (1989): *Proc. Natl. Acad. Sci. USA,* 86:3847–3851.
24. Hofmann, S. L., Eaton, D. L., Brown, M. S., McConathy, W. J., Goldstein, J. L., and Hammer, R. E. (1990): *J. Clin. Invest.,* 85:1542–1547.
25. Kondo, I., and Berg, K. (1990): *Clin. Genet.,* 37:132–140.
26. Maartmann-Moe, K., and Berg, K. (1981): *Clin. Genet.,* 20:352–362.
27. McLean, J. W., Tomlinson, J. E., Kuang, W.-J., et al. (1987): *Nature,* 330:132–137.
28. Miles, L. A., Fless, G. M., Levin, E. G., Scanu, A. M., and Plow, E. F. (1989): *Nature,* 339:301–303.
29. Mohr, J., and Berg, K. (1963). *Acta Genet.,* 13:343–348.
30. Morton, N. E., Berg, K., Dahlén, G., Ferrell, R. E., and Rhoads, G. G. (1985): *Genet. Epidemiol.,* 2:113–121.
31. Pedersen, J. C., and Berg, K. (1988): *Clin. Genet.,* 34:306–312.
32. Rath, M., Niendorf, A., Reblin, T., Dietel, M., Krebber, H.-J., and Beisiegel, U. (1989): *Arteriosclerosis,* 9:579–592.
33. Rhoads, G. G., Dahlén, G., Berg, K., Morton, N. E., and Dannenberg, A. L. (1986): *JAMA,* 256:2540–2544.
34. Rittner, C. (1971): *Vox Sang.,* 20:526–532.
35. Schultz, J. S., Shreffler, D. C., and Sing, C. F. (1974): *Ann. Hum. Genet.,* 38:39–46.
36. Seed, M., Hoppichler, F., Reaveley, D., et al. (1990): *N. Engl. J. Med.,* 322:1494–1499.
37. Sing, C. F., Schultz, J. S., and Shreffler, D. C. (1974): *Ann. Hum. Genet.,* 38:47–56.
38. Utermann, G. (1990): In: Scanu, A. M., ed. *Lipoprotein(a).* San Diego: Academic Press, pp. 75–85.
39. Utermann, G., Duba, C., and Menzel, H. (1988): *Hum. Genet.,* 78:47–50.
40. Utermann, G., Hoppichler, F., Dieplinger, H., Seed, M., Thompson, G., and Boerwinkle, E. (1989): *Proc. Natl. Acad. Sci. USA,* 86:4171–4174.
41. Utermann, G., Menzel, H. J., Kraft, H. G., Duba, H. C., Kemmier, H. G., and Seitz, C. (1987): *J. Clin. Invest.,* 80:458–65.
42. Walton, K. W. (1972): In: Peeters, H., ed. *Protides of the biological fluids, 19th colloquium 1971.* Oxford: Pergamon, pp. 225–226.
43. Weitkamp, L. R., Guttormsen, S. A., and Schultz, J. S. (1988): *Hum. Genet.,* 79:80–82.

Atherosclerosis Reviews, Volume 23,
edited by P. C. Weber and A. Leaf.
Raven Press, Ltd., New York © 1991.

Lipoprotein Lipase: The Molecule and Its Regulation

Thomas Olivecrona and Gunilla Bengtsson-Olivecrona

*Department of Medical Biochemistry and Biophysics,
University of Umeå, S-901 87 Umeå, Sweden*

The focus in atherosclerosis research is presently on cholesterol transport and on how cholesterol-rich lipoproteins are involved in development of lesions. However, the main lipid transported with lipoproteins is triglyceride and the cholesterol-rich lipoproteins, low-density lipoprotein (LDL) and high-density lipoprotein (HDL), can be viewed as remnants from triglyceride-transporting primary lipoproteins. Moreover, it is the turnover of triglyceride-rich lipoproteins (TGRLP) that is directly linked to dietary lipid intake and to energy metabolism—factors that the epidemiologic evidence tells us are of prime importance for atherosclerosis. A main determinant of TG transport is the activity of lipoprotein lipase (LPL) at endothelial sites in various tissues. In this paper, we first review some of the aspects of the molecular structure and properties of LPL. We then integrate these aspects with current information on regulation of LPL synthesis and turnover. Our goal is to understand how lipolysis of TGRLP is regulated *in vivo*.

MOLECULAR STRUCTURE AND EVOLUTION

LPL is a member of a protein family that also includes hepatic lipase and pancreatic lipase (16). There are extensive homologies throughout the amino acid sequences of the three lipases. This indicates that the molecule has retained its overall structure through evolution; there have been no major deletions or addition of pieces from other genes (Fig. 1).

Pancreatic lipase (4) and LPL have reciprocal functions in the quantitatively major pathway of fat transport-digestion and deposition of dietary lipids. These lipases share the ability to hydrolyze TG very rapidly; their turnover numbers are 1,000/sec or more. They are, however, highly specialized for their respective functions. Pancreatic lipase is unable to hydrolyze lipoprotein TG in the plasma environment, and LPL is not active at the high bile salt concentration in the intestine. The two lipases require different activator proteins for their physiological functions—colipase and apolipoprotein (apo) C-II, respectively. These activator

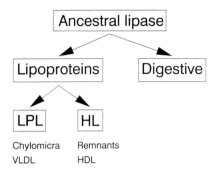

FIG. 1. The evolutionary relationship between the lipases. Recent studies in several laboratories have established that lipoprotein lipase (LPL), hepatic lipase, and pancreatic lipase must have evolved from a common ancestor. Even though the evolutionary relationship is not clear, it appears likely that a first gene duplication gave a digestive lipase (pancreatic lipase) and a lipoprotein-metabolizing lipase. The latter then further specialized into LPL and hepatic lipase by a second gene duplication.

proteins may represent a clue to how the two lipases have adapted to the different physicochemical environments in which they act.

The activator for LPL, apoC-II, is a member of an apolipoprotein family that also comprises apoC-I, C-III, A-I, A-II, A-IV, and E. ApoC-II is a single polypeptide chain of 79 amino acids with flexible conformation (26). Model studies indicate that the N-terminal part of the molecule serves to attach it to phospholipid surfaces by formation of amphipathic helixes. The ability to bind to and activate LPL is located in the C-terminal part of the molecule. Colipase has a similar size, around 100 amino acids (4). In contrast to apoC-II, it is a tightly folded protein with several disulfide bonds. There is wide cross-reaction for members of each lipase-activator pair. For instance, human and bovine LPL are activated by the chicken analogue to apoC-II; colipase from fish and birds activates porcine pancreatic lipase. Despite these wide cross-reactions within each system, colipase cannot substitute for apoC-II, and apoC-II cannot substitute for colipase. No sequence homologies have been found between apoC-II and colipase. It thus appears that the two activators have evolved separately.

Hepatic lipase does not require an activator protein. Other differences between LPL and hepatic lipase are more subtle. Both lipases act on lipoproteins in a plasma environment. However, they prefer different types of lipoprotein particles as substrate. The derangements of plasma lipoproteins in patients with genetic deficiencies of one of the enzymes, and results from many model experiments, indicate that LPL acts on the TGRLP, chylomicra (CYM), and very-low-density lipoprotein (VLDL), whereas hepatic lipase acts on HDL and on remnants of CYM and VLDL formed by LPL. This particle selection probably reflects differences in the "lipid binding" or "interface recognition" sites on the two lipases. In addition, there are differences in how the enzymes select substrate molecules after they have bound to the lipoprotein particles.

In a current study, Deckelbaum et al. have compared hydrolysis of phospholipids and TG in isolated lipoproteins by the two enzymes (7). For each type of lipoprotein used, hepatic lipase always hydrolyzed more phospholipid for a given amount of TG hydrolysis. To obtain a model system in which substrate selection could be directly studied, Rojas et al. (20) incorporated trace amounts of triolein in liposomes of egg yolk phosphatidylcholine. Hamilton and Small have demonstrated that up to about 3% triolein can be accommodated in a phospholipid bilayer (12). Hence, in our model system, the lipase would see a few TG molecules exposed among many phospholipid molecules at the surface of the liposomes. Using identical liposomes as substrate for LPL and hepatic lipase, we found that hepatic lipase hydrolyzed more phosphatidylcholine molecules for each triolein molecule hydrolyzed than LPL did. This is the same result as with lipoproteins and demonstrates more directly that the difference resides in how the enzymes select substrate molecules at the interface. Other studies have also shown differences in action between the lipases. For instance, hepatic lipase appears to have a relatively higher activity against monoglycerides and a relatively higher activity against ester bonds involving long polyunsaturated fatty acids (10). Hence, the two lipases not only select different lipoproteins as substrates, they do somewhat different things to the lipoproteins.

LOCALIZATION AND TURNOVER OF ENDOTHELIAL LPL

LPL displays high activity in adipose tissue and some muscles, but the enzyme is also present in many other tissues (6). Recent studies have shown that LPL mRNA is present in a wide variety of tissues in humans, guinea pigs, rats, and mice, albeit at very different levels. Quantitation showed that in rats and mice, the highest amounts of LPL mRNA are found in adipose tissue, heart, and some red muscles (13,25). The sites of LPL synthesis have been further explored by *in situ* hybridization using labeled RNA probes (2,11,29) and compared to the distribution of LPL protein as revealed by immunohistochemistry (2,29). In white and brown adipose tissue, heart and skeletal muscle, and in lactating mammary gland, there was positive hybridization over all members of the major cell types, indicating that mature and immature adipocytes, muscle cells, and mammary epithelial cells are main sources of LPL. These tissues also showed strong immunoreaction for LPL protein at the vascular endothelium. No LPL mRNA was detected in endothelial cells in any of the tissues studied.

Nevertheless, there was immunoreaction for LPL protein at the endothelial surface of all blood vessels—even in tissue with little or no LPL mRNA. For instance, in the lung, LPL mRNA was present in scattered cells—probably macrophages—but there was LPL protein all along the capillaries. In the glomeruli of the kidney, there was strong immunofluorescence for LPL protein, despite a lack of LPL mRNA in the surrounding cells. These observations suggest the following model for LPL transport (Fig. 2): Initially, the enzyme moves from synthesis in parenchymal cells to binding sites in adjacent capillaries. It then moves along the vascular endothelium from one binding site to the next, carried by blood. The concentration of LPL in the general circulation is kept low by avid uptake in the liver (3). Hence, the system is not in equilibrium, but there is a concentration gradient from areas with LPL synthesis to other parts of the vascular mesh, and there is net flow of LPL to the liver.

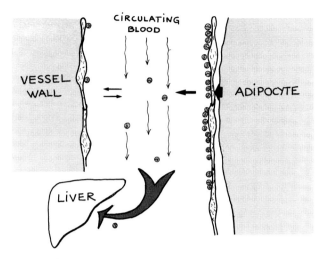

FIG. 2. The transport of lipoprotein lipase (LPL). The enzyme is produced by parenchymal cells, illustrated here by a lipase-producing cell to the right. LPL is released from these cells and moves to binding sites at the luminal side of the endothelial cells in adjacent capillaries. The lipase then moves slowly along the endothelial surface from one binding site to the next, carried by blood. When it enters larger vessels and the general circulation, it can spread to binding sites in other tissues, including those which do not produce LPL. This spreading is counteracted by avid uptake of LPL in the liver. Hence, the system is not in equilibrium, but there is continuous supply of new LPL molecules from sites of synthesis, resulting in high concentration at these capillary segments. There is also continuous net uptake and degradation of LPL by the liver. (From ref. 14.)

REGULATION OF LPL SYNTHESIS AND SECRETION

There are several examples of transcriptional regulation of LPL during development, differentiation, and activation of cells (reviewed in 16). It is less clear whether changes in LPL mRNA are involved in regulation of LPL activity in adipose tissue and in muscles during feeding-fasting and exercise. Taken together, available studies show, on one hand, that there can be rapid and large changes in adipose tissue LPL activity without corresponding changes in LPL mRNA, indicating that additional, posttranslational mechanisms operate. On the other hand, there appears to be a potential for down-regulation of adipose LPL mRNA during prolonged fasting (16,23).

A general finding in pulse-chase experiments with adipocytes is that LPL is transported rapidly out from the cell, reaching the medium within 40 min of synthesis (5,23,28). This is similar to times noted for other proteins that are rapidly secreted by the so-called default, or constitutive, pathway. Another general finding is that only a fraction of newly synthesized LPL (0–30%) is released. The rest is rapidly degraded intracellularly; after 1 to 2 hr of chase, less than 40% of the pulse-labeled LPL remains in the cell (Fig. 3). These studies do not give any indication for buildup of an intracellular store of (active or inactive) LPL that can be drawn upon by hormonal signals.

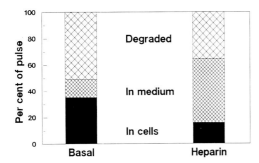

FIG. 3. Effect of heparin on the fate of pulse-labeled lipoprotein lipase (LPL) in guinea pig adipocytes. The adipocytes were pulse-labeled for 10 min with ^{35}S-methionine and then chased in medium with or without heparin (100 μg/ml). After 2 hr, cells and media were harvested, and LPL was immunoprecipitated. The amount degraded was calculated by difference compared to cells harvested at the end of the 10-min pulse-labeling period. (Adapted from ref. 23.)

Earlier studies have shown that there are two aspects to regulation of LPL activity in adipose tissue and heart. One is changes in total tissue activity; the other is redistribution of the enzyme toward the vascular endothelium in the up-regulated states, e.g., in adipose tissue after a meal. An attractive hypothesis is that hormonal or other signals shift the transport of LPL such that more is secreted and less is degraded. This would explain the observed redistribution and at the same time explain the observations that total adipose tissue LPL activity increases even though LPL mRNA and synthesis do not increase, or increase less than LPL activity. There is some evidence for such a mechanism from labeling experiments with adipose tissue pieces (9,17). The only way that increased secretion has been obtained *in vitro* is through addition of heparin to the medium. With heparin, more than half (5,23)—and in one case all (28)—of newly synthesized LPL was released to the medium. Most investigators agree that heparin does not change the rate at which LPL is transported to the cell surface, but it increases the fraction released to the medium at the expense of the fraction degraded.

It has been demonstrated that treatment with a phosphatidylinositol (PI)-specific phospholipase C causes enhanced release of LPL in some cell systems (5) and that such cleavage can be stimulated by insulin (21). It has also been shown that some heparan sulfate proteoglycans are linked to the plasma membrane via a PI-anchor. Hence, one exciting possibility is that insulin activation of a PI-specific phospholipase C releases PI-linked heparan sulfate proteoglycans from the cell surface, and thereby enhances LPL release and transfer to the endothelium.

REGULATION OF LPL ACTION AT THE VASCULAR ENDOTHELIUM

The mechanisms described above regulate the amount of LPL delivered to the vascular endothelium. The amount of LPL there sets an upper limit to the amount of lipoprotein TG that can be hydrolyzed, and thus made available for cellular metabolic reactions. The massive hypertriglyceridemia in patients deficient in LPL or in its activator, apoC-II, demonstrate that LPL is needed for normal catabolism of TGRLP. It is not so clear whether LPL is rate-limiting in normal individuals (for discussion, see ref. 27). Recent studies show weak or nonsignificant correlations between LPL activity and the concentration or fractional catabolic rate of plasma TG (1,8). A few years ago, Cryer reviewed data from animal studies (6) and concluded that endothelial LPL activity in tissues generally exceeds the rate of TG uptake as measured *in vivo* or during tissue perfusion.

This brings up the question of whether there is any regulation of the activity exerted by LPL at the endothelium and takes us back to the molecular properties of LPL. Model studies have shown that the enzyme can bind fatty acids and that this has a marked effect on some of its interactions (14,19). Specifically, fatty acids impede or abolish the interaction of the enzyme with model lipoproteins, with its activator protein (apoC-II), and with heparin/heparan sulfate. Although it is true that fatty acids generally cause some product inhibition of lipase action, these effects are not nearly as marked with most other lipases. A dramatic demonstration of this effect is that the action of pancreatic lipase on its physiological substrates is enhanced, rather than impeded, by fatty acids (4).

These *in vitro* observations led us to speculate that fatty acids could disrupt the binding of LPL both to lipoproteins and to endothelial binding sites. This could provide a fine-tuned regulation of LPL action by the ability of the underlying tissue to assimilate the fatty acids.

To create an experimental overloading of the TG clearing system, Peterson et al. (18) infused Intralipid to fasted volunteers. The dose given, 0.3 g/kg body weight per hr, was close to the potential rate of endothelial LPL hydrolysis, but well above immediate energy needs. The infusion caused progressive rise of plasma TG in all study subjects and increases of plasma free fatty acids (FFA) that varied between individuals. Plasma LPL activity also rose; this increase correlated to FFA but not to TG, both with respect to the levels reached and to the time course. At the same time, Saxena et al. (22) found that physiological concentrations of fatty acids dissociate LPL from cultured endothelial cells. This finding suggests the following sequence of events: Sometimes fatty acids are released by LPL at endothelial sites more rapidly than the underlying tissue can transport and metabolize them. This results in spillage of fatty acids into blood and to formation of LPL–fatty acid complexes with inhibition of continued hydrolysis and dissociation of LPL from endothelial heparan sulfate. The implication is that LPL may (sometimes? often? usually?) be present in excess, and the real limitation of TG transport lies in the metabolism of fatty acids by the underlying tissue. Feedback control of LPL by its fatty acid products may create a direct link between the regulation of tissue energy metabolism and lipoprotein turnover.

ACKNOWLEDGMENT

Our studies on lipoprotein lipase are supported by grant 13X-727 from the Swedish Medical Research Council.

REFERENCES

1. Applebaum-Bowden, D., McLean, P., Steinmetz, A., et al. (1989): *J. Lipid Res.,* 30:1895–1906.
2. Camps, L., Reina, M., Llobera, M., Vilaró, S., and Olivecrona, T. (1990): *Am. J. Physiol.,* 258: C673–C681.
3. Chajek-Shaul, T., Ziv, E., Friedman, G., Bar-On, H., and Bengtsson-Olivecrona, G. (1988): *Biochim. Biophys. Acta,* 963:183–191.
4. Chapus, C., Rovery, M., and Verger, R. (1988): *Biochimie,* 70:1233–1244.
5. Cisar, L. A., Hoogewerf, A. J., Cupp, M., Rapport, C. A., and Bensadoun, A. (1989): *J. Biol. Chem.,* 264:1767–1774.
6. Cryer, A. (1987): In: Borensztajn, J., ed. *Lipoprotein lipase.* Chicago: Evener, pp. 277–327.
7. Deckelbaum, R. J., Ramakrishnan, S., Eisenberg, S., Olivecrona, T., and Bengtsson-Olivecrona, G. (1991): Unpublished data.
8. Després, J. P., Ferland, M., and Moorjani, S., et al. (1989): *Arteriosclerosis,* 9:485–492.
9. Doolittle, M., Ben-Zeev, O., Elovson, J., Martin, D., and Kirchgessner, T. G. (1990): *J. Biol. Chem.,* 265:4570–4577.
10. Ekström, B., Nilsson, Å., and Åkesson, B. (1989): *Eur. J. Clin. Invest.,* 19:259–264.
11. Goldberg, I. J., Soprano, D. R., Wyatt, M. L., Vanni, T. M., Kirchgessner, T. G., and Schotz, M. C. (1989): *J. Lipid Res.,* 30:1569–1577.
12. Hamilton, J. A., and Small, D. M. (1981): *Proc. Natl. Acad. Sci. USA,* 78:6878–6882.
13. Kirchgessner, T. G., Leboeuf, R. C., and Langner, C. A., et al. (1989): *J. Biol. Chem.,* 264:1473–1482.
14. Olivecrona, T., and Bengtsson-Olivecrona, G. (1987): In: Borensztajn, J., ed. *Lipoprotein lipase,* Chicago: Evener, pp. 15–58.
15. Olivecrona, T., and Bengtsson-Olivecrona, G. (1989): In: Lane, D. A., and Lindahl, U., eds. *Heparin.* London: Edward Arnold, pp. 335–361.
16. Olivecrona, T., and Bengtsson-Olivecrona, G. (1989): *Curr. Opin. Lipidol.,* 1:116–121, 222–230.
17. Olivecrona, T., Price, S. R., and Pekala, P. H., et al. (1987): In: Paoletti, R., Kritchevsky, D., and Holmes, W. R., eds. *Drugs affecting lipid metabolism.* Berlin: Springer, pp. 88–93.
18. Peterson, J., Bihain, B. E., Bengtsson-Olivecrona, G., Deckelbaum, R. J., Carpentier, Y. A., and Olivecrona, T. (1990): *Proc. Natl. Acad. Sci. USA,* 87:909–913.
19. Posner, I., and DeSanctis, J. (1987): *Biochemistry,* 26:3711–3717.
20. Rojas, C., Olivecrona, T., and Bengtsson-Olivecrona, G. (1991): *Eur. J. Biochem.,* 197:315–321.
21. Saltiel, A. R. (1989): *Trends Endocrinol. Metab.,* 1:158–163.
22. Saxena, U., Witte, L. D., and Goldberg, I. J. (1989): *J. Biol. Chem.,* 264:4349–4355.
23. Semb, H., and Olivecrona, T. (1987): *Biochim. Biophys. Acta,* 921:104–115.
24. Semb, H., and Olivecrona, T. (1989): *Biochem. J.,* 262:505–511.
25. Semenkovich, C. F., Chen, S.-H., Wims, M., Luo, C.-C., Li, W.-H., and Chan, L. (1989): *J. Lipid Res.,* 30:423–432.
26. Smith, L. C., and Pownall, H. J. (1984): In: Borgström, B., and Brockman, H., eds. *Lipases.* Amsterdam: Elsevier, pp. 263–328.
27. Taskinen, M. R. (1987): In: Borensztajn, J., ed. *Lipoprotein lipase.* Chicago: Evener, pp. 201–228.
28. Vannier, C., and Ailhaud, G. (1989): *J. Biol. Chem.,* 264:13206–13216.
29. Vilaró, S., Camps, L., Reina, M., Perez-Clausell, J., Llobera, M., and Olivecrona, T. (1990): *Brain Res.,* 506:249–253.

Atherosclerosis Reviews, Volume 23,
edited by P. C. Weber and A. Leaf.
Raven Press, Ltd., New York © 1991.

Postprandial Triglycerides, High-Density Lipoproteins, and Coronary Artery Disease

Josef R. Patsch and Herbert Braunsteiner

*Division of Clinical Atherosclerosis Research, Department of Medicine,
University of Innsbruck, A-6020 Innsbruck, Austria*

The interrelationship among high-density lipoprotein (HDL) cholesterol, plasma levels of triglyceride (TG)-rich lipoproteins, and the risk of coronary artery disease (CAD) has been well established. There is a strong negative association between levels of HDL cholesterol and CAD risk and a weaker association between TG and CAD risk, while HDL and TG-rich lipoproteins exhibit a strong inverse association.

Two major hypotheses have been proposed for the role of HDL in the development of CAD: (a) The so-called causalist view assigns HDL a protective effect against atherosclerosis. According to this theory, HDL trap excess cholesterol from cellular membranes by esterification and transfer the esterified cholesterol to TG-rich lipoproteins that are subsequently removed by hepatic receptors. This reverse cholesterol transport from peripheral cells to the liver counteracts the deposition of cholesterol at sites where an excessive cholesterol load produces atherosclerosis. Thus, high HDL cholesterol levels signify a high rate of reverse cholesterol transport. (b) In the so-called noncausalist view, HDL do not interfere directly with cholesterol deposition in the arterial wall but instead reflect the metabolism of TG-rich lipoproteins and their conversion to atherogenic remnants. According to this view, high HDL cholesterol levels indicate an efficient metabolism of TG-rich lipoproteins and a low production rate of atherogenic remnants.

HDL AND TRIGLYCERIDES AS CARDIOVASCULAR RISK INDICATORS

Several major prospective epidemiologic studies have established a strong inverse and independent relationship between HDL cholesterol and CAD risk. In their analysis of the Framingham Heart Study (FHS), the Lipid Research Clinics Prevalence Mortality Follow-up Study (LRCF), the control groups of the Coronary Primary Prevention Trial (CPPT), and the Multiple Risk Factor Intervention Trial (MRFIT), Gordon et al. (7,8) came to the conclusion that HDL cholesterol represents a strong independent risk factor for CAD and that a 1-mg/dl increment in HDL cholesterol is associated with decrease in CAD risk of 2% in men and 3% in women.

In contrast to HDL cholesterol, TG are not generally accepted as a risk factor for CAD. Although the association of elevated TG levels with CAD usually withstands significance tests using univariate analyses, the relationship tends to break down when multivariate analyses are employed. Here, TG are eliminated by HDL cholesterol as a risk factor (2). This fact, however, does not necessarily mean that TG or TG-rich lipoproteins are not causative agents for CAD. Over a wide range, HDL cholesterol levels are determined largely by the metabolism of TG-rich lipoproteins. The influence of TG-rich lipoproteins on HDL is particularly pronounced in the postprandial state, when chylomicrons enter the circulation. Therefore, HDL cholesterol can be viewed as an integrative marker of TG transport in all states of absorption; this fact tends to eliminate the rapidly fluctuating TG as a risk factor (10).

INTERRELATIONSHIP BETWEEN HDL
AND TG-RICH LIPOPROTEINS

HDL are secreted into the circulation not as mature spherical lipoproteins but as discoidal precursor particles devoid of cholesteryl esters (CE). The action of the cholesterol-esterifying plasma enzyme lecithin:cholesterol acyltransferase (LCAT) transforms nascent HDL into mature spherical HDL. Spherical HDL exist as two major subfractions: the small, lipid-poor, and dense HDL_3 and the larger, more lipid-rich, and less dense HDL_2. HDL_3 plasma levels are generally constant among individuals, whereas HDL_2 levels vary greatly and thus account for most of the variability of total HDL cholesterol. Therefore, the more interesting HDL subfraction in terms of CAD risk assessment is HDL_2.

TG-rich lipoproteins affect HDL_2 levels in two ways: (a) Rapid lipolysis of TG-rich lipoproteins by the enzyme lipoprotein lipase (LPL) generates excess surface material, predominantly phospholipids, which is assimilated by HDL. This uptake of lipid promotes the formation of the large HDL_2, thereby raising the cholesterol-carrying capacity of HDL. The assimilation of lipolytic surface remnants by HDL not only affects the formation of HDL_2 but may also protect arterial wall cells. Surface remnants, when not incorporated into HDL, are cytotoxic to macrophages in culture (4). (b) Delayed lipolysis of TG-rich lipoproteins increases the opportunity for the reciprocal transfer of TG from TG-rich lipoproteins into HDL and of CE from HDL into TG-rich lipoproteins. This neutral lipid exchange reaction is catalyzed by lipid transfer protein–I (LTP-I) (1,13). Triglycerides transferred to HDL are hydrolyzed by the enzyme hepatic lipase (12). In this way, HDL cholesterol is transferred into TG-rich lipoproteins, large HDL are converted into small HDL and the cholesterol-carrying capacity of HDL decreases. Hence, rapid lipolysis of TG-rich lipoproteins keeps HDL_2 levels (and thus HDL cholesterol) high by promoting the formation of the larger HDL_2 as well as by preventing their catabolism. The response of HDL cholesterol to the rapid fluctuations of the concentrations of TG-rich lipoproteins is comparably slow and truncated; it constitutes the biochemical basis for the "memory" of HDL with respect to TG transport (10).

Lipolysis as a determinant of HDL_2 levels may be the mechanism linking low HDL cholesterol to the cardiovascular risk constellation of obesity, hyperinsulinemia, and insulin resistance. In 146 healthy subjects of both sexes, 41% of the HDL_2 variance was explained by the combined effect of the waist-to-hip ratio as a measure of truncal obesity, the plasma insulin level, and the degree of glucose intolerance (11). In a different study, weight reduction and its maintenance lowered fasting TG levels, increased HDL cholesterol, and raised the concentration of HDL_2. The HDL_2:HDL_3 cholesterol ratio was strongly correlated to the insulin responsiveness of adipose tissue LPL but not to postheparin plasma LPL. This suggests a tissue-specific regulation of LPL—and of HDL_2 levels— by insulin (6). Both studies show that insulin resistance limits LPL action of adipose tissue and thereby decreases HDL_2.

HDL levels are determined not only by the metabolism of TG-rich lipoproteins but also by the secretion of HDL precursors. Overexpression of human apolipoprotein (apo) A-I in transgenic mice greatly augmented the concentration of this apolipoprotein in the animals' plasma. The apoA-I pool size was directly related to HDL cholesterol levels. The slope of the regression line indicated that the apoA-I/cholesterol mass ratio of the particles was 0.26, equaling that of human HDL_3 (14). Provided that apoA-I is secreted in association with phospholipids, the enhanced biosynthetic rate of apoA-I can be equated with an increased availability of HDL precursors. In this experimental situation, plasma apoA-I levels correlated with HDL cholesterol. However, the elevation was confined to small particles such as HDL_3, while the concentration of HDL_2 remained unaffected (14). This result suggests that another factor—presumably the supply of surface remnants released from TG-rich lipoproteins through lipolysis—is rate-limiting for the formation of HDL_2.

THE ROLE OF LIPID TRANSFER IN CHOLESTEROL TRANSPORT

According to the causalist reverse cholesterol transport hypothesis, one essential component of reverse cholesterol transport is the transfer of CE from HDL to TG-rich lipoproteins. In this way, cholesterol transported with HDL can enter the final leg in its tour from peripheral cells to the liver. In the noncausalist view, however, the role of the LTP-I reaction is diametrically opposed to that in reverse cholesterol transport: A loss of HDL cholesterol into TG-rich lipoproteins is considered potentially harmful because cholesterol would be redistributed from the system of antiatherogenic to the one of atherogenic particles. LTP-I would thus provide a mechanism for switching "good" cholesterol into "bad" cholesterol. Therefore, absence of LTP-I should be a decisive test for the two metabolic models under discussion. If the reverse cholesterol transport hypothesis were correct, the deficiency should disrupt this pathway and thus *predispose* to CAD. Alternatively, if HDL were an indicator for TG transport, LTP-I deficiency should prevent the additional enrichment of TG-rich lipoproteins with HDL-derived cholesterol and thus *protect against* CAD.

A genetic LTP-I deficiency has indeed been described in two Japanese siblings (9). The disorder is caused by substitution of adenine for guanine at the 5' splice donor site of intron 14 of the LTP-I gene (3). Because of the absence of LTP-I, HDL fail to become enriched in TG, which prevents their degradation by hepatic lipase. The result is a vast elevation of HDL cholesterol (248 mg/dl and 175 mg/dl, respectively) and an overwhelming preponderance of the large HDL subfractions. Plasma levels of low-density lipoproteins (LDL) are decreased, presumably because the reciprocal transfer of HDL CE into CYM and very-low-density lipoproteins (VLDL)—and ultimately into LDL—is blocked also. LTP-I deficiency segregates as a familial trait of longevity and resistance to cardiovascular disorders. Therefore, this "experiment of nature" argues strongly against the causalist notion of reverse cholesterol transport.

More recently, attempts have been made to delineate the influence of neutral lipid transfer on the reaction partner of HDL, the TG-rich lipoproteins. In one study in rabbits, monoclonal antibody inhibition of LTP-I produced the expected compositional changes of both lipoprotein reaction partners. HDL CE rose significantly with a concomitant fall in HDL TG, and the CE to TG ratio of VLDL declined significantly (15). This result provides direct evidence that part of the CE transported with TG-rich lipoproteins originate from HDL. Another study investigated the effect of postprandial lipemia on distribution of CE in plasma lipoproteins in humans (5). In going from the postabsorptive to the postprandial state, the fraction of CE transported in TG-rich lipoproteins rose 25-fold while that in LDL and HDL fell by 15% each. Although the transfer of CE from LDL to TG-rich lipoproteins leaves these CE in the same metabolic cascade, the CE transferred from HDL to TG-rich lipoproteins are translocated from the pool of "good" to that of "bad" cholesterol.

The biochemical and clinical data regarding HDL cholesterol and CAD reviewed here support the noncausalist hypothesis, which holds that the negative association between HDL cholesterol and CAD does not depend solely on a direct antiatherogenic action of HDL. The noncausalist theory, however, cannot be interpreted to suggest that HDL are unrelated to atherogenesis and are only passively affected by the truly atherogenic events. On the contrary, the LTP-I mechanism for switching "good" into "bad" cholesterol assigns HDL a central role in the pathogenesis of atherosclerosis. The driving force behind the switch, however, is the metabolism of TG-rich lipoproteins. Rapid clearance of TG-rich lipoproteins promotes the formation of HDL_2, and low levels of TG-rich lipoproteins do not allow excessive transfer of HDL CE into TG-rich lipoproteins.

This keeps the cholesterol-carrying capacity of HDL—i.e., HDL cholesterol—high, and the net effect is antiatherogenic. Delayed clearance and accumulation of TG-rich lipoproteins do not allow the formation of HDL_2 and lead to excessive loss of CE from HDL into lipoprotein fractions associated with high CAD risk. HDL cholesterol is reduced and the net effect is atherogenic.

ACKNOWLEDGMENT

This work was supported by grant HL-27341 from the National Institutes of Health and by grant S-46/06 from the Austrian Fonds zur Förderung der wissenschaftlichen Forschung.

REFERENCES

1. Albers, J. J., Tollefson, J. H., Chen, C.-H., and Steinmetz, A. (1984): Isolation and characterization of human plasma lipid transfer proteins. *Arteriosclerosis,* 4:49–58.
2. Austin, M. E. (1989): Plasma triglyceride as a risk factor for coronary heart disease. The epidemiologic evidence and beyond. *Am. J. Epidemiol.,* 129:249–259.
3. Brown, M. L., Inazu, A., and Hesler, C. B., et al. (1989): Molecular basis of lipid transfer protein deficiency in a family with increased high-density lipoproteins. *Nature,* 342:448–451.
4. Chung, B. H., Segrest, J. P., Smith, K., Griffin, F. M., and Brouillette, C. G. (1989): Lipolytic surface remnants of triglyceride-rich lipoproteins are cytotoxis to macrophages but not in the presence of high density lipoprotein. A possible mechanism of atherogenesis? *J. Clin. Invest.,* 83: 1363–1374.
5. Dullaart, R. P. F., Groener, J. E. M., V Wijk, H., Sluiter, W. J., and Erkelens, D. W. (1989): Alimentary lipemia-induced redistribution of cholesteryl ester between lipoproteins. Studies in normolipidemic, combined hyperlipidemic, and hypercholesterolemic men. *Arteriosclerosis,* 9: 614–622.
6. Eckel, R. H., and Yost, T. J. (1989): HDL subfractions and adipose tissue metabolism in the reduced-obese state. *Am. J. Physiol.,* 256:E740–E746.
7. Gordon, D. J., Probstfield, J. L., and Garrison, R. J., et al. (1989): High-density lipoprotein cholesterol and cardiovascular disease. Four prospective American studies. *Circulation,* 79:8–15.
8. Gordon, D. J., and Rifkind, B. M. (1989): High-density lipoprotein—the clinical implications of recent studies. *N. Engl. J. Med.,* 321:1311–1316.
9. Koizumi, J., Mabuchi, H., and Yoshimura, A., et al. (1985): Deficiency of serum cholesteryl-ester transfer activity in patients with familial hyperalphalipoproteinemia. *Atherosclerosis,* 58: 175–186.
10. Miesenböck, G., and Patsch, J. R. (1990): Relationship of triglyceride and high-density lipoprotein metabolism. *Atherosclerosis Rev.,* 18:119–128.
11. Ostlund, R. E. Jr., Staten, M., Kohrt, W. M., Schultz, J., and Malley, M. (1990): The ratio of waist-to-hip circumference, plasma insulin level, and glucose intolerance as independent predictors of the HDL_2 cholesterol level in older adults. *N. Engl. J. Med.,* 322:229–234.
12. Patsch, J. R., Prasad, S., Gotto, A. M. Jr., and Bengtsson-Olivecrona, G. (1984): Postprandial lipemia: A key for the conversion of high-density lipoprotein₂ into high-density lipoprotein₃ by hepatic lipase. *J. Clin. Invest.,* 74:2017–2023.
13. Tall, A. R. (1986): Plasma lipid transfer proteins. *J. Lipid Res.,* 27:361–367.
14. Walsh, A., Ito, Y., and Breslow, J. L. (1989): High levels of human apolipoprotein A-I in transgenic mice result in increased plasma levels of small high density lipoproteins (HDL) comparable to human HDL_3. *J. Biol. Chem.,* 264:6488–6494.
15. Whitlock, M. E., Swenson, T. L., and Ramakrishnan, F. L., et al. (1989): Monoclonal antibody inhibition of cholesteryl ester transfer protein activity in the rabbit. *J. Clin. Invest.,* 84:129–137.

Atherosclerosis Reviews, Volume 23,
edited by P. C. Weber and A. Leaf.
Raven Press, Ltd., New York © 1991.

Morphological Characteristics of the Developing Atherosclerotic Plaque

Animal Studies and Studies of Lesions from Young People

Robert W. Wissler

*Department of Pathology and the Specialized Center of Research on Atherosclerosis,
University of Chicago Medical Center, Chicago, Illinois 60637*

The advanced atherosclerotic plaque has two major components (Fig. 1). First there is the cholesterol- and lipid-rich acellular part of the plaque, where much of the lipid is deposited. This is a major portion of the *atheroma,* a term derived from the Greek stem meaning "soft, grumous, or porridge-like." The surrounding *sclerotic* area of the plaque is composed of collagen and compressed cells, as well as elastin and other matrix elements. This part often forms a firm, fibrous cap over the advanced atherosclerotic plaque (33).

Chemical analyses of severe atherosclerotic plaques from humans and from the best animal models of the human disease indicate that on the average, fully developed plaques are composed of about one-half lipid components and one-half protein, including the protein of the cells and the extracellular fiber proteins that they produce (see Fig. 1). Obviously, there are great variations in these elements. The pathobiological factors controlling the variations in the relative quantities of the different components are still not entirely understood. They may be the result of changes in the numerous risk factors that influence atherogenesis in humans either in youth or during later years, or they may be due to genetic metabolic differences endogenous to the individual.

Our knowledge of atherosclerosis has increased rapidly in recent years. We know that most of the cells that accumulate in the progressive atherosclerotic plaque in rhesus monkeys, Yorkshire swine (31,38), and humans (14,32) are modified smooth muscle cells (SMC). These are cells that have migrated from the media and proliferated in the arterial intima. They have undergone changes that have made them more likely than the usual contractile cells in the media of the artery to continue to divide and synthesize collagen and to take up lipid (6). At present, cell proliferation and blood lipid infiltration are known to be two of the main processes of atherogenesis (33).

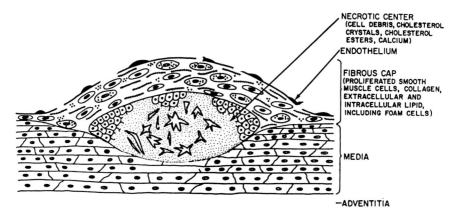

FIG. 1. Major components of advanced atheromatous plaque in people. The average plaque shows about 50% lipid and about 50% protein, the latter derived from cells, collagen, elastin, proteoglycans, etc. (From ref. 33.)

The important role of endothelial cell injury in the atherosclerotic processes has also been recognized. We are now able to evaluate the two main types of active cells derived from mononuclear invasion of the artery from the bloodstream—namely, monocytes and T lymphocytes (12,44). They also vary greatly in number from one developing atherosclerotic lesion to another.

MAJOR PATHOGENIC PROCESSES AT THE ARTERY WALL LEVEL

Lipid (Lipoprotein) Deposition

For many years, evidence has supported the hypothesis that low-density lipoprotein (LDL) and very-low-density lipoprotein (β-VLDL), both of which are rich in apoB, are the main transporters of cholesterol from the bloodstream into the arterial intima (9,11). Recently, it has been shown that under some conditions, LDLs—and perhaps some of the VLDLs—are rather remarkably changed when they enter the artery wall (30). It has been reported that oxidative changes substantially alter the effects of the LDL on the cells of the artery and the types of cells in which the altered LDL is deposited. Recent studies have also shown that oxidized LDL can cause severe injury to both endothelial and arterial SMC and that this damage intensifies atherosclerotic plaque development (15). Cell injury during atherogenesis includes endothelial cell death and desquamation, SMC death, and a shortened life span of the lipid-laden macrophages (monocyte-derived "foam" cells) (20,21,30).

Furthermore, it has now been reported that several of the epitopes of LDL that result from oxidation (22) or glycosylation (45,46) are likely to be recognized as antigenic. These altered lipoproteins may provide additional mechanisms for accelerated atherogenesis when they stimulate both humoral and cellular autoimmune reactions. In some cases, they provide the stimulus for the development of a type of "atheroarteritis" that several studies of both human and experimental animal atherosclerosis have reported when there are substantial levels of circulating immune complexes (41).

Endothelial Transport Vesicles as Regulators of Lipoprotein Infiltration

Arterial endothelium is an imperfect barrier to lipoprotein transport. LDLs, high-density lipoproteins (HDL), and some of the remnants of both VLDLs and chylomicrons (CYM) can gain entrance to the intima by means of endothelial cell transport vesicles (26). Evidence indicates that circulating LDLs can pass through these transport vesicles at a regulated rate and on into the artery wall

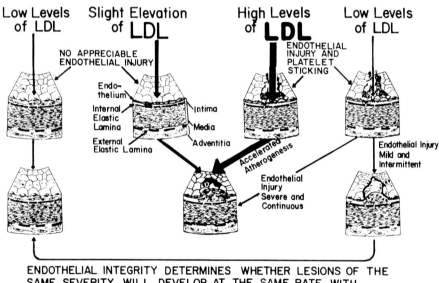

ENDOTHELIAL INTEGRITY DETERMINES WHETHER LESIONS OF THE SAME SEVERITY WILL DEVELOP AT THE SAME RATE WITH DIFFERENT LIPOPROTEIN LEVELS

FIG. 2. Several pathogenetic sequences recognized as influencing the prevention or the development of progressive atherosclerosis in the human and nonhuman primate. In most instances of sustained low levels of LDL, the areas that are not subject to endothelial injury or have only rare intermittent endothelial injury are protected from the progression of atherosclerosis. The usual cases of advanced disease develop with slight elevations of LDL and little sustained endothelial injury, whereas advanced disease can develop very rapidly in individuals with homozygous familial hypercholesterolemia. Some individuals who present exceptional or paradoxical development of accelerated atherosclerosis without evidence of the presence of any classical risk factors (hyperlipidemia, hypertension, or cigarette smoking) may most likely be the victims of chronic sustained endothelial damage due to the effects of circulating immune complexes, free radicals, and the production of epitopes of oxidized LDL or other as yet unrecognized causes. In muscular arteries, these lesions are often concentric, transmural, and the site of rather intense inflammation, or a condition we have termed "atheroarteritis" (33).

and the adventitial lymph. Movement, although regulated, is accomplished without the apoB or LDL receptors that are needed for endocytosis of lipoproteins for cell growth and metabolism.

Much of the recent work both in human and experimental animal studies indicates that the endothelium is intact when fatty streaks and fatty plaques develop in the more vulnerable parts of the arterial tree. Nevertheless, there is increasing evidence that changes in the arterial cell surface, accompanied by or independent of changes in the composition of the monocyte, lymphocytes, and platelets, may constitute an important part of the atherogenic process, especially when sustained low-grade injury from circulating immune complexes or other long-term chemical injuries are involved (16).

Some investigators consider atherosclerosis to be partly the result of a mild inflammatory process with signs of subacute to chronic inflammation, i.e., inflammatory cells (mainly monocytes and lymphocytes), edema, etc. (13). Furthermore, some of the early studies on the role of platelet-derived growth factor (PDGF) in the development of atherosclerosis assumed that endothelial injury with endothelial cell loss, followed by platelet adhesion and platelet spreading, was an important trigger of smooth muscle cell proliferation (23,25). It now appears that this is a major pathogenetic process when atherogenesis follows obvious endothelial cell destruction by mechanical factors such as balloon catheter injury or in the advanced stages of progression of the complicated plaque. But it does not appear to be a dominant mechanism when atherogenesis is primarily a result of sustained low-grade hypercholesterolemia (33) (Fig. 2).

The Major Contribution of Smooth Muscle Cell Proliferation to Atherosclerotic Plaque Formation

One may regard atherogenesis as largely a reaction to injury or as a process primarily due to an oversupply and an underutilization of lipoproteins in the artery wall. Both of these processes are involved. The lipid deposition in the early stages appears to be largely intracellular and to occur mainly in SMC that have migrated into the intima and proliferated there (44). These SMC make up the second major component of the developing plaque. The two processes of lipid infiltration and SMC proliferation may be viewed as an interaction between an inflammatory process and the effects of prolonged hyperlipidemia (29). As illustrated in Fig. 3, these two major processes reinforce each other to support the development of a progressive atherosclerotic plaque. For plaques that appear to be accelerated in their development and appear to be at least partially the result of a low-grade nondestructive inflammatory reaction to injury, there are numerous possibilities for sustaining this kind of long-term endothelial damage. A number of the prolonged endothelial injurious processes that may produce increased permeability to lipoproteins and thus promote atherogenesis are listed in Table 1.

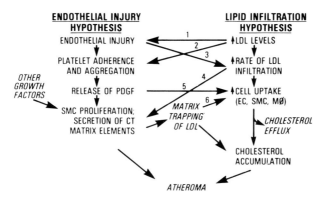

FIG. 3. Some of the interactions between endothelial injury and lipid infiltration in the pathogenesis of atherosclerosis. They indicate that (1) hyperlipidemia—especially as oxidized LDL—may injure endothelium; (2) platelet aggregation and release of platelet-derived growth factor may be initiated; (3) sustained injury of the endothelium as produced by immune complexes or by autoimmune reactions to oxidized LDL may increase the rate of lipoprotein infiltration; (4) LDL from hypercholesterolemic serum can stimulate proliferation of arterial smooth muscle cells under many types of conditions; (5) LDL receptors on smooth muscle cells are increased when growth factors are present; and (6) the synthetic state smooth muscle cells make more proteoglycans, which in turn can bind more LDL in the subintimal space. (From ref. 29.)

Monocyte Sticking and the Macrophage/Foam Cell Components of the Developing Plaque

Studies of experimental animals fed atherogenic diets have shown that the number of monocytes sticking to the endothelium are increased, especially in those areas most susceptible to atherosclerotic development. Studies have also shown that the monocyte-derived macrophages common in many types of subacute and chronic inflammatory processes are capable of being overloaded with cholesterol, cholesteryl esters, and fatty acids. These scavenger cells resemble the foam cells commonly seen in the lesions of animals that develop fatty streaks and fatty plaques when fed high-cholesterol diets. In other words, the scavenger

TABLE 1. *Factors producing prolonged or repeated injury to arterial endothelium*

Sustained mechanical injury	Chronic endotoxemia
Prolonged hemodynamic	Anoxia and CO
Repeated trauma	Cigarettes (CO and NO_2)
Sustained angiotensin effects	Severe anoxia
Norepinephrine and other vasoactive amines	Prolonged stasis
Cigarette smoking	Chronic uremia
High-dosage cocaine use	Homocystinemia
Ag-Ab reactions, autoimmunity, and immune	Hypercholesterolemia (especially of LDL and
complexes	β-VLDL)
Leukotrienes and other "free radical"	Thromboxane
mechanisms	

cells demonstrate the uptake of cholesterol by means of the scavenger pathway originally described by Goldstein et al. (10).

In contrast to arterial SMC, which are generally fairly well regulated in terms of their lipid storage, these monocyte-derived macrophages can take up very large amounts of modified lipoproteins, including those which are subjected to oxidation (30). Although these cells are rarely very numerous in the developing atheromatous lesions in young people, small numbers of them are frequently present in small clusters just under the endothelium. There is also evidence that these cells may transfer lipids to SMC, which can then be overloaded so that they too can become foam cells (47). Under these circumstances, one may regard the macrophage as a "nurse cell," since it may provide a major route by which cholesterol and cholesteryl ester in large quantities can accumulate in the arterial intima and particularly within the cytoplasm of "modulated" SMC.

The macrophage and its functions are complex. It is most likely that its principal role as a scavenger inhibits lesion progression by generating lipases, removing excess lipid from developing plaques, as well as by furnishing collagenases and elastases to counteract the sclerotic part of the plaque. On the other hand, in some circumstances it may greatly facilitate lipid accumulation both inside and around the SMC and stimulate SMC proliferation by means of its growth factors (17,24).

Most of the studies on monocyte sticking have included an element of chronic endothelial damage that may not be present in many of the slowly developing atherosclerotic lesions in the human disease process produced by hypercholesterolemia. Just as the SMC fits the criteria of a multifunctional cell type in relation to atherogenesis, it is at least equally true that the monocyte-derived macrophage can be considered a multifunctional cell. Its role in human atherogenesis needs to be better defined since few if any studies implicate this cell type in human atherogenesis. In fact, recent evidence indicates that in young people in the United States, the numbers of these cells are inversely related to lesion progression (44).

Table 2 presents some of the functions of the macrophage that may be particularly relevant to its role in atherosclerosis. All of the secretory products listed in this table could be important in either atherogenesis or the regression of atherosclerotic lesions. The first four classes of secretory products may be of some importance in terms of lipid deposition, smooth muscle cell proliferation, and angiogenesis. The next four elements listed—including collagenase, elastase, hydrolases, and lysozymes—might be better considered as protective processes to counteract plaque progression.

The list of macrophage surface receptors that have been identified on the surface of the cell is equally important to the processes of atherogenesis and regression. If we consider modified LDL, including oxidized LDL, as the end products of LDL metabolism, the vulnerability of altered LDL to macrophage disposal can certainly be regarded as a step toward the elimination of worn-out LDL that is no longer useful in furnishing a regulated supply of cholesterol for

TABLE 2. *Macrophage features and functions related to either atherogenesis or to prevention of atherosclerotic plaque progression*

Secretory products	Surface receptors	Additional functions
Lipoprotein lipase	Acetyl-LDL	Phagocytosis
ApoE	Malondialdehyde-LDL	Immunologic-antigen processing
Angiogenesis factor	Dextran sulfate-LDL	and presentation
Macrophage-derived growth	β-VLDL	Cytolysis
factor	ApoB-containing lesion	Lipid metabolism (acid and neutral
Lysozyme	complexes and	lipid hydrolases and
Collagenase	epitopes of	synthetases)
Elastase	oxidized LDL	
Lysosomal acid hydrolases	Chylomicron remnants	
Superoxides and hydrogen	Fc fraction of	
peroxide	immunoglobulins	
Complement factors	Complement factor C-3	
Prostaglandins	Mannose	
Prostacyclin (PGI$_2$)	Insulin	
Thromboxane		
Leukotrienes		
Platelet-activating factor		
Interferons		

cell membranes in the artery wall, or in the liver or spleen, or for other cellular components of the reticuloendothelial system and the mesenchyme membranes.

The additional functions listed in the table (as well as many others not included here) emphasize the potential these cells have for either progression of or protection against the atherosclerotic process. Further study is needed to augment our knowledge and clarify the role of the multifunctional monocyte-derived macrophages in the artery wall in relation to atherosclerosis.

Smooth Muscle Cell Migration, Proliferation, Phenotypic Modulation, and Connective Tissue Matrix Synthesis (Collagen, Elastin, and Proteoglycans)

For many years, there has been general agreement that the intimal modified SMC population, derived largely from the arterial media by means of migration and then greatly augmented by proliferation, makes up the principal cells of the atherosclerotic plaque at almost every stage of its development (40). It is true that some early fatty streaks in humans, principally those found in infancy and early childhood, may show a predominance of monocyte-derived macrophages filled with lipid (28). It is also true that some animal models, notably the cholesterol-fed rabbit and fowl, have a major population of foam cells that are probably not derived from SMC. However, when they have been studied extensively and quantitatively, most other true plaques in humans and animals show a predominance of SMC, many of which are lipid-laden. In fact, many of them are converted to greatly overloaded lipophages that can only be distinguished from monocyte-derived macrophage foam cells by using suitable cell markers. As was mentioned earlier, there is now some tantalizing *in vitro* evidence that

SMC can be overloaded with lipid by the neighboring macrophage foam cells (47).

There also appears to be general agreement that the SMC found in the intima of developing lesions with or without lipid droplets are quite different in their morphology and metabolism from those found in the more or less quiescent underlying media (6). Although neither the cause, development, nor fundamental nature of these modified SMC is completely clear, there are many investigators who look upon these changes as a fundamental characteristic of the cells that migrate and proliferate and presumably pass on their synthetic and enzymatic properties to all of the SMC in that area. This view of a somatic mutation from a sterol- or virus- or carcinogen-induced shift in the artery wall cells' metabolic and genetic machinery is strengthened by the recent identification of virus and viral products in the atherosclerotic plaque cells and the presence of appropriate proto-oncogenes in some of the human plaques (1,2).

On the other hand, some evidence suggests that the phenotypic shift of this cell type from a contractile form to more of an embryonic synthetic form—a phenomenon termed "phenotypic modulation"—is a potentially reversible shift in the cells' metabolism and therefore best regarded as a natural selection response to a stimulus (Fig. 4) (6).

These issues are important because the reversibility of the cell types after removal of the stimuli toward atherosclerosis may depend to some extent on the fundamental nature of these cell changes and may influence whether the lesions are reversible. The modified SMC in the lesions do appear to be more synthetic, to take up lipid more actively, and to proliferate more readily in response to stimuli. These changes also appear to be reversible (37,39).

What stimulates the proliferation of the SMC in the lesion or *in vitro?* A few years ago, the answer to this question appeared much simpler than it does now. Reports from a number of laboratories have shown that some property of hyperlipidemic serum, localized in a rather narrow cut of the LDL fraction labeled LDL-1, was a potent stimulator of SMC proliferation (7,35), especially for cells from primary cultures that had reached a quiescent phase as they grew out from the primary explant. Further investigations have shown that this reaction is successfully blocked by sufficient quantities of HDL from normolipidemic animals (48).

Several laboratories have identified a different mechanism involving the recently identified platelet-derived growth factor (PDGF), which can be isolated from the platelets' α granules. This appears to be an essential growth factor for SMC (25). This growth factor, or a very similar one, is also found in a number of other locations—namely, in the monocyte-derived macrophage, the endothelial cell, and particularly the proliferating endothelial cell or the injured endothelial cell (24). Even the SMC appears to be able to synthesize this growth factor (16).

Furthermore, many other growth factors have been isolated. At present, investigators trying to keep up to date on the mechanisms by which SMC proliferate are surfeited with numerous sources and types of growth factors from which to

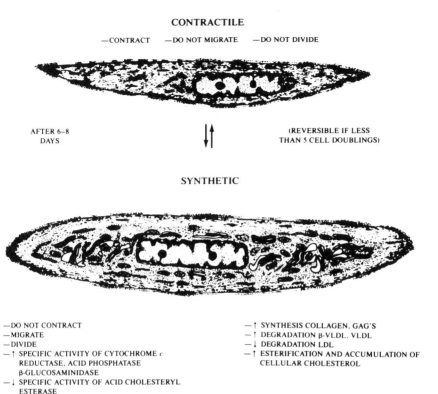

FIG. 4. Differences between the smooth muscle cells that are converted to a synthetic form and become quite different in form and function in the developing intimal lesions of atherosclerosis as compared to their appearance and their site of metabolic activity in the media of the artery. (From ref. 6.)

choose. All that can be said with certainty is that the SMC can undergo sustained migrations and proliferation under a number of circumstances, including sustained hyperlipidemia, endothelial injury and regeneration, platelet adhesion and PDGF infiltration of an injured area of the artery, as well as monocyte infiltration into the artery wall, even when the endothelium is apparently intact (24).

The SMC that make up the major population of the atherosclerotic plaque apparently synthesize more collagen, elastin, and probably more proteoglycans than they were synthesizing in the media of the artery. These changes to a synthetic metabolic mode probably have a very strong influence on the development of the fibrous cap and the binding of hyperlipidemic LDL and its excess of cholesterol in the arterial intima (5).

It is obvious from this brief summary that much work still needs to be done in order to understand fully the stimuli and the responses of the SMC under conditions that simulate atherogenesis in the whole organism.

Cell Necrosis in Advancing Atherosclerosis

Just as intracellular lipid deposition, SMC proliferation, and synthesis of many connective tissue elements are the hallmarks of developing atherosclerosis in many species, including humans, cell necrosis is also an important component of the progressive lesion. Necrosis may be the result of poor cell nutrition, because as the plaque becomes larger, thicker, and richer in cholesterol and cholesteryl esters, the cell population in the deeper parts of the plaque cannot receive sufficient oxygen and food by diffusion (31). Now we have evidence that oxidized LDL is a major constituent of the developing atherosclerotic plaque, which is capable of producing necrosis of both SMC and endothelium (30). Clearly, the mechanisms of cell death—especially the necrosis of cells overloaded with lipid in human atherosclerotic plaques—need more study. Several toxic substances from the bloodstream are being investigated. Until we understand how these substances correlate with cell breakdown, the role of cell necrosis in the development of atherosclerotic plaques will be shrouded in mystery.

Microthrombi

For many years, a number of investigators have believed that a substantial part of the atherogenic process evolves from small mural thrombi, collecting on almost normal artery walls, particularly in some areas of increased susceptibility to atherosclerosis. Most of the evidence for this type of pathogenesis in humans is circumstantial, but recent searches in the developing lesions in human and animal subjects have documented such microthrombi (27). Usually, they are rather few in number, and the full transition to a lipid-containing small plaque has rarely been observed on the systemic arterial side of the human circulation. Data from ongoing studies should help to elucidate how frequently this pathogenetic sequence is found in seemingly healthy young individuals who are nonetheless developing atherosclerosis (34).

THE INTERACTION OF PATHOGENETIC PROCESSES— OLD AND NEW RISK FACTORS

Almost all of the epidemiological evidence indicates that risk factors such as hyperlipidemia, cigarette smoking, hypertension, and diabetes reinforce each other and that they have at the very least an additive effect in human lesions. Early results from our PDAY study indicate that this effect holds true for young people 15 to 34 years of age (18). Similarly, a number of experimental studies have shown the same kind of reinforcement of one risk factor by another in relation to the types and severity of lesions documented by well-controlled studies. Perhaps the most important interaction is that between hyperlipidemia and factors engendering arterial endothelial damage and inflammation.

Hyperlipidemia and Immune Complexes

If we agree that the additive association between circulating immune complexes and hyperlipidemia is likely to accelerate the atherosclerotic process, then we can explain the accelerated atherogenesis seen in young women with lupus erythematosus (4) or the accelerated and accentuated atheroarteritis that develops in heart transplant subjects (3) or in the excellent laboratory animal model of serum sickness in the rabbit (19). We recently reported that atherosclerotic lesions in animals or people who have circulating immune complexes are generally concentric and are likely to be transmural and inflamed (41). This condition, which can be defined as atheroarteritis, contrasts with the condition of plaques seen in humans or in rhesus monkeys without immune complexes and in whom the lesions are almost always eccentric and largely limited to the intima, with very little evidence of inflammatory reaction (42,43).

Cigarette Smoking and Hyperlipidemia

We recently reported that lesions in young men in the United States, starting at age 15, are much more severe where the patient's background includes cigarette smoking as well as hyperlipidemia (44). There are potentially many ways in which cigarette smoking may influence atherogenesis. Several of these involve the sustained stimulation of the adrenergic system, producing excessive quantities of epinephrine and norepinephrine, and its effects of tachycardia, pressor effects, vasoconstriction, and direct damage to the endothelium, with resulting increased permeability to lipoproteins.

If tobacco hypersensitivity is as widespread as has been reported (8), then some of the augmentation of the development of atherosclerosis by cigarette smoking might be the result of endothelial injury and a hypersensitivity type of inflammation. This, too, is likely to increase endothelial permeability for lipoproteins.

FACTORS THAT AUGMENT AND ACCELERATE THE DEVELOPMENT OF ATHEROSCLEROSIS BY INTENSIFYING THE CLASSICAL RISK FACTORS

A developing body of evidence suggests that heretofore unrecognized immunological factors that alter the microarchitecture of the atherosclerotic plaque present a hidden risk responsible for some of the paradoxical cases of severe accelerated atherosclerosis.

We have presented evidence from several types of pathological studies. These include experimental studies in cynomologus and rhesus monkeys (36), advanced human lesions in older people (41), and developing lesions in younger individuals (42,43).

It is possible to conclude from the results of our studies thus far that there are additional causes for this pattern of lesion microarchitecture. Only about half of the concentric and transmural lesions found in almost 10% of the otherwise chronic disease-free young people had severely elevated immune complexes by either the ELISA or the PEG method. On the other hand, these elevated levels are rarely found in individuals who have the usual eccentric coronary artery lesions. There is a need for further investigation of the nature of sustained endothelial injury that supports this pattern of lesion development. We intend to focus on this question as we continue our studies of the pathobiological determinants of atherosclerosis in youth.

ACKNOWLEDGMENT

This work was supported in part by National Institutes of Health grants HL 14164 and HL 33740. It is a part of the U.S.A. Multicenter Cooperative Study of the Pathobiological Determinants of Atherosclerosis in Youth (PDAY). The author is grateful to Gertrud Friedman and Alexander Arguelles for their skilled assistance in preparing this manuscript.

REFERENCES

1. Benditt, E. P. (1977): *Sci. Am.*, 236:74–84.
2. Benditt, E. P. (1988): *Arch. Pathol. Lab. Med.*, 112:997–1001.
3. Billingham, M. E. (1989): *Transplant. Proc.*, 21:3665–3666.
4. Bulkley, B. H., and Roberts, W. C. (1975): *Am. J. Med.*, 58:243–265.
5. Campbell, G. R., Campbell, J. H., Manderson, J. A., Horrigan, S., and Rennick, R. E. (1988): *Arch. Pathol. Lab. Med.*, 112:977–986.
6. Campbell, J. H., and Campbell, G. R. (1985): *Exp. Mol. Pathol.*, 42:139–162.
7. Fless, G. M., Kirchhausen, T., Fischer-Dzoga, K., Wissler, R. W., and Scanu, A. M. (1982): *Arteriosclerosis*, 41:171–183.
8. Francus, T., Klein, R. F., Staiano-Coico, L., Becker, C. G., and Siskind, G. W. (1988): *J. Immunol.*, 140:1823–1829.
9. Getz, G. S., Vesselinovitch, D., and Wissler, R. W. (1969): *Am. J. Med.*, 46:657–673.
10. Goldstein, J. L., Ho, Y. K., Basu, S. K., and Brown, M. S. (1979): *Proc. Natl. Acad. Sci.*, 76: 333–337.
11. Gould, R. G., Wissler, R. W., and Jones, R. J. (1964): In: Jones, R. J., ed. *Evolution of the atherosclerotic plaque*. Chicago: University of Chicago Press, pp. 205–214.
12. Hansson, G. K., Jonasson, L., Lojsthed, B., Stemme, S., Kocher, O., and Gabbiani, G. (1988): *Atherosclerosis*, 72:135–141.
13. Haust, D. (1983): In: Silver, M. D., ed. *Cardiovascular pathology*. New York: Churchill Livingstone, pp. 191–316.
14. Haust, M. D., More, R. H., and Movat, H. Z. (1960): *Am. J. Pathol.*, 37:377.
15. Jurgens, G., Hoff, H. F., Chisolm, G. M. III, and Esterbauer, H. (1987): *Chem. Phys. Lipids*, 45:315–336.
16. Libby, P. (1987): *Mol. Aspects Med.*, 9:499–567.
17. Liebovich, S. J., and Ross, R. (1976): *Am. J. Pathol.*, 84:501–513.
18. McGill, H. C. Jr., and PDAY Research Group (1990): *JAMA*, 264:3018–3024.
19. Minick, C. R., Murphy, G. E., and Campbell, W. G. (1966): *J. Exp. Med.*, 124:635–651.
20. Morel, D. W., Hessler, J. R., and Chisolm, G. M. (1983): *J. Lipid Res.*, 24:1070.
21. Morel, D. W., Hessler, J. R., and Chisolm, G. M. (1983): *FASEB*, 42:771.
22. Palinski, W., Yla-Herttuala, S., and Rosenfeld, M. E., et al. (1990): *Arteriosclerosis*, 10:325–335.

23. Ross, R. (1976): *N. Engl. J. Med.,* 295:420–425.
24. Ross, R. (1981): *Arteriosclerosis,* 1:293–311.
25. Ross, R., and Glomset, J. (1976): *N. Engl. J. Med.,* 295:369–377.
26. Simionescu, M., and Simionescu, N. (1983): *Physiol. Rev.,* 63:1536–1579.
27. Spurlock, B. O., and Chandler, A. B. (1987): *Scanning Microsc.,* 1:1359–1365.
28. Stary, H. C. (1989): *Arteriosclerosis,* 9(suppl. I):19–32.
29. Steinberg, D. (1983): *Arteriosclerosis,* 3:283–301.
30. Steinberg, D., Parthasarathy, S., Carew, T. E., Khoo, J. C., and Witztum, J. L. (1989): *NEJM,* 320:915–924.
31. Thomas, W. A., Kim, D. N., Lee, K. T., Reiner, J. M., and Schmee, J. (1983): *Exp. Mol. Pathol.,* 39:257–270.
32. Wissler, R. W. (1968): *J. Athero. Res.,* 8:201–213.
33. Wissler, R. W. (1984): In: Braunwald, E., ed. *Heart disease: a textbook of cardiovascular medicine.* Philadelphia: W.B. Saunders, pp. 1183–1204.
34. Wissler, R. W. (1991): *Ann. NY Acad. Sci.,* 623:26–39.
35. Wissler, R. W., Fischer-Dzoga, K., Bates, S. R., Chen, R. M., and Eisele, B. (1980): *Folia Angiol.,* 28:32–36.
36. Wissler, R. W., and Vesselinovitch, D. (1983): *Am. J. Cardiol.,* 52:2A–7A.
37. Wissler, R. W., and Vesselinovitch, D. (1984): In: Malinow, M. R., and Blaton, V. H., eds. *Regression of atherosclerotic lesions.* New York: Plenum, pp. 21–41.
38. Wissler, R. W., and Vesselinovitch, D. (1987): In: Gallo, L. L., ed. *Cardiovascular disease.* New York: Plenum, pp. 337–357.
39. Wissler, R. W., and Vesselinovitch, D. (1990): *Am. J. Cardiol.,* 65:33F–40F.
40. Wissler, R. W., Vesselinovitch, D., and Davis, H. R. (1987): In: Olsson, A. G., ed. *Atherosclerosis: biology and clinical science.* Edinburgh: Churchill Livingstone, pp. 57–73.
41. Wissler, R. W., Vesselinovitch, D., Davis, H. R., Lambert, P. H., and Bekermeier, M. (1985): *Ann. NY Acad. Sci.,* 454:9–22.
42. Wissler, R. W., Vesselinovitch, D., Davis, H. R., and Yamada, T. (1987): In: Strandness, D., Didisheim, P., Clowes, A., and Watson, J., eds. *Vascular diseases: current research and clinical applications.* Orlando, FL: Grune & Stratton, pp. 241–256.
43. Wissler, R. W., Vesselinovitch, D., and Ko, C. (1989): *Transplant. Proc.,* 21:3707–3708.
44. Wissler, R. W., Vesselinovitch, D., and Komatsu, A. (1990): *Ann. NY Acad. Sci.,* 598:418–434.
45. Witztum, J. L., Mahoney, E. M., Branks, M. J., Fisher, M., Elam, R., and Steinberg, D. (1982): *Diabetes,* 31:283–291.
46. Witztum, J. L., Steinbrecher, U. P., Kesaniemi, Y. A., and Fisher, M. (1984): *Proc. Natl. Acad. Sci. USA,* 81:3204–3208.
47. Wolfbauer, G., Glick, J. M., Minor, L. K., and Rothblat, G. H. (1986): *Proc. Natl. Acad. Sci. USA,* 83:7760–7764.
48. Yoshida, Y., Fischer-Dzoga, K., and Wissler, R. W. (1984): *Exp. Mol. Pathol.,* 41:258–266.

Atherosclerosis Reviews, Volume 23,
edited by P. C. Weber and A. Leaf.
Raven Press, Ltd., New York © 1991.

The Role of Endothelial Denudation Injury, Plaque Fissuring, and Thrombosis in the Progression of Human Atherosclerosis

M. J. Davies, *N. Woolf, and *D. R. Katz

*St. George's Hospital Medical School, British Heart Foundation Cardiovascular
Pathology Unit, and Department of Histopathology, London, SW17 ORE, England;
and *University College and Middlesex School of Medicine, Histopathology
Department, Middlesex Hospital, London, WIN 8AA, England*

The raised fibrolipid plaque is the substrate on which clinical symptoms develop in human atherosclerosis either by causing chronic obstruction to flow or by the complication of superimposed thrombosis causing acute arterial obstruction. When compared with populations with a lower risk, the aorta and coronary arteries in populations with a high risk of ischemic heart disease have more of the intima involved by raised plaques at necropsy (24). The mean intimal involvement by plaques in populations with hypertension is higher than in normotensive populations (27). The Pathological Determinants of Atherosclerosis in Youth study (PDAY) has confirmed the direct relation of the degree of intimal involvement by plaques to the level of the blood pressure, smoking, and the plasma low-density lipoprotein (LDL) levels in young subjects dying of nonvascular causes such as trauma or suicide (25). Thus, the number of raised plaques is a major determinant of the risk of developing atherosclerotic cardiac and cerebral disease.

The major components, by volume, of human raised plaques are lipid, either contained within foam cells or deposited as an extracellular pool (30), and connective tissue matrix proteins (33). The cells containing lipid are either macrophages of monocytic origin or smooth muscle cells (SMC). The great majority of cells completely distended by lipid (foam cells) are of monocytic origin (3,18), as demonstrated by immunohistochemistry using antibodies to a range of monocyte/macrophage-specific antigens such as EBMII and HAM 56. The use of two cell-specific immune markers in one histological section allows differential counts of the numbers of macrophage and SMC to be made in different areas of the plaque (Fig. 1). Use of immunocytohistochemistry also shows that a significant population of T lymphocytes is present within many plaques (20,21). The connective tissue matrix protein present in the largest amount is collagen, which is responsible for the tensile strength of the tissue; but elastin and glycosoaminogly-

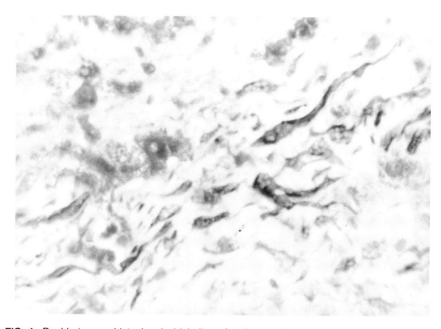

FIG. 1. Double immunohistochemical labeling of actin-containing smooth muscle cells (brown) and EMBII expression in macrophages (red) on human plaque cap tissue. The smooth muscle cells are predominantly, but not exclusively, spindle-shaped. Some contain lipid droplets. The macrophages containing the cytoplasmic antigen EMBII are polygonal and surround some extracellular crystalline cholesterol.

cans (GAG) also contribute to the mechanical properties of the tissue (33). The connective tissue matrix is synthesized by SMC (7). Calcium is deposited within both the collagenous matrix and as nodular masses within lipid; calcium thus may make a major contribution to the mass of the plaque although not to its volume.

Human fibrolipid plaques have a characteristic microanatomy (Fig. 2). The central core of the plaque contains a pool of extracellular lipid, including cholesteryl ester and cholesterol crystals. Foam cells surround the lipid core. The lipid core is separated from the lumen of the artery by a cap of fibromuscular tissue in which SMC lie in oval lacunae within a collagen-rich stroma. The surface of the plaque is covered by an endothelial layer; but because it is only one cell thick, this will not contribute to the mechanical strength of the cap tissue.

Analysis of the constituents of human raised plaques by volume (Table 1) shows a very considerable heterogeneity even within an individual coronary artery. At one extreme, a plaque may contain very little lipid; at the other extreme, there may be a large pool of extracellular lipid making up over 50% of the plaque volume. Even when large amounts of lipid are present, collagen must remain a

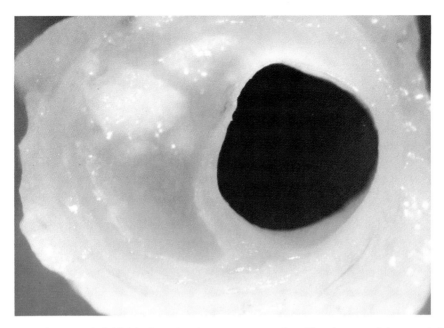

FIG. 2. An eccentric lipid-rich plaque in a human coronary artery. The plaque contains a central area of lipid that is separated from the lumen by the fibromuscular cap. The cap is thick at one end but much thinner at the other; this thin area indicates a point of potential weakness.

major component to maintain plaque integrity. In general, the more lipid present, the greater the number of macrophages. The developmental relation between predominantly fibrous and lipid-rich plaques in humans is unknown; however, regression trials in animal models indicate that a change from lipid-rich to fibrous forms can occur following lowering of plasma lipids (5).

The predominant components in the early growth of a plaque and hence the progression of human atherosclerosis are lipid accumulation and collagen synthesis. However, the heterogeneity of human raised lesions suggests the two processes are not inevitably directly linked. The progression of human disease as

TABLE 1. *Percent volume composition of eight plaques in one right coronary artery*

	Lipid content	Connective tissue	Smooth muscle	Macrophages
A	2.6	72.5	19.8	5.1
B	5.6	76.1	17.2	1.1
C	6.9	71.2	18.6	3.3
D	10.5	60.6	22.3	6.6
E	20.8	52.2	23.4	3.6
F	32.6	48.6	6.9	11.9
G	44.5	41.0	2.4	12.1
H	54.3	33.5	4.2	8.0

documented by angiography is not linear (6). High-grade stenoses appear in segments of apparently normal coronary artery in the time between two angiographic examinations, and it is impossible to predict the sites of new lesions or future acute occlusions causing myocardial infarction (MI) (1,19). Coronary arteries containing plaques dilate to preserve the lumen size (17); an apparently normal angiogram can therefore conceal a large fibrolipid plaque, and a new angiographic lesion cannot be equated with a recently formed plaque but is one that has entered an accelerated growth phase. The human angiographic data show that these later stages of plaque growth are episodic and unpredictable.

The episodic sudden growth of human coronary plaques can be shown to be due to thrombosis both within and on the plaque (9). The relation of type B unstable angina and acute MI to coronary thrombosis has been established by detailed autopsy studies (11), by angiography (2), and angioscopy (15,29), in life, and by the success of thrombolytic therapy in reopening occluded vessels. The angiographic recognition that eccentric stenoses with a ragged outline (type II lesions) represented an unstable plaque undergoing thrombosis (16) was a major advance in the clinical understanding of acute myocardial ischemia.

THROMBOSIS AND ATHEROSCLEROSIS

Animal models of atherosclerosis clearly demonstrate that the endothelial surface is intact in the initial stages of plaque development. Once raised lesions are present, endothelial denudation develops, and platelet reactions with the underlying exposed connective tissue matrix occur (13,14,28). Such endothelial denudation is associated with the presence of lipid-filled macrophages within the intima immediately beneath the endothelium. Studies of human coronary arteries taken from the explanted heart at cardiac transplantation and perfused instantly to preserve the endothelial structure for scanning electron microscopy show that endothelial denudation is common over raised plaques, is associated with platelet deposition, is associated with intense foam cell infiltration of the adjacent intima, and does not occur in normal vessels without atherosclerosis taken from subjects undergoing transplantation for cardiomyopathies (12).

Thrombi demonstrated by scanning electron microscopy are microscopic in scale, but the process of deposition of fibrinogen-related material in the intima is a major factor in plaque progression (4). More widespread endothelial loss allows the formation of larger thrombi that can cause acute symptoms and are demonstrable by angiography. Up to one-third of coronary thrombi large enough to be detected by angiography at necropsy in subjects dying from coronary atherosclerosis are due to this process of endothelial denudation and superficial intimal injury (9). The characteristic feature of this form of thrombus is that it is superimposed on the surface of an otherwise intact plaque (Fig. 3).

Two-thirds of major coronary thrombi are due to a deeper intimal injury caused by the process known variously as "plaque fissuring," "rupture," "crack-

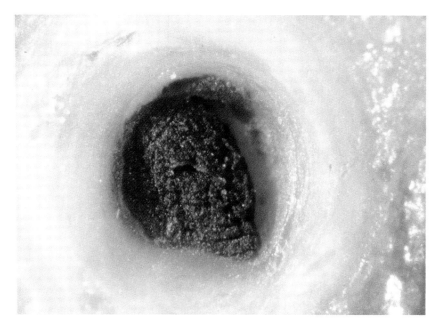

FIG. 3. Dissecting microscopic appearance of a large thrombus due to superficial intimal injury. The thrombus is superimposed on an otherwise intact concentric plaque, and there is no intraplaque thrombus.

ing," or "ulceration." In this process, clearly described by Constantinides in 1966 (8), a tear extends from the arterial lumen through the endothelial surface and plaque cap to enter the central lipid core of the plaque. A subsequent event is that blood enters the plaque itself and forms a thrombus within the intima. Thrombus forms rapidly due to the reaction of platelets with both exposed collagen and with tissue factor (34) present in significant amounts in the lipid core. The plaque volume is significantly increased, and the degree of stenosis rapidly increases. The plaque shape is also altered, producing the characteristic eccentric stenosis with an irregular edge (type II stenosis) seen in unstable angina (16).

The next event is either that the fissure heals by smooth muscle proliferation and the thrombus within the plaque organizes to be replaced by collagen, or that thrombosis continues to extend through the tear to project into the lumen. Thrombosis is initially mural still allowing antegrade flow but later may develop into acute occlusion (Fig. 4).

The factors determining whether intraluminal thrombosis does, or does not, develop must include the magnitude of the tearing of the plaque cap. The break in the cap ranges from fissures 100 to 200 μ across to spiral tears extending over many millimeters with elevation of an intimal flap and extrusion of the lipid contents of the plaque into the lumen. Tears at this latter extreme of magnitude must be followed inevitably by intraluminal thrombosis and are probably difficult

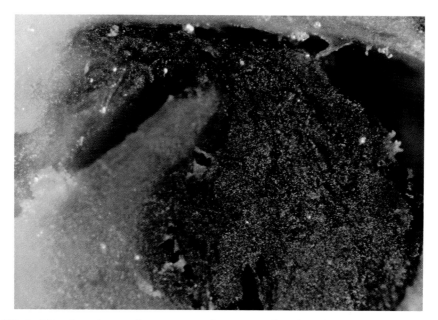

FIG. 4. Dissecting microscopic appearance of a coronary thrombus due to deep intimal injury and plaque fissuring. The cap of the lipid-rich plaque is broken. There is a thrombus that is partially within the plaque and projects through the fissure to form a polypoid mass within the lumen.

to reopen with fibrinolytic therapy. Intraluminal thrombus formation following more minor tears is probably determined by the innate thrombotic and fibrinolytic status of the patient at the time.

Review of angiographic data on human coronary atherosclerosis shows that many stenoses increase abruptly without a recognized episode of acute myocardial ischemia (6). These silent episodes of thrombosis predominantly occurring within, rather than on, the plaque are an important cause of progression in the later stages of the disease. Recently healed fissures can be recognized histologically by the presence of thrombus within the plaque and new connective tissue within the cap. The process by which spontaneous cap tears heal is identical to that which occurs following angioplasty tears in plaques and is mediated by smooth muscle proliferation. Analysis of the coronary arteries of subjects with atherosclerosis, but who have died of noncardiac causes such as trauma, suicide, or stroke, shows that 8% of individuals have a recently healed fissure whereas subjects with a history of hypertension, diabetes, or previous infarction have twice that frequency (10). Such data underscore the role of clinically silent fissuring in plaque growth and highlight the need to understand the mechanisms by which plaques enter an unstable phase with a risk of fissuring.

THE PATHOGENESIS OF PLAQUE FISSURING

Reconstruction of human coronary thrombi shows that the plaques that develop fissuring contain a central core of lipid deficient in collagen bundles supporting the cap from beneath (9,26,31). The most common site where tears develop is at the insertion of the cap into the adjacent, more normal vessel wall (26). A small number of intimal tears occur in the absence of a lipid-rich pool, either developing between layers of collagen or at the interface between plates of calcified collagen and noncalcified adjacent tissue. Such events may be more common as a precipitator of thrombosis in the ectatic calcified arteries of old age.

The original descriptions of plaque fissuring noted an accumulation of foam cells in the cap (8)—an observation which has been confirmed by quantification (23). The caps of intact coronary artery plaques show focal areas in which the collagen is reduced in amount; these areas are associated with foam cell infiltration and are potential points of weakness in the tissue (Fig. 2). The presence of pools of extracellular lipid within the intima will alter the distribution of the hemodynamic stress across the vessel wall in systole. In a computer model of plaques with a pool of lipid occupying an arc of the vessel wall (i.e., eccentric rather than concentric), circumferential wall stress in systole was shown to be elevated and concentrated on the plaque cap (26) as a consequence of the inability of the lipid-rich areas to carry a load.

In the aorta and major vessels such as the carotid artery, plaque fissuring leads to the formation of ulcerated lesions covered by thrombus that can persist for longer periods of time than in the coronary arteries. This provides the opportunity at necropsy to compare the structure of plaques that are still intact with those that have undergone recent fissuring. However, plaques in which the cap has been completely destroyed cannot be analyzed. In a comparison of ulcerated with intact plaques, evaluations have been performed that included mechanical testing of the cap tissue, analysis of the volume of the plaque occupied by lipid, the monocyte/macrophage and SMC density, and the biochemical composition of the plaque cap.

Plaque caps that have ulcerated have a significantly reduced stress at fracture and greater extension ratio than the caps of intact plaques (22). Biochemical

TABLE 2. *Biochemical analysis (% dry wt.) of cap tissue in human aortic plaques*

	Ulcerated plaques (*n* = 24)	Nonulcerated plaques (*n* = 31)
Total protein	54.8 (1.2)	57.2 (2.2)
Collagen	35.4 (8.4)	56.8 (1.4)[a]
Elastin	0.87 (.27)	1.17 (.31)
GAG	0.9 (.20)	1.9 (.2)[a]

[a] $p < 0.05$. Figures are shown as mean and SEM.

TABLE 3. *Characteristics of lipid and cellular content of ulcerated and intact human aortic plaque caps*

	Ulcerated ($n = 24$)	Nonulcerated ($n = 62$)
Extracellular lipid		
(% of plaque volume)	54.9% (3.8)	22.1% (2.4)
Density of SMC	65.2 (13.2)	174.0 (11.9)
Density of MO	122.1 (13.3)	62.2 (8.8)
SMC/MO ratio	1.2/1.0	5.8/1.0

SMC, smooth muscle cells; MO, monocytes.
All parameters different at $p < 0.001$. Figures are shown as mean and SEM.

analysis of the cap tissue shows that the collagen and GAG content of cap tissue from ulcerated plaques is significantly lower than that in intact plaques (Table 2). The concentrations of elastin and the ratio of collagen types are not significantly different. Cap tissue in which the macrophage population is high has a reduced resistance to fracture under tensile stress (23). The cap tissue of ulcerated plaques shows an absolute increase in the number of monocytes/macrophages and an absolute decrease in the concentration of SMC (Table 3). These changes result in very different ratios of the numbers of smooth muscle cells as compared with monocytes in the two types of plaque. In intact plaques, SMC predominate; whereas in ulcerated plaques, the ratio of SMC to monocytes is less than one.

Plaque fissuring can thus be seen in part to be due to an increase of mechanical stress on the cap tissue in systole, and in part due to a weakening of the cap tissue itself. The main biochemical alteration is a loss of collagen and GAG, both of which are significant contributors to the mechanical strength of the tissue. The loss of connective tissue matrix is associated with an increase in the number of macrophages. It remains to be ascertained whether the connective tissue matrix changes are caused actively by the macrophages, which are capable of producing enzymes active against both collagen and GAG, or whether they represent a simple loss of the synthetic capacity of the SMC.

REFERENCES

1. Ambrose, J., Tannenbaum, M., and Alexopoulos, D., et al. (1988): *J. Am. Coll. Cardiol.,* 12:56–62.
2. Ambrose, J., Winters, S., and Arora, R. (1986): *J. Am. Coll. Cardiol.,* 7:472–478.
3. Aqel, N., Ball, R., Waldmann, H., and Mitchinson, M. (1984): *Atherosclerosis,* 53:265–271.
4. Bini, A., Fenoglio, J., Mesa-Tejada, M., Kudryk, B., and Kaplan, K. (1989): *Arteriosclerosis,* 9: 109–121.
5. Blankenhorn, D., and Kramsch, D. (1989): *Circulation,* 79:1–7.
6. Bruschke, A., Kramer, J., Bal, E., Haque, I., Detranto, R., and Goormastic, M. (1989): *Am. Heart J.,* 117:296–305.
7. Campbell, J., Reardon, M., Campbell, G., and Nestel, P. (1985): *Arteriosclerosis,* 5:318–328.
8. Constantinides, P. (1966): *J. Athero. Res.,* 6:1–17.
9. Davies, M. (1990): *Circulation,* 82(suppl. III):1138–1146.
10. Davies, M., Bland, J., Hangartner, J., Angelini, A., and Thomas, A. (1989): *Eur. Heart J.,* 10: 203–208.

11. Davies, M., and Thomas, A. (1985): *Br. Heart J.,* 53:363–373.
12. Davies, M., Woolf, N., Rowles, P., and Pepper, P. (1988): *Br. Heart J.,* 60:459–464.
13. Faggiotto, A., and Ross, R. (1984): *Arteriosclerosis,* 4:341–356.
14. Faggiotto, A., Ross, R., and Harker, L. (1984): *Arteriosclerosis,* 4:323–340.
15. Forrester, J., Litvak, F., Grundfest, W., and Hickey, A. (1987): *Circulation,* 75:505–513.
16. Fuster, V., Badimon, L., Cohen, M., Ambrose, J., Badimon, J., Chesebro, J. (1988): *Circulation,* 77:1213–1220.
17. Glagov, S., Weisenberd, W., Zarins, C., Stankunavicius, R., Kolettis, G. *N. Engl. J. Med.,* 316: 1371–1375.
18. Gown, A., Tsukakda, T., and Ross, R. (1986): *Am. J. Pathol.,* 125:191–207.
19. Hackett, D., Davies, G., and Maseri, A. (1988): *Eur. Heart J.,* 9:1317–1323.
20. Hansson, G., Jonasson, L., Seifert, P., and Stemme, S. (1989): *Arteriosclerosis,* 9:567–578.
21. Jonasson, L., Holm, J., Skalli, O., Bondjers, G., and Hansson, K. (1986): *Arteriosclerosis,* 6: 131–138.
22. Lendon, C., Briggs, A., Born, G., Burleigh, M., and Davies, M. (1988): *Biochem. Soc. Trans.,* 16:1032–1033.
23. Lendon, C., Davies, M., Born, G., and Richardson, P. (1991): *Atherosclerosis,* 87:87–90.
24. McGill, H. (1968): *The geographic pathology of atherosclerosis.* Baltimore: Williams & Wilkins.
25. PDAY Research Group. (1991): *J. Am. Med. Assoc.,* 264:3018–3024.
26. Richardson, P., Davies, M., and Born, G. (1989): *Lancet,* 2:941–944.
27. Robertson, W., and Strong, J. (1968): *Lab. Invest.,* 18:538–551.
28. Ross, R., Faggiotto, A., Bowenpope, D., and Raines, E. (1984): *Eur. Heart J.,* 5:77–82.
29. Sherman, C., Litvak, F., and Grundfest, W. (1986): *N. Engl. J. Med.,* 315:913–919.
30. Stary, H. (1989): *Arteriosclerosis,* 9:1–19.
31. Tracy, R., Devaney, K., and Kissling, G. (1985): *Virchows Arch. [A],* 405:411–427.
32. Tracy, R., and Kissling, G. (1988): *Arch. Pathol. Lab. Med.,* 112:1056–1065.
33. Wight, T. (1989): *Arteriosclerosis,* 9:1.
34. Wilcox, J., Smith, K., Schwartz, S., and Gordon, D. (1989): *Proc. Natl. Acad. Sci. USA,* 86: 2839–2843.

Atherosclerosis Reviews, Volume 23,
edited by P. C. Weber and A. Leaf.
Raven Press, Ltd., New York © 1991.

Lipoprotein Modification and Atherogenesis

Daniel Steinberg

*Department of Medicine, University of California, San Diego,
La Jolla, California 92093*

Atherosclerosis is a multifaceted disorder that probably has multiple causes. In this chapter, we discuss atherosclerotic lesions that are induced primarily, if not exclusively, by elevation of plasma lipoprotein levels. This is certainly the case in individuals with low-density lipoprotein (LDL) receptor defects, in whom the grossly accelerated atherosclerosis must be directly attributable to the single gene defect—a gene defect that has as its immediate consequence a rise in plasma LDL levels (4). The same reasoning applies to the atherosclerosis seen in Watanabe heritable hyperlipidemic (WHHL) rabbits, in whom the gene defect has also been identified (41).

LDL is not the only lipoprotein present at higher concentrations when the LDL receptor is defective. Recent studies show that there is also an increase in intermediate-density lipoproteins (IDL) rich in apolipoprotein E and resembling β-very-low-density lipoprotein (β-VLDL) in some properties (21). However, there is a human disease in which elevation of LDL is the *only* abnormality. Patients with a specific mutation at amino acid residue 3,500 have normal LDL receptors, but they fail to clear LDL at a normal rate because the apolipoprotein B is defective (19,39). Since IDL rich in apoE are recognized by the LDL receptor based on their apoE content rather than their apoB, removal of LDL remnants is normal in these subjects. Recent studies show that these patients do have premature atherosclerosis and may clinically closely resemble patients with heterozygous familial hypercholesterolemia (38). Thus, we can say with confidence that an elevation of plasma LDL alone is enough to induce atherosclerosis. Most people with "garden-variety" hypercholesterolemia have predominantly an elevation of the LDL fraction. Consequently, it behooves us to understand as much as we can about the interactions between LDL particles and the vascular wall.

CURRENT VIEWS ON THE INITIATION OF FATTY-STREAK LESIONS AND THEIR PROGRESSION

The earliest grossly visible lesion of atherosclerosis is the fatty streak. This lesion is characterized by the accumulation of lipid-laden foam cells that arise in part from circulating monocytes that have entered the subendothelial space and in part from smooth muscle cells (SMC) that have migrated from the media into the intima. The identification of foam cells as derived from monocyte/ macrophages can now be made conclusively by using monoclonal antibodies that specifically recognize these cell types and distinguish them from SMC. The mechanism by which SMC become foam cells is not understood. Incubation of SMC with even very high concentrations of LDL *in vitro* fails to convert them to foam cells. Recent evidence suggests that under the proper conditions rabbit smooth muscle cells can begin to express the acetyl LDL receptor; this could play a role in converting them to foam cells (30). In the case of the monocyte/ macrophage, the evidence is conclusive that these cells do express the acetyl LDL receptor. Their uptake of modified forms of lipoprotein could account for their conversion to foam cells (13). Exactly what modifications are necessary and the evidence that some of these occur *in vivo* will be discussed subsequently.

First, let us continue with the natural history of the atherosclerotic lesion. The fatty streak develops under an anatomically unbroken endothelial lining. There is now a consensus that physical "stripping" of endothelial cells is not a prerequisite to the development of the atherosclerotic lesion either in experimental animals or in humans. Although the accumulation of lipid is the hallmark of the early lesion, the progression of the lesion is characterized most notably by growth of cells and deposition of connective tissue matrix components.

THE LDL PARADOX

There is no doubt that LDL is atherogenic, and there is no doubt that the lipid accumulating in the artery wall during the genesis of the atherosclerotic lesion is ultimately derived from circulating atherogenic lipoproteins. Yet we find the same kinds of lipid-laden foam cells in developing lesions of humans and animals that lack the LDL receptor. How do these cells acquire LDL lipids? One possibility is that they take up LDL by nonspecific mechanisms when the LDL concentration is very high. Another possibility is that the macrophages used in our *in vitro* studies do not reflect the properties of the macrophages resident in the artery wall. A final possibility is that the LDL taken up by the cells is not the same as the LDL circulating in the plasma. In other words, it is possible that modifications of the LDL occur in the artery wall and that it is the modified form that is taken up readily by the arterial macrophages.

The first clue that modification of LDL structure might be the answer came from the studies of Goldstein and co-workers (13). They showed that chemical treatment of LDL with acetic anhydride converted it to a form that was recognized by a specific, saturable receptor on mouse peritoneal macrophages. However, there was no evidence that any significant amount of acetylated LDL could be generated *in vivo*. Beginning with the work of Henriksen et al. (16), a series of studies carried out at the Specialized Center of Research on Arteriosclerosis in La Jolla, California, established that oxidative modification of LDL can mimic the change induced by acetylation [reviewed by Steinberg et al. in 1989 (35)]. It was first shown (16) that incubation of LDL with cultured cells under appropriate conditions converts it to a form recognized by the same receptor described by Goldstein et al. in 1979 (13). This was surprising but in retrospect becomes readily understandable. During oxidative modification of LDL, the polyunsaturated fatty acids undergo fragmentation, and the aldehydic fragments generated conjugate with the epsilon amino groups of lysine residues. This is very closely analogous to what happens with chemical acetylation—i.e., the amino groups of lysine residues are the target. However, it is not known exactly how the configuration recognized by the acetyl LDL receptor is generated. The acetyl LDL receptor has now been cloned in the laboratory of Krieger (24). Oxidized LDL, while taken up in part by way of the acetyl LDL receptor, appears to be recognized also by one or more additional receptors on mouse peritoneal macrophages (34) but purification and characterization of the postulated additional receptors have not been accomplished.

OXIDATIVE MODIFICATION OF LDL

In retrospect, it is surprising that it took so long to become aware of the possible importance of oxidative modification of LDL. It has been known for a long time that purified LDL fractions are extremely labile to denaturation and oxidative damage (32). On the other hand, as long as the LDL is in whole plasma, it is much more stable. This made it seem improbable that any significant oxidative damage would occur *in vivo*. Now, however, there is a considerable body of evidence indicating that oxidative modification does in fact occur *in vivo* (this evidence is reviewed in the following section).

Once purified from plasma, LDL undergoes auto-oxidation very readily in the presence of even very low concentrations of transition metals (iron or copper). In the presence of cultured cells, oxidation can proceed even when only truly trace quantities of metal ion are present (36). The events during cell-catalyzed oxidation do not appear to be significantly different from those that occur during auto-oxidation. In both cases, there is extensive peroxidation of polyunsaturated fatty acids, which begins slowly but accelerates markedly once the indigenous antioxidant compounds in LDL have been exhausted (α-tocopherol, β-carotene and others) (9). There is extensive breakdown of lecithin to yield lysolecithin (36) and fragmentation of the apoB (10). The latter appears to be not a proteolytic process but an oxidative degradation. Without going into further detail, suffice it to say that the chemical changes are complex and manifold and that what we refer to as "oxidized LDL" is almost certainly heterogeneous and far from a recognizable single entity. The reproducibility from experiment to experiment is not good. This fact must be recognized when trying to evaluate a rapidly growing body of literature on oxidative modification of LDL. It is important to note that any of the three major cell types in the artery wall can oxidatively modify LDL (7,15–17,25,28).

EVIDENCE THAT OXIDATIVE MODIFICATION OCCURS *IN VIVO*

The evidence that LDL is oxidized *in vivo* has been reviewed recently (35). It has been shown that (a) LDL gently extracted from atherosclerotic lesions, both human and rabbit, has physical, chemical, and biological properties like those of LDL oxidized *in vitro* (27,42). In addition, (b) immunohistochemical approaches show that atherosclerotic lesions (but not normal segments of the artery) stain positively with antibodies generated against oxidized LDL or so-called models of oxidized LDL, such as malondialdehyde-conjugated LDL (33); and (c) autoantibodies against oxidized LDL have been demonstrated both in human and rabbit plasma (27). Most important, (d) three laboratories have reported now that treatment of rabbits with antioxidant compounds slows the progression of atherosclerosis (3,6,22).

The issue of whether or not oxidation of LDL can take place in the plasma is not settled. Certainly its oxidation *in vitro* is inhibited even by relatively low concentrations of serum. On the other hand, oxidation can be effected if a free radical generator is added to whole plasma (12). It should be stressed that the liver sinusoidal endothelial cells and Kuppfer cells express the acetyl LDL receptor and rapidly remove any LDL that has been modified to the point where it is recognized by these receptors. The half-life of injected acetyl LDL or oxidized LDL is measured in minutes (26). Thus, one would not expect ever to find in plasma a significant concentration of LDL oxidized to the point that it is a ligand for the acetyl LDL receptor. On the other hand, LDL that has been conjugated with a limiting amount of malondialdehyde (or has undergone oxidation for only a very brief period) is no longer recognized by the receptor for native LDL and is not yet modified sufficiently to be recognized by the acetyl LDL or scavenger receptors (14). Such LDL particles could be generated away from the artery wall, circulate for an extended time, and eventually enter the artery, there to become more fully oxidized and promote atherogenesis. Studies by Avogaro and co-workers (1) suggest that some LDL of this kind is present in normal plasma.

ADDITIONAL WAYS IN WHICH OXIDATIVELY MODIFIED LDL IS POTENTIALLY MORE ATHEROGENIC THAN NATIVE LDL

The fact that oxidized LDL is recognized by the scavenger receptors facilitates the generation of foam cells. In addition, however, oxidized LDL can contribute to atherogenesis in other ways:

1. It is itself a chemotactic agent for circulating monocytes (30) and could therefore contribute to the recruitment of monocytes into the site of a developing arterial lesion.
2. When minimally oxidized, it can stimulate the release of monocyte chemotactic protein-1 from endothelial cells (8).

3. It inhibits the motility of tissue macrophages and could thus contribute to a "trapping" phenomenon (30).
4. It is cytotoxic (18) and could account for some of the inflammatory processes occurring during the history of the lesion. Most specifically, it could contribute to the loss of endothelial cells as lesions become more complex.
5. It has the potential of releasing macrophage colony stimulating factor from endothelial cells (31), which could lead to expansion of the macrophage population in a developing lesion.

OTHER POTENTIALLY RELEVANT MODIFICATIONS

Studies by Khoo et al. in 1988 (20) showed that self-aggregates of LDL are taken up much more rapidly by peritoneal macrophages than is native LDL. Interestingly, the uptake occurred not by way of the scavenger receptors but by way of the LDL receptor itself. Aggregation in these studies was induced by simply violently agitating the solution of LDL. Treatment of LDL with phospholipase C can also induce aggregation (37). Such phospholipase-induced aggregates behave very much like aggregates induced by surface denaturation (vortexing). Whether or not aggregation plays a role *in vivo* remains uncertain. There is circumstantial evidence, however, in the form of electron micrographs demonstrating the presence in the intima of cholesterol-fed animals of aggregates of lipid that could very well represent aggregates of LDL (11).

Complexes of LDL with immunoglobulins can be taken up into macrophages by way of the F_c receptor; this could be another mechanism for inducing foam cells. Modified lipoproteins are highly immunogenic (36), and autoantibodies against LDL or glycosylated LDL have been demonstrated (2,23,40).

Finally, complexes of LDL with connective tissue elements have been recognized for some time. One of the best studied of these is the complex of LDL with proteoglycans (5). The proteoglycan content of artery wall increases markedly during atherogenesis. Thus, these complexes could very well be involved.

The *in vivo* evidence regarding the importance of these alternative forms of modified LDL remains limited, but we look forward to further studies in the near future to assess their possible importance.

SUMMARY

Evidence supporting the oxidative modification hypothesis has accumulated rapidly in the past several years. We now have a number of lines of evidence indicating that oxidative modification does in fact occur *in vivo* and that prevention of it slows the progression of atherosclerotic lesions. Ultimately, it will require a clinical intervention trial in humans before we can be certain of its relevance to clinical disease, but the evidence in hand suggests that the time for such a clinical intervention trial may be soon.

REFERENCES

1. Avogaro, P., Bon, G. B., and Cazzoloto, G. (1988): *Arteriosclerosis,* 8:79–87.
2. Beaumont, J. L., Jacotot, B., and Beaumont, V. (1967): *Presse Med.,* 75:2315–2320.
3. Björkhem, I., Henriksson-Freyschuss, A., Breuer, O., Diczfalusy, U., Berglund, L., and Henriksson, P. (1991): *Arterio. Thromb.,* 11:15–22.
4. Brown, M. S., and Goldstein, J. L. (1986): *Science,* 232:34–47.
5. Camejo, G. (1982): *Adv. Lipid Res.,* 19:1–51.
6. Carew, T. E., Schwenke, D. C., and Steinberg, D. (1987): *Proc. Natl. Acad. Sci. USA,* 84:7725–7729.
7. Cathcart, M. K., Morel, D. W., and Chisolm, G. M. III (1985): *J. Leukocyte Biol.,* 38:341–350.
8. Cushing, S. D., Berliner, J. A., Valente, A. J., et al. (1990): *Proc. Natl. Acad. Sci. USA,* 87:5134–5138.
9. Esterbauer, H., Jürgens, G., Quehenberger, O., and Koller, E. (1987): *J. Lipid Res.,* 28:495–509.
10. Fong, L. G., Parthasarathy, S., Witztum, J. L., and Steinberg, D. (1987): *J. Lipid Res.,* 28:1466–1477.
11. Frank, J. S., and Fogelman, A. M. (1989): *J. Lipid Res.,* 30:967–978.
12. Frei, B., Stocker, R., and Ames, B. N. (1988): *Proc. Natl. Acad. Sci. USA,* 85:9748–9752.
13. Goldstein, J. L., Ho, Y. K., Basu, S. K., and Brown, M. S. (1979): *Proc. Natl. Acad. Sci. USA,* 76:333–337.
14. Haberland, M. E., Fogelman, A. M., and Edwards, P. A. (1982): *Proc. Natl. Acad. Sci. USA,* 79: 1712–1716.
15. Heinecke, J. W., Rosen, H., and Chait, A. (1984): *J. Clin. Invest.,* 74:1890–1894.
16. Henriksen, T., Mahoney, E. M., and Steinberg, D. (1981): *Proc. Natl. Acad. Sci. USA,* 78:6499–6503.
17. Henriksen, T., Mahoney, E. M., and Steinberg, D. (1983): *Arteriosclerosis,* 3:149–159.
18. Hessler, J. R., Robertson, A. L., Jr., and Chisolm, G. M. (1979): *Atherosclerosis,* 32:213–219.
19. Innerarity, T. L., Mahley, R. W., Weisgraber, K. H., et al. (1990): *J. Lipid Res.,* 3:1337–1349.
20. Khoo, J. C., Miller, E., McLoughlin, P., and Steinberg, D. (1988): *Arteriosclerosis,* 8:348–358.
21. Kita, T., Brown, M. S., Bilheimer, D. W., and Goldstein, J. L. (1982): *Proc. Natl. Assoc. Sci. USA,* 79:5693–5697.
22. Kita, T., Nagano, Y., Yokode, M., et al. (1987): *Proc. Natl. Acad. Sci. USA,* 84:5928–5931.
23. Klimov, A. N., Denisenko, A. D., Vinogradov, A. G., et al. (1988): *Atherosclerosis,* 74:41–46.
24. Kodama, T., Freeman, M., Rohrer, L., Zabrecky, J., Matsudaira, P., and Krieger, M. (1990): *Nature,* 343:531–535.
25. Morel, D. W., DiCorleto, P. E., and Chisolm, G. M. (1984): *Arteriosclerosis,* 4:357–364.
26. Nagelkerke, J. F., Havekes, L., van Hinsbergh, V. W., and van Berkel, T. J. (1984): *Arteriosclerosis,* 4:256–264.
27. Palinski, W., Rosenfeld, M. E., Ylä-Herttuala, S., et al. (1989): *Proc. Natl. Acad. Sci. USA,* 86: 1372–1376.
28. Parthasarathy, S., Printz, D. J., Boyd, D., Joy, L., and Steinberg, D. (1986): *Arteriosclerosis,* 6: 505–510.
29. Pitas, R. E. (1990): *J. Biol. Chem.,* 265:12722–12727.
30. Quinn, M. T., Parthasarathy, S., Fong, L. G., and Steinberg, D. (1987): *Proc. Natl. Acad. Sci. USA,* 84:7725–7729.
31. Rajavashisth, T. B., Andalibi, A., Territo, M. C., et al. (1990): *Nature,* 344:254–257.
32. Ray, B. R., Davisson, E. O., and Crespi, H. L. (1954): *J. Phys. Chem.,* 58:841–846.
33. Rosenfeld, M. E., Palinski, W., Ylä-Herttuala, S., Butler, S., and Witztum, J. L. (1989): *Arteriosclerosis,* 10:336–349.
34. Sparrow, C. P., Parthasarathy, S., and Steinberg, D. (1989): *J. Biol. Chem.,* 264:2599–2604.
35. Steinberg, D., Parthasarathy, S., Carew, T. E., Khoo, J. C., and Witztum, J. L. (1989): *N. Engl. J. Med.,* 320:915–924.
36. Steinbrecher, U. P., Parthasarathy, S., Leake, D. S., Witztum, J. L., and Steinberg, D. (1984): *Proc. Natl. Acad. Sci. USA,* 81:3883–3887.
37. Suits, A. G., Chait, A., Aviram, M., and Heinecke, J. W. (1989): *Proc. Natl. Acad. Sci. USA,* 86: 2713–2717.
38. Tybjaerg-Hansen, A., Gallagher, J., Vincent, J., et al. (1990): *Atherosclerosis,* 80:235–242.

39. Vega, G. L., and Grundy, S. M. (1986): *J. Clin. Invest.,* 78:1410–1414.
40. Witztum, J. L., Steinbrecher, U. P., Kesaniemi, Y. A., and Fisher, M. (1984): *Proc. Natl. Acad. Sci. USA,* 81:3204–3208.
41. Yamamoto, T., Bishop, R. W., Borwn, M. S., Goldstein, J. L., and Russell, D. N. (1986): *Science,* 232:1230–1237.
42. Ylä-Herttuala, S., Palinski, W., Rosenfeld, M. E., et al. (1989): *J. Clin. Invest.,* 84:1086–1095.

Atherosclerosis Reviews, Volume 23,
edited by P. C. Weber and A. Leaf.
Raven Press, Ltd., New York © 1991.

The Acetylated Low-Density Lipoprotein Receptor or Macrophage Scavenger Receptor

Lucia Rohrer

Preclinical Research, Sandoz Pharma Ltd., CH-4002 Basel, Switzerland

In atherosclerosis, the endocytosis of plasma cholesterol by monocytes/macrophages results in the formation of foam cells (4,15). Surprisingly, normal macrophages express very few low-density lipoprotein (LDL) receptors of the classical type (15); therefore, they take up native LDL sparingly. Brown and Goldstein could demonstrate that chemically modified LDL loses the ability to bind to the classical receptor, but is now recognized by another high-affinity receptor on macrophages, the acetylated LDL (AcLDL) receptor (4,15).

This receptor recognizes the increased negative charges that are unmasked on the apoB-100 protein in LDL when the ϵ-amino group of lysine residues are abolished by acetylation (4,15). Uptake of AcLDL is inhibited competitively by a wide variety of polyanions (4), from which it is concluded that the receptor recognizes charge as well as conformation. In this regard, its ability to distinguish single-stranded polynucleotides is striking; polyinosinic acid binds to it, but polycytidylic acid does not (4). Another more physiologically relevant modification of LDL was discovered by Steinberg and collaborators (37): oxidized LDL (OxLDL) competes for binding of AcLDL and delivers sufficient cholesterol to produce foam cells. Due to its broad but limited set of ligands, the AcLDL receptor became known as the scavenger receptor.

STRUCTURE

Following the original chemical identification by Via et al. (41), we isolated the scavenger receptor from bovine lung, determined a partial amino acid sequence, and cloned two closely related cDNAs from a lung library (24,25,32). The scavenger receptor sequence predicts an oligomeric structure: each monomer contains seven putative N-glycosylation sites, one membrane-spanning domain, its N-terminal 50 amino acids are in the cytoplasm, and its C-terminus is extracellular. The type I sequence predicts a 453 amino acid protein with the following domain structure: (a) N-terminal cytoplasmic (amino acid residues 1–50), (b) transmembrane (51–76), (c) spacer (77–108), (d) α-helical coiled-coil (109–271), (e) collagenous (272–343), and (f) C-terminal cysteine-rich (344–453). The type II bovine scavenger receptor is identical to the type I receptor, except that the 110–amino acid cysteine-rich C-terminal domain is replaced by a 6 amino acid C-terminus. The external region of both receptors contains the only portion with significant similarity to other proteins (domain V, the collagenous domain). The scavenger receptor is the first known cell membrane receptor containing a collagen-like domain.

Based on the primary structure of both types, it is possible that the scavenger receptor assembles into a trimer. This model assumes that the α-helical coiled-coil domain forms a single triple-stranded left-handed superhelix that merges with the right-handed collagen-like triple helix to form a single long fibrous stalk of about 400 Å in length. Alternative models based on aggregation of subunits are possible, e.g., it could be similar to hexameric complement factor C1q (31). There it would be two trimeric collagen-like domain contagions with three dimeric coiled-coil domains. The finding of a second type of receptor raises the possibility that hetero-oligomers could form *in vitro*.

BINDING SPECIFICITY

The novel characteristic of the scavenger receptor is its unusual binding specificity for a broad but limited set of ligands. This receptor binds a wide variety of polyanions, including chemically modified proteins and lipoproteins, acidic phospholipids, and certain polynucleotides (4). The type II receptor lacking the cysteine domain can mediate endocytosis of AcLDL and its activity is remarkably similar to that of the type I receptor (32) and it exhibits the same broad ligand specificity. This clearly indicates that one or both of the extracellular fibrous domains are the binding domain for AcLDL rather than the cysteine-rich domain. The collagenous domain seems ideal for this role; specifically, it is reminiscent of collagen binding of a wide variety of molecules. Examples include asymmetric acetylcholinesterase binding to proteoglycans (3), lung surfactant-associated apoproteins binding to lipids (35), mannose-binding protein association with hydrophobic surfaces (6), and strikingly the binding of complement factor C1q to DNA (33). Collagen can bind lipids (10) and many macromolecules (40), including fibronectin, fibrinogen, thrombospondin, laminin, and von Willebrand factor. LDL binds to type I collagen and its binding is enhanced by modification that converts LDL into a ligand of the scavenger receptor (20). The predicted net positive charge of the collagenous domain could contribute to polyanionic ligand binding, but more subtle structural features are probably responsible for the specificity of polynucleotide binding. The α-helical coiled-coil structure could also be involved in the unique specificity of the receptor. In addition, posttranslational modifications are probably involved in ligand binding as well as receptor assembly, stability, intracellular sorting, and endocytosis.

FOAM CELL FORMATION

Numerous studies suggest that OxLDL may play a key role in atherogenesis (37–39,41). OxLDL is cytotoxic to endothelial cells, vascular smooth muscle cells, and fibroblasts (19). Furthermore, it is chemotactic for monocytes (30), capable of stimulating macrophage differentiation (13), and has been detected in atherosclerotic plaques (2,8,16–18,27,29,34,42). These and other studies have led to the proposal that OxLDL and the macrophage scavenger receptor may play a critical role in initiating atherosclerotic lesions (23,37–39). It has been assumed that oxidation of LDL in the subendothelial space converts LDL into a ligand of the scavenger receptor and that receptor-mediated endocytosis of OxLDL may be a primary pathway for cholesterol deposition in macrophages during plaque development *in vivo*. In cultured macrophages, scavenger-receptor-mediated uptake of modified LDL can result in massive lipid accumulation and these lipid-rich cells resemble the macrophage foam cells in atherosclerotic plaques (4,5). Examination of modified LDL binding to cultured macrophages has shown that AcLDL and OxLDL do not bind identically, raising the possibility that there may be more than one class of scavenger receptor or receptor binding site for modified LDL (1,9,28,36).

Incubation of stable Chinese hamster ovary (CHO) cell transfectants, expressing high levels of either type I or type II bovine scavenger receptor with AcLDL, results in cytoplasmic lipid droplet accumulation similar to that in macrophage foam cells whereas untransfected cells do not (11). Macrophage-specific gene products other than the scavenger receptor are not required for modified LDL-induced lipid accumulation. The type I and type II bovine scavenger-receptor-transfected cell lines independently mediate high-affinity OxLDL endocytosis and there are no substantial differences in their binding specificities. Both types of receptor exhibited nonreciprocal cross-competition: AcLDL efficiently competes for both its own endocytosis and OxLDL endocytosis by the transfected cells, whereas OxLDL competes efficiently for its own endocytosis but only poorly for the endocytosis of AcLDL. There are several possible explanations for these findings. For example, the scavenger receptor might have different binding sites for OxLDL and AcLDL (1), or the receptor may have different conformations, similar to allosteric enzymes. Further analyses will have to be performed to elucidate these unusual findings.

The nonreciprocal cross-competition observed in the transfected cells differs from that found in cultured murine macrophages (1,28). It is not clear if species or cell type differences or differences in lipoprotein preparations are responsible for these discrepant observations. The synthesis of a heteromeric receptor might explain some of these observations. Alternatively, the expression in macrophages of some other, as yet unknown type of scavenger receptor that exhibits its own distinctive binding properties (1,28) may account for the different affinities observed for ligand cross-competition.

CONSERVED STRUCTURE IN BOVINE, MURINE, AND HUMANS

Isolation of type I and type II cDNAs from the murine macrophage cell line P388D-1 [by Freeman et al. (12)] and from a stimulated human monocytic cell line THP-1 [by Matsumoto et al. (26)] showed the presence of mRNAs encoding both types of receptors in a single cell. Comparison of the bovine, human, and murine sequences indicates that most of the structural characteristics of the scavenger receptor type I and type II are conserved, except for the C-terminal domain of the type II receptor. In mouse and cow, the type II C-terminal domain is 6 amino acid residues long; in humans, it contains 17 amino acids. In all three species, the transiently expressed receptors were shown to mediate the endocytosis of AcLDL with similar affinities and the same distinct broad specificity (12,24,26,32).

Studies with the bovine type I and type II scavenger receptor showed that the cysteine-rich domain is not required for the distinctive broad ligand specificity (12,24,26,32). The finding that this domain is also observed in the human and murine receptor suggests that it has some as yet undefined independent function.

Northern blot analysis showed the expression of the human gene in brain in addition to the previously known organs: liver, lung, and placenta (24,26,32). Independent chromosomal mapping of the murine and the human scavenger-receptor genes showed that they are located in the proximal half of chromosome 8 (12,26), suggesting that a single gene encodes for both mRNAs.

HIGHLY CONSERVED FAMILY OF CYSTEINE-RICH PROTEIN DOMAINS

Protein sequence analysis by Krieger (12) showed that the type I scavenger-receptor cysteine-rich (SRCR) domain helps to define a previously unrecognized family of highly conserved domains that are found in three classes of proteins: (i) the human T- and specialized B-lymphocyte differentiation antigen CD5 (22) and the murine homologue Ly-1 (21); (ii) human complement factor I, which proteolytically regulates the complement cascade (14); and (iii) the sea urchin sperm speract receptor, which mediates the activation of sperm by egg peptides (7).

SUMMARY

Interest in the scavenger receptor has been focused mainly on its possible role in macrophage lipoprotein metabolism and atherosclerosis. Both types of scavenger receptor expressed by CHO transfectants show high-affinity and saturable endocytosis of both AcLDL and OxLDL and the broad binding specificity that is the hallmark of macrophage scavenger receptors (31). Incubation of this cell lines with AcLDL, but not LDL, also results in substantial cytoplasmic lipid-droplet accumulation similar to those in macrophage foam cells whereas un-transfected cells do not. Further studies of the lipid-laden CHO cells are necessary before it is possible to conclude that the transfected cells precisely mimic foam-cell formation by cultured macrophages. Nevertheless, other macrophage-specific gene products than the scavenger receptor are not required for modified LDL-dependent intracellular lipid accumulation. Due to the broad binding specificity and collagen-like domain, the scavenger receptor could be involved in other physiological systems, for e.g., cell-to-cell or cell-to-extracellular matrix inter-actions, inflammation, and macrophage-associated immune responses. The pos-sible involvement in the immune system is underlined by the current finding of a similarity between the cysteine domain of the scavenger receptor type I and the SRCR domains in CD5 (22).

REFERENCES

1. Arai, H., Kita, T., Yokode, M., Narumiya, S., and Kawai, C. (1989): Multiple receptors for modified low density lipoproteins in mouse peritoneal macrophages: different uptake mechanisms for acetylated and oxidized low density lipoproteins. *Biochem. Biophys. Res. Commun.,* 159: 1375–1382.
2. Boyd, H. D., Gown, A. M., Wolfbauer, G., and Chait, A. (1989): Direct evidence for a protein recognized by a monoclonal antibody against oxidatively modified LDL in atherosclerotic lesions from Watanabe heritable hyperlipidemic rabbit. *Am. J. Pathol.,* 135:815–825.
3. Brandan, E., Maldonado, M., Garrido, J., and Inestrosa, N. C. (1985): Anchorage of collagen-tailed acetylcholinesterase to the extracellular matrix is mediated by heparan sulfate proteoglycans. *J. Cell Biol.,* 101:985–992.
4. Brown, M. S., and Goldstein, J. L. (1983): Lipoprotein metabolism in the macrophage: implications for cholesterol deposition in atherosclerosis. *Annu. Rev. Biochem.,* 52:223–261.
5. Brown, M. S., Goldstein, J. L., Krieger, M., Ho, Y. K., and Anderson, R. G. (1979): Reversible accumulation of cholesteryl esters in macrophages incubated with acetylated lipoproteins. *J. Cell Biol.,* 82:597–613.
6. Colley, K. J., and Baentziger J. U. (1987): Biosynthesis and secretion of the rat core-specific lectin. Relationship of binding activity. *J. Biol. Chem.,* 262:3415–3421.
7. Dangott, L. J., Jordan, J. E., Bellet, R. A., and Grabers, D. L. (1989): Cloning of the mRNA for the protein that crosslinks to the egg peptide speract. *Proc. Natl. Acad. Sci. USA.,* 86:2128–2132.
8. Daugherty, A., Zweifel, B. S., Sobel, B. E., and Schonfeld, G. (1988): Isolation of low density lipoprotein from atherosclerotic vascular tissue of Watanabe heritable hyperlipidemic rabbits. *Arteriosclerosis,* 8:768–777.
9. Dresel, H. A., Friedrich, E., Via, D. P., Sinn, H., Ziegler, R., and Schettler, G. (1987): Binding of acetylated low density lipoprotein and maleylated bovine serum albumin to the rat liver: one or two receptors? *EMBO J.,* 6:319–326.
10. Frank, J. S., and Folgelman, A. M. (1989): Ultrastructure of the intima in WHHL and cholesterol-fed rabbit aortas prepared by ultra-rapid freezing and freezing-etching. *J. Lipid Res.,* 30:967–978.
11. Freeman, M., Ekkel, Y., Rohrer, L., Penman, M., Freedman, N. J., Chisolm, G. M., and Krieger, M. (1991): Expression of type I and type II bovine scavenger receptors in Chinese hamster ovary cells: lipid droplet accumulation and nonreciprocal cross competition by acetylated and oxidized low density lipoprotein. *Proc. Natl. Acad. Sci. USA,* (in press).
12. Freeman, M., Ashkenas, J., Rees, D. J., Kingsley, D. M., Copeland, N. G., Jenkins, N. A., and Krieger, M. (1990): An acient, highly conserved family of cysteine-rich protein domains revealed by cloning type I and type II murine macrophage scavenger receptors. *Proc. Natl. Acad. Sci. USA.,* 87:8810–8814.
13. Frostegrad, J., Nilsson, J., Haegerstrand, A., Hamsten, A., Wigzell, H., and Gidlund, M. (1990):

Oxidized low density lipoprotein induces differentiation and adhesion of human monocytes and the monocytic cell line U937. *Proc. Natl. Acad. Sci. USA.*, 87:904–908.

14. Goldberg, G., Bruns, G. A. P., Rits, M., Edge, M. D., and Kwiatkowski, D. J. (1987): Human complement factor. I: Analysis of cDNA-derived primary structure and assignment of its gene to chromosome 4. *J. Biol. Chem.*, 262:10065–10081.

15. Goldstein, J. L., Ho, Y. K., Basu, S. K., and Brown, M. S. (1979): Binding site on macrophages that mediates uptake and degradation of acetylated low density lipoprotein, producing massive cholesterol deposition. *Proc. Natl. Acad. Sci. USA.*, 76:333–337.

16. Haberland, M. E., Fong, D., and Cheng, L. (1988): Malondialdehyde-altered protein occurs in atheroma of Watanabe heritable hyperlipidemic rabbits. *Science,* 241:215–218.

17. Henriksen, T., Mahoney, E. M., and Steinberg, D. (1981): Enhanced macrophage degradation of low density lipoprotein previously incubated with cultured endothelial cells: recognition by receptors for acetylated low density lipoproteins. *Proc. Natl. Acad. Sci. USA.*, 78:6499–6503.

18. Henriksen, T., Mahoney, E. M., and Steinberg, D. (1983): Enhanced macrophage degradation of biologically modified low density lipoprotein. *Arteriosclerosis,* 3:149–159.

19. Hessler, J. R., Morel, D. W., Lewis, L. J., and Chisolm, G. M. (1983): Lipoprotein oxidation and lipoprotein-induced cytotoxicity. *Atherosclerosis,* 32:213–229.

20. Hoover, G. A., McCormick, S., and Kalant, N. (1988): Interaction of native and cell-modified low density lipoprotein with collagen gel. *Atherosclerosis,* 8:525–534.

21. Huang, H. J. S., Jones, N. H., Strominger, J. L., and Herzenberg, L. A. (1987): Molecular cloning of Ly-1, a membrane glycoprotein of mouse T lymphocytes and a subset of B cells: molecular homology to its human counterpart Leu-1/T1 (CD5). *Proc. Natl. Acad. Sci. USA.*, 84:204–208.

22. Jones, N. H., Clabby, M. L., Dialynas, D. P., Huang, H. J. S., Herzenberg, L. A., and Strominger, J. L. (1986): Isolation of complementary DNA clones encoding the human lymphocyte glyco-protein T1/Leu-1. *Nature (Lond.),* 323:346–349.

23. Juergens, G., Hoff, H. F., Chisolm, G. M., and Esterbauer, H. (1987): Modification of human serum low density lipoprotein by oxidation—characterization and pathophysiological implications. *Chem. Phys. Lipids,* 45:315–336.

24. Kodama, T., Freeman, M., Rohrer, L., Zabrecky, J., Matsudaira, P., and Krieger, M. (1990): Type I macrophage scavenger receptor contains alpha-helical and collagen-like coiled coils. *Nature (Lond.),* 343:531–535.

25. Kodama, T., Reddy, P., Kishimoto, C., and Krieger, M. (1988): Purification and characterization of a bovine acetyl low density lipoprotein receptor. *Proc. Natl. Acad. Sci. USA.*, 85:9238–9242.

26. Matsumoto, A., Naito, M., Itakura, H., et al. (1990): Human macrophage scavenger receptors: primary structure, expression, and localisation in atherosclerotic lesions. *Proc. Natl. Acad. Sci. USA.*, 87:9133–9137.

27. Mowri, H., Ohkuma, S., and Takamo, T. (1988): Monoclonal DLR1a/104G antibody recognizing peroxidized lipoproteins in atherosclerotic lesions. *Biochim. Biophys. Acta.,* 963:208–214.

28. Ottnad, E., Via, D. P., Sinn, H., Friedrich, E., Ziegler, R., and Dresel, H. A. (1990): Binding characteristics of reduced hepatic receptors for acetylated low-density lipoprotein and maleylated bovine serum albumin. *Biochem. J.,* 265:689–698.

29. Palinski, W., Rosenfeld, M. E., Yla-Herttuala, S., et al. (1989): Low density lipoprotein undergoes oxidative modification in vivo. *Proc. Natl. Acad. Sci. USA.*, 86:1372–1376.

30. Quinn, M. T., Parthasarathy, S., Fong, L. G., and Steinberg, D. (1987): Oxidatively modified low density lipoproteins: a potential role in recruitment and retention of monocyte/macrophages during atherogenesis. *Proc. Natl. Acad. Sci. USA.*, 84:2995–2998.

31. Reid, K. B. M. (1982): Proteins involved in the activation and control of the two pathways of human complement. *Biochem. Soc. Trans.,* 11:1–12.

32. Rohrer, L., Freeman, M., Kodama, T., Pennman, M., and Krieger, M. (1990): Coiled-coil fibrous domains mediate ligand binding by macrophage scavenger receptor type II. *Nature (Lond.),* 343: 570–572.

33. Rosenberg, A. M., Prokopchuk, P. A., and Lee, J. S. (1988): The binding of native DNA to the collagen-like segment of C1q. *J. Rheumatol.,* 15:1091–1096.

34. Rosenfeld, M. E., Palinski, W., Ylan-Herttuala, S., Butler, S., and Witztum, J. L. (1990): Dis-tribution of oxidation specific lipid-protein adducts and apolipoprotein B in atherosclerotic lesions of varying severity from WHHL rabbits. *Arteriosclerosis,* 10:336–349.

35. Ross, G. F., Notter, R. H., Meuth, J., and Whitsett, J. A. (1986): Phospholipid binding and biophysical activity of pulmonary surfactant-associated protein (SAP)-35 and its non-collagenous COOH-terminal domains. *J. Biol. Chem.,* 261:14283–14291.

36. Sparrow, C. P., Parthasarathy, S., and Steinberg, D. J. (1989): A macrophage receptor that recognizes oxidized low density lipoprotein but not acetylated low density lipoprotein. *J. Biol. Chem.*, 264:2599–2604.
37. Steinberg, D., Parthasarathy, S., Carew, T. E., Khoo, J. C., and Witztum, J. L. (1989): Beyond cholesterol. Modification of low-density lipoprotein that increase its atherogenicity. *New Engl. J. Med.*, 320:915–924.
38. Steinbrecher, U. P., Lougheed, M., Kwan, W. C., and Dirks, M. (1989): Recognition of oxidized low density lipoprotein by the scavenger receptor of macrophages results from derivatization of apoprotein B by products of fatty acid peroxitation. *J. Biol. Chem.*, 264:15216–15223.
39. Steinbrecher, U. P., Zhang, H., and Lougheed, M. (1990): Role of oxidatively modified LDL in atherosclerosis. *Free Radical Biol. Med.*, 9:155–168.
40. Takagi, J., Kasahara, K., Sekiya, F., Inada, Y., and Saito, Y. (1988): Subunit B of factor XIII is present in bovine platelets. *Thromb. Res.*, 50:767–774.
41. Via, D. P., Dresel, H. A., Cheng, S. L., and Gotto, A. M. (1985): Murine macrophage tumors are source of a 260,000-dalton acetyl-low density lipoprotein receptor. *J. Biol. Chem.*, 260:7386–7397.
42. Yla-Herttuala, S., Palinski, W., Rosenfeld, M. E., et al. (1989): Evidence for the presence of oxidatively modified low density lipoprotein in atherosclerotic lesions of rabbit and man. *J. Clin. Invest.*, 84:1086–1095.

Atherosclerosis Reviews, Volume 23,
edited by P. C. Weber and A. Leaf.
Raven Press, Ltd., New York © 1991.

Aortic Smooth Muscle Cells Heterogeneity

Effects of Thyroid Hormone, Cholesterol Feeding, and Nifedipine Treatment

Paolo Pauletto, Gianluigi Scannapieco, and *Saverio Sartore

*Institute of Clinical Medicine, *Institute of General Pathology and National Research Council Unit for Muscle Biology and Physiopathology, University of Padova, 35100 Padova, Italy*

A panel of monoclonal antibodies specific for smooth muscle (SM) and non-muscle (NM) myosin, immunocytochemical procedures, and Western blotting experiments were used to study myosin isoform composition and distribution in smooth muscle cells (SMC) of rabbit aorta *in vivo* and *in vitro* (2,13). The SM-E7 antibody reacted with both myosin heavy chain (MHC) isoforms of SM type (SM-MHC-1 and -2) present in the adult rabbit aorta. The NM-G2 antibody recognized the NM myosin heavy chains present in platelets, fibroblasts, macrophages, and lymphocytes (2,13). Using these antibodies, different SMC populations were identified in the aortic media of the normal adult rabbit aorta. The majority of medial SMC contained SM myosin exclusively, whereas a few SMC were characterized by the expression of both SM and NM myosin isoforms.

During experimental atherogenesis in rabbits, the size of this latter SMC population markedly increased in the media and represented the predominant SMC type in the atherosclerotic plaque. In the earlier stages of development, SMC of rabbit aorta coexpress SM and NM myosin (13). Thus, SMC showing an "immature" pattern of myosin expression are present in the normal media, increase in the media underlying the atherosclerotic plaque, and represent the main cell type in the plaque. In rabbits, the number of these SMC of "immature" type seems to be influenced by such different stimuli as the thyroid hormone level and nifedipine, a calcium-channel blocker.

In the aortic media of thyroxine-treated rabbits, the size of the SMC population expressing an "immature" pattern of myosin was markedly increased in comparison to controls. Propylthiouracil (PTU) treatment resulted in decrease of these SMC. On the other hand, nifedipine was able to prevent atherogenesis in rabbits when the treatment was started along with cholesterol feeding but not when it was started after the development of atherosclerotic lesions. Prevention of the development of lesions was accompanied by marked reduction of the

SMC of "immature" type in the media. A similar reduction was found in the media of control nifedipine-treated rabbits and of animals in which the treatment did not induce regression of already established lesions. Moreover, in primary SMC cultures, nifedipine reduces the expression of NM myosin.

MYOSIN ISOFORM EXPRESSION IN VASCULAR SMOOTH MUSCLE THROUGHOUT DEVELOPMENT

In analogy with the adult bovine aorta (12), Western blotting experiments on crude extracts from New Zealand White (NZW) rabbit aortas showed that this tissue is composed of two different MHC, SM-MHC-1 (Mr = 205 kDa) and SM-MHC-2 (Mr = 200 kDa). In the fetal/neonatal stage of development, aortic SM was found to contain SM-MHC-1 but not SM-MHC-2. NM-MHC showed the same electrophoretic mobility as the faster-migrating SM isoform. Moreover, NM-MHC was expressed in an inverse manner with respect to SM-MHC-2. In fact, it was detectable in the early stages of development but absent in adulthood (2).

Double immunofluorescence experiments were carried out on cryosections of fetal/neonatal aorta using SM-E7 conjugated with fluorescein isothiocyanate and

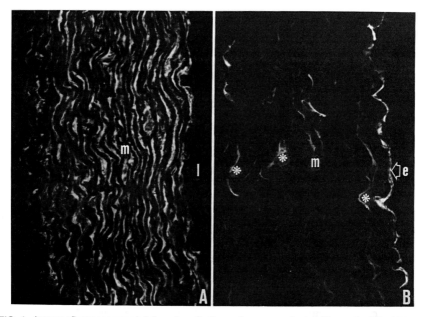

FIG. 1. Immunofluorescence staining of aortic tissue from normal adult (3-month-old) rabbit with anti-myosin antibodies. Note that in (**A**) all medial (m) SMC are labeled by SM-E7, whereas in (**B**) rare, scattered (asterisks) medial SMC are stained with NM-G2 antibody. e, endothelium. (×525.)

NM-G2 indirectly labeled with rodamine isothiocyanate (13). In those experiments, all SMC of the aortic media were reactive with both antibodies.

Thus, at this stage of development all SMC of rabbit aorta coexpress SM and NM myosin isoforms (2,13).

Cryosections from aortic tissue of normal adult (3-month-old) rabbit were also tested. All medial SMC appeared to be labeled by SM-E7 (Fig. 1A), whereas rare medial cells stained with NM-G2, particularly beneath the intimal elastic lamina (Fig. 1B). These cells were double-labeled by both SM-E7 and NM-G2 (13). Because these cells show the same immunostaining properties peculiar to the fetal/neonatal stage, we concluded that a specific SMC subpopulation showing an "immature" pattern of myosin isoform expression is present in the aortic media of adult NZW rabbit (13). Similar results were obtained in the bovine aorta (12).

The existence of structural and functional similarities between neonatal SMC and adult proliferating SMC has been reported in several studies (6). In light of these results, we evaluated myosin isoform expression of aortic SMC in NZW rabbits subjected to such stimuli as changes in thyroid hormone and cholesterol levels. We also employed calcium-channel blockers, which are capable of promoting or inhibiting vascular SMC proliferation.

INFLUENCE OF THYROID HORMONE ON MYOSIN ISOFORM EXPRESSION IN VASCULAR SMOOTH MUSCLE

A 1-month course of administration of L-thyroxine (100 μg/kg/day) to adult NZW rabbits resulted in hyperthyroidism. A marked intimal thickening was noted in the animals' thoracic aorta. The thickened intima was composed of a large number of homogeneous, well-organized cells negative for Sudan black and oil red O.

The cellular composition of the intima from hyperthyroid animals was further analyzed using a panel of antibodies specific for cytocontractile proteins (myosin isoforms), cytoskeletal proteins (desmin and vimentin), and monocytes/macrophages. Immunostaining of the aortic cryosections with NM-G2 showed that all the intimal cells and the large majority of the medial cells were reactive to this antibody (Fig. 2C, D). A similar pattern of immunoreactivity was found using the SM-E7 anti-SM myosin antibody (Fig. 2A, B). Double immunofluorescence experiments showed that although the large majority of SMC are labeled by both antibodies, a few cells in the media underlying the intimal thickening are labeled exclusively by SM-E7 or by NM-G2 (not illustrated).

The anti-vimentin antibody stained all the medial cells of the normal media as well as those of the thickened intima of hyperthyroid rabbits and the underlying media. By contrast, the anti-desmin antibody did not react with cells present in the intimal thickening and recognized a few cells in the media (not illustrated). Finally, very rare cells were positive to the anti-macrophage antibody in thickened

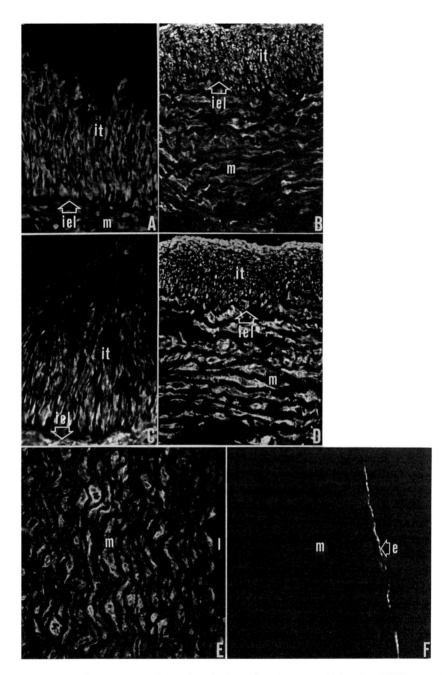

FIG. 2. Immunofluorescence staining of aortic tissue from hyperthyroid (**A–D**) and PTU-treated (**E–F**) adult (3-month-old) rabbit with anti-myosin antibodies. Note that thyroxine administration to rabbits induces an intimal thickening (it) for the presence of SMC that are stained by SM-E7 (**A, B**) and NM-G2 (**C, D**) antibodies. SMC positive with NM-G2 antibody are also numerous in the underlying media (m). In PTU-treated animals, medial NM-G2 immunoreactivity (**F**) completely disappears, whereas staining with SM-E7 is still seen (**E**). iel, internal elastic lamina; e, endothelium. (×525.)

intima whereas no cells stained in the media. Thus, we conclude that the cells in the aortic intima of hyperthyroid animals are almost exclusively SMC showing an "immature" pattern of myosin isoform expression. Compared to controls, the size of this SMC population is markedly increased also in the media.

Treatment of hyperthyroid rabbits with PTU induced normalization of thyroid hormone levels within 1 month. This normalization was accompanied by marked reduction of intimal thickening and decrease of the SMC population with an "immature" pattern of myosin isoform expression. The effect of PTU treatment on the aortic wall of control euthyroid rabbits is shown in Fig. 2E, F. Although NM-G2 stains a few SMC in the normal aorta (Fig. 1B) (13), this antibody recognized the vascular endothelium alone in PTU-treated animals, since cells positive with NM-G2 had completely disappeared (Fig. 2F). The immunoreactivity of these cryosections with SM-E7 is comparable to that found in control rabbits—i.e., almost all medial SMC are reactive (Fig. 2E; for comparison, see Fig. 1A).

In vitro experiments showed that thyroxine is able to promote, in a dose-dependent manner, the [^{3}H]thymidine incorporation in cultured vascular SMC (not shown).

On the whole, our findings are consistent with a specific role for thyroid hormone in modulating the proliferation/migration activity of a specific medial SMC subpopulation in the absence of significant changes of the serum cholesterol levels.

EFFECTS OF CHOLESTEROL FEEDING AND NIFEDIPINE TREATMENT ON VASCULAR SMOOTH MUSCLE

Three-month-old NZW rabbits were kept on a 1% cholesterol-enriched diet for 3 months. Plasma cholesterol levels ranged between 1,600 and 2,000 mg/dl throughout the study period. After the animals were killed, their aortas were processed for computerized morphometry, which was carried out on serial histological sections. Specimens were frozen for immunocytochemistry, and Western blotting experiments were carried out on atherosclerotic and control tissue. Because atherosclerotic plaque is composed of different cell populations of NM type such as monocytes/macrophages and lymphocytes, Western blotting and immunocytochemical techniques were used to test the specificity of SM-E7 and NM-G2. All the above cell types were recognized by NM-G2 but not by SM-E7.

In cryosections from the atherosclerotic aorta of cholesterol-fed rabbits, the media underlying the plaque was recognized by SM-E7 in a manner similar to the normal media (Fig. 3A; for comparison, see Fig. 1A). In the atherosclerotic plaque, a specific reactivity with this antibody was also found (Fig. 3A). NM-G2 recognized a larger number of cells in the plaque than SM-E7. Moreover, this antibody recognized more medial cells in the atherosclerotic aorta than in the normal aorta (Fig. 3B; for comparison, see Fig. 1B). In particular, NM-G2–

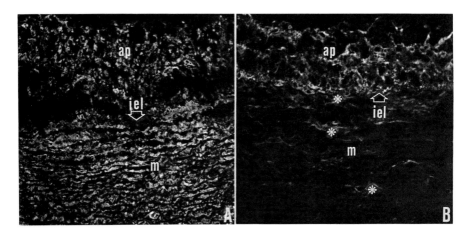

FIG. 3. Immunofluorescence staining of atherosclerotic rabbit aorta after 2 months of cholesterol feeding with anti-myosin antibodies. Note that in the plaque (ap) numerous SMC are labeled with SM-E7 (**A**) and NM-G2 (**B**). In the underlying media (m), all SMC are stained with SM-E7, whereas only a few cells, mainly localized close to the internal elastic lamina (iel), are recognized by NM-G2 antibody (asterisks). (×525.)

positive cells were more numerous beneath the atherosclerotic plaque (Fig. 3B). Almost all intimal and medial cells recognized by NM-G2 were double-labeled by SM-E7. However, some cells are recognized by NM-G2 alone (13). In the plaque, but not in the underlying media, part of these cells were also reactive with the OKM* 1 monoclonal antibody, which is specific for human monocytes/granulocytes and NK cells but cross-reacts with the rabbit system (13). Because careful morphological examinations on hematoxylin–eosin–stained histological sections did not reveal the presence of lymphocytes, it seems reasonable to assume that the medial SMC recognized only by NM-G2 represent a distinct SMC population. Conversely, some of these cells in the plaque seem to be macrophages or lymphocytes.

The effects of nifedipine on atherogenesis and myosin isoform expression of aortic cells was evaluated in hypercholesterolemic NZW rabbits following two different protocols. Animals were maintained on 1% cholesterol-enriched diet for 12 weeks. After 4 weeks, some rabbits were given the drug (20 mg twice daily) for another 8 weeks without discontinuing the cholesterol-enriched diet. In this experiment, we tried to induce some regression in the extent of atherosclerotic lesions ("regression experiment"). In another set of experiments, NZW rabbits were treated with nifedipine for the entire course of the 12-week cholesterol-enriched diet. The aim of this study was to prevent the development of atherosclerotic lesions ("prevention experiment").

Other NZW rabbits maintained on a standard diet were given nifedipine for 12 weeks to test whether the drug had any direct effect on SMC heterogeneity. Nifedipine treatment modified neither blood pressure nor plasma cholesterol levels throughout the study. Appreciable plasma levels of the drug were detected in the animals of each treatment group.

Compared to findings in the controls, a marked increase in intimal surface was observed in the aortas from rabbits kept on cholesterol-rich diet for 12 weeks (1.49 ± 0.53 mm^2 versus 0.05 ± 0.02 mm^2; $p < 0.001$ by analysis of variance).

In the "regression experiment," no significant difference in the area of intimal thickening was observed in the aortas from the cholesterol-fed, nifedipine-treated

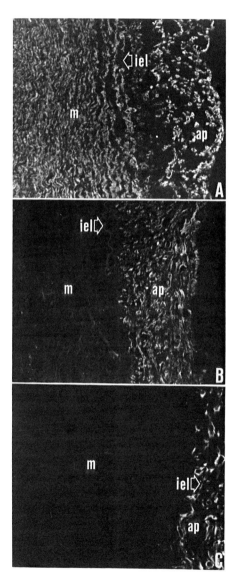

FIG. 4. Immunofluorescence staining of atherosclerotic, nifedipine-treated rabbit aorta with anti-myosin antibodies. In the aortic tissue from these animals, medial SMC reactive with NM-G2 antibody disappear (**B, C**), whereas staining with SM-E7 antibody is still present. No change in the immunoreactivity with anti-myosin antibodies was observed in the plaque (ap). iel, internal elastic lamina; m, aortic media. (A, B: ×525; C: ×800.)

rabbits as compared to the hypercholesterolemic untreated animals (1.38 ± 0.56 mm^2). Conversely, in the "prevention experiment," the area of intimal thickening was about fivefold smaller than that found in hypercholesterolemic untreated animals (0.33 ± 0.11 mm^2 versus 1.49 ± 0.53 mm^2; $p < 0.01$ by analysis of variance).

Figure 4 shows the immunocytochemical pattern observed in the aorta of hypercholesterolemic, nifedipine-treated rabbits in the "regression experiment." The cells present in the plaque showed the same immunostaining pattern with SM-E7 and NM-G2 as the hypercholesterolemic untreated animals (Fig. 3)— i.e., the majority of cells were labeled with both antibodies, whereas a minority of cells were stained either by SM-E7 or NM-G2 (Fig. 3). As far as the media underlying the plaque is concerned, the SM-E7 reactivity was unchanged but the NM-G2–positive cells disappeared (Fig. 4B, C).

In the "prevention experiment," the majority of animals displayed a near-normal intima. In some cases where a thin intimal thickening was noted, most intimal cells were double-reactive with SM-E7 and NM-G2. In all animals, the reactivity of the aortic media to the NM-G2 was almost absent. Absence of NM-G2–positive cells was also evident in the nifedipine-treated animals who were kept on a standard diet.

Thus, in all three sets of experiments performed with nifedipine, the SMC of "immature" type disappeared from the aortic media.

When preconfluent primary cultures of rabbit aorta were studied using SM-E7 and NM-G2, most cells were double-labeled. Only very rare cells were reactive with SM-E7 or NM-G2 alone. After nifedipine was added to the culture medium (final concentration, 10^{-5} M) for 5 days, a different immunostaining pattern was observed—i.e., almost all SMC were labeled by SM-E7 alone and very rare cells were double-labeled or labeled by NM-G2. This indicates that nifedipine has a marked effect on the expression of NM myosin.

CONCLUSIONS

In previous studies, cytoskeletal and cytocontractile proteins such as desmin, vimentin, actin, and myosin have been proposed as markers of SMC differentiation (1,3,5). These markers provided evidence for SMC heterogeneity in the normal media as well as in the atherosclerotic plaque and intimal thickening. So far, data on SMC heterogeneity in the media underlying the plaque are mainly morphological. In particular, the use of actin as a marker of SMC differentiation during atherogenesis at the single-cell level is hampered by the lack of antibodies specific for all the actin isotypes.

The combined use of monoclonal antibodies specific to either SM or NM myosin allowed us to define precisely the differentiation pattern of SMC during development as well as during atherogenesis at the single-cell level. In fetal rabbit aorta, the SMC of the aortic media coexpress SM and NM myosin. This "immature" pattern of myosin isoform expression is found in a few SMC present in the aortic media of the adult animal. In hyperthyroid animals (Fig. 5) and after cholesterol feeding (Fig. 6), the size of this cell population is greatly increased in the thickened intima and even in the underlying media.

Functional and structural similarities between fetal/neonatal and adult proliferating SMC are well established (6). It might be that under hypercholesterolemic diet (or with hyperthyroidism), some differentiated SMC of the media, expressing SM myosin alone, undergo a phenotypic modulation toward the "immature" phenotype, expressing both SM and NM myosin, with enhanced replicative properties. Alternatively, one could posit (9) the existence of a stem-like cell compartment composed of "immature" SMC that could be selectively recruited by different stimuli for intimal thickening.

Regression of intimal thickening will occur if the inciting stimulus is suppressed, as in the case with thyroid hormone, or after discontinuation of a cholesterol-rich diet (10), but not if the stimulus persists, as in the case with the "regression experiment" in our cholesterol-fed animals. However, prevention of intimal thickening can be achieved when the atherogenic stimulus is counterbalanced from the beginning, as in the "prevention experiment" (Fig. 6). The differential effect of nifedipine in the above experiments can be explained by the immunocytochemical studies reported here.

The medial SMC of "immature" type, which may represent the main source of SMC found in the plaque, virtually disappeared when rabbits were treated from the beginning of the cholesterol feeding (Fig. 6). A marked decrease in the

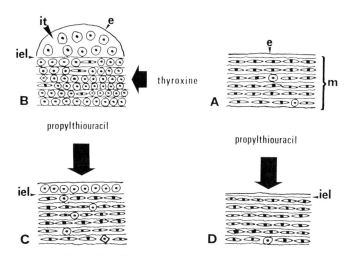

FIG. 5. Vascular smooth muscle cell populations in euthyroid, hyperthyroid, and propylthiouracil-treated rabbits. (**A**) normal euthyroid; (**B**) hyperthyroid; (**C**) hyperthyroid, propylthiouracil-treated; (**D**) propylthiouracil-treated. it: intimal thickening; m: aortic media; iel: internal elastic media; e: endothelium. ⊙ : SMC reactive with SM-E7 antibody; ⊙: SMC reactive with both SM-E7 and NM-G2 antibodies; ◇ : SMC reactive with NM-G2 antibody.

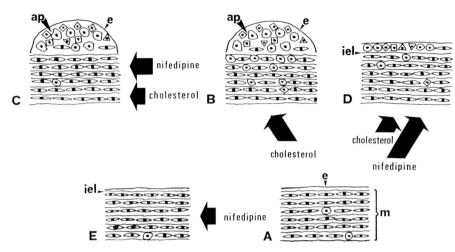

FIG. 6. Effect of nifedipine on the atherosclerotic lesions induced in rabbits by cholesterol feeding. **(A)** normocholesterolemic; **(B)** cholesterol-fed; **(C)** nifedipine-treated + cholesterol-fed (nifedipine administered along with cholesterol after inducing atherosclerosis); **(D)** nifedipine-treated + cholesterol-fed (nifedipine and cholesterol given concomitantly from the beginning of the experiment); **(E)** nifedipine-treated. ap: atherosclerotic plaque; m: aortic media; e: endothelium. ⊂⊃ : SMC reactive with SM-E7 antibody; ⊙: SMC reactive with both SM-E7 and NM-G2 antibodies; ◊ : SMC reactive with NM-G2 antibody. ▽ △ ▫: other cells of nonmuscle type (inflammatory cells).

size of the SMC population was also observed in the media of the animals in the "regression experiment," but the change was not accompanied by a reduction of the intimal lesions. The different effects of nifedipine on both intima and media are related to distinct functional properties of the SMC of these two vascular layers. Indeed, cultured SMC from rabbit atherosclerotic lesions display a higher proliferation rate than SMC from the normal media (8). Different levels of PDGF-like activity have been found in the media and in the intima of normal arterial wall (11). Moreover, we cannot rule out the possibility that nifedipine concentration within the atherosclerotic lesions is not sufficient to induce any quantitative or qualitative effect.

On the other hand, we can hypothesize that nifedipine is effective only when administered in the early phase of atherogenesis and SMC "activation." In fact, in balloon injury experiments, nifedipine is effective in preventing SMC intimal proliferation within 48 hr after injury but not if the treatment is delayed by 7 days (4). Aside from the antiproliferative effect of the drug on SMC (7), the results of our tissue culture experiments suggest that nifedipine has a direct effect on the differentiation pattern of aortic SMC. Changes of reactivity with the NM-G2 antibody observed *in vivo* and *in vitro* are probably not due to conformational changes of the myosin molecule, since treatment with different detergents does not modify the NM-G2 staining pattern in aortic cryosections.

We believe that the decreased reactivity of vascular SMC with the NM-G2 antibody reported here is related to inhibition of the synthesis or to an accelerated catabolism of the NM myosin isoform and, thus, to the induction of the differentiated SMC phenotype. It remains to be established whether changes in the differentiation state are also accompanied by changes in the proliferative properties.

REFERENCES

1. Benzonana, G., Skalli, O., and Gabbiani, G. (1988): Correlation between the distribution of smooth muscle or non-muscle myosins and alfa-smooth muscle actin in normal and pathological soft tissues. *Cell Motil. Cytoskeleton,* 11:260–274.
2. Borrione, A. C., Zanellato, A. M. C., Scannapieco, G., Pauletto, P., and Sartore, S. (1989): Myosin heavy-chain isoform in adult and developing rabbit vascular smooth muscle. *Eur. J. Biochem.,* 183:413–417.
3. Gabbiani, G., Kocher, O., Bloom, W. S., Vandekerchove, J., and Weber, K. (1984): Actin expression of rat aortic intimal thickening, human atheromatous plaque, and cultured rat aortic media. *J. Clin. Invest.,* 73:148–152.
4. Jackson, C. L., Bush, R. C., and Bowyer, D. E. (1988): Inhibitory effect of calcium antagonists on balloon catheter–induced arterial smooth muscle cell proliferation and lesion size. *Atherosclerosis,* 69:115–122.
5. Kocher, O., Skalli, O., Cerutti, D., Gabbiani, F., and Gabbiani, G. (1985): Cytoskeletal features of rat aortic cells during development. An electron microscopic, immunohistochemical, and biochemical study. *Circ. Res.,* 56:829–838.
6. Nilsson, J. (1986): Growth factors and the pathogenesis of atherosclerosis. *Atherosclerosis,* 62: 185–199.
7. Nilsson, J., Sjolund, M., Palmberg, L., von Euler, A. M., Jonzon, B., and Thyberg, J. (1985): The calcium antagonist nifedipine inhibits arterial smooth muscle cell proliferation. *Atherosclerosis,* 58:109–122.
8. Pietila, K., and Nikkari, T. (1980): Enhanced growth of smooth muscle cells from atherosclerotic rabbit aortas in culture. *Atherosclerosis,* 36:241–248.
9. Schwartz, S. M., Reidy, M. R., and Clowes, A. W. (1985): Kinetics of atherosclerosis: a stem cell model. *Ann. N.Y. Acad. Sci.,* 454:292–304.
10. Thiery, J., Niedmann, P. D., and Seidel, D. (1987): The beneficial influence of nifedipine on the regression of the cholesterol-induced atherosclerosis in rabbits. *Res. Exp. Med.,* 187:359–367.
11. Walker, N. N., Bowen-Pope, D. F., Ross, R., and Reidy, M. A. (1986): Production of platelet-derived growth factor-like molecules by cultured arterial smooth muscle cells accompanies proliferation after injury. *Proc. Natl. Acad. Sci. USA,* 83:7311–7315.
12. Zanellato, A. M. C., Borrione, A. C., Giuriato, L., et al. (1990): Myosin isoforms and cell heterogeneity in vascular smooth muscle. I. Developing and adult bovine aorta. *Dev. Biol.,* 141: 431–446.
13. Zanellato, A. M. C., Borrione, A. C., Tonello, M., Scannapieco, G., Pauletto, P., and Sartore, S. (1990): Myosin isoform expression and smooth muscle cell heterogeneity in normal and atherosclerotic rabbit aorta. *Arteriosclerosis,* 10:996–1009.

Atherosclerosis Reviews, Volume 23,
edited by P. C. Weber and A. Leaf.
Raven Press, Ltd., New York © 1991.

Mechanisms of Plaque Formation

Cellular Changes and the Possible Role of Growth-Regulatory Molecules

Elaine W. Raines and Russell Ross

Department of Pathology, University of Washington, Seattle, Washington 98195

Advanced lesions of atherosclerosis that result in clinical sequelae are smooth muscle proliferative lesions that occlude the affected artery by increasing the thickness of the innermost layer of the artery, the intima. Because of the silent and slow progression of the disease in humans, examination of the evolution of lesions of atherosclerosis has been difficult. Our understanding of the cellular constituents of lesions and the early changes that result in the formation of fatty streaks and their progression to advanced lesions is the result of observations of atherosclerosis in animal models. Induction of hypercholesterolemia, the most common risk factor for atherosclerosis, in nonhuman primates and swine (3,4,7,8,19,20), as well as models of hypertension (1,17) have demonstrated a similar series of cellular interactions and changes in the development of lesions of atherosclerosis. These studies have supported the hypothesis that the earliest phases of atherosclerosis represent a specialized form of chronic inflammation (22,29). The following overview outlines our understanding of the cellular changes observed in hypercholesterolemic animal models of atherosclerosis. In addition, we also discuss the potential roles of these cells in the initiation and progression of lesions of atherosclerosis.

CELLULAR CHANGES OBSERVED IN EXPERIMENTAL MODELS OF ATHEROSCLEROSIS

Morphologic examination of the arterial trees of a series of *Macaca nemestrina* maintained on a low- (19,20) or high-cholesterol diet (3,4) for 2 weeks to $3\frac{1}{2}$ years has revealed the cellular changes involved in lesion development. Within 7 to 12 days after inducing high levels of hypercholesterolemia (plasma levels of 500–1,000 mg/dl) or within 6 to 8 months after lower levels (plasma levels of 200–400 mg/dl), the first cellular response that can be observed is that clusters of leukocytes attach to the endothelium of the artery wall throughout the aorta, iliac, coronary, and carotid arteries. These leukocytes consist principally of monocytes together with some lymphocytes, primarily CD4- and CD8-positive T cells. The attached cells migrate along the surface of the endothelium, penetrate between the endothelial cells, and accumulate subendothelially within the intima. The monocytes take up lipid that has accumulated in the intima due to trans-endothelial transport from the hypercholesterolemic plasma. Data in cholesterol-fed rabbits suggest that focal increases in LDL observed in lesion-susceptible sites before fatty-streak formation are due to localized differences in LDL retention and diminished fractional rates of LDL degradation, not to selectively increased permeability (34). Within a short period of time, the monocytes become filled with large lipid droplets. These collections of foam cells, or fatty streaks, enlarge by the process of continued chemoattraction of additional monocytes that attach to the surface of the developing lesion and enter and expand the lesion.

With increasing duration of hypercholesterolemia, smooth muscle cells (SMC) are attracted from the underlying media into the intima, where they also begin to take up lipid and become foam cells. Some of the SMC may also be present in preexisting intimal cushions. Within the intima, the SMC proliferate and synthesize new connective tissue, resulting in a mixed macrophage, T-cell, smooth muscle–proliferative lesion. Studies in WHHL rabbits and comparably hypercholesterolemic fat-fed rabbits to determine the proliferating cells by administration of [^{3}H]thymidine prior to their death, demonstrate that approximately 30% of cells incorporating thymidine were identified as macrophages and approximately 45% were SMC (28). Thus, both macrophage and smooth muscle proliferation may contribute to lesion development.

Observations in the hypercholesterolemic animals suggest that most fatty streaks progress to fibrous plaques by a continuing process of attraction of SMC and monocytes into the lesion. However, in humans, the relationship of fatty streaks to advanced lesions is more controversial (18,22). However, it is clear that in both humans and nonhuman primates that the period of time required for this evolution depends on many factors, including the degree and duration of hypercholesterolemia, the anatomic site involved, and the genetic susceptibility of the host. At some branches and bifurcations opposite the flow divider, junctional separations between individual endothelial cells overlying the fatty streak are accompanied by retraction of these endothelial cells. Many of the lipid-filled macrophages are uncovered and in many cases are swept into the bloodstream, where they can be found in the circulation (3). Some remain *in situ,* and platelets may be found adherent to some of the exposed macrophages as well as to exposed connective tissue. In both low- and high-level hypercholesterolemia, these changes temporally precede the formation of advanced proliferative smooth muscle lesions at similar anatomic sites. In these animals, platelet-macrophage interactions were first observed in the iliac arteries. After longer periods, similar changes occurred at higher levels in the abdominal and thoracic aorta. The cellular changes observed in animals with low-level hypercholesterolemia were similar to those observed in animals with high-level hypercholesterolemia, but the cellular changes progress more slowly (19,20).

THE ROLE OF GROWTH-REGULATORY MOLECULES IN THE PATHOGENESIS OF ATHEROSCLEROSIS

Advanced lesions that occlude the affected artery are responsible for the clinical sequelae associated with cardiovascular disease. The intima is thickened because of a large increase in SMC, formation of new connective tissue matrix by these SMC, and, in hyperlipidemic individuals, by the presence of both intracellular and extracellular lipid. Although atherosclerosis does not represent the response of the artery wall to a single initiating event, similar cellular changes have been described in experimental models of hyperlipidemia (3,4,7,8,19,20) and hypertension (1,17). Any attempt to determine the mechanisms of lesion formation must account for the multiplicity of initiating factors, the focal nature of lesion formation, the increased adhesion and attraction of monocytes into the artery, the accumulation and proliferation of SMC within the intima, and the formation of connective tissue.

Directed cell migration and proliferation have been shown to be induced by a number of peptide growth factors and cytokines. In addition to stimulating directed cell migration and cell growth, these growth-regulatory molecules, regulate many other critical cell functions, including lipid metabolism and connective tissue formation. Table 1 lists peptide growth factors and cytokines that may be delivered by infiltrating leukocytes or activation of cells within the artery wall. The multifunctionality of peptide growth factors is illustrated by their ability to induce molecular events characteristic of processes as diverse as inflammation, angiogenesis, tissue repair, and cancer [reviewed in Sporn and Roberts (36)]. By binding to specific cell surface receptors on responsive cells, these growth-regulatory molecules induce signals that evoke a large number of biological responses, dependent on the factor, the responsive cell, and its environment (35). Both the factors and their cell surface receptors appear to be tightly regulated. For example, platelet-derived growth factor (PDGF), a potent growth factor and chemoattractant for SMC, can be synthesized and secreted by macrophages, endothelium, and smooth muscle in addition to platelets (26,29,32). However, PDGF is not expressed or secreted by normal cells except following activation or injury. In human and nonhuman primate lesions of atherosclerosis, PDGF-B chain expression is increased, and PDGF-B chain has been localized to approximately 20% of the macrophages present in lesions at all stages of lesion development (31). The β-subunit of the PDGF receptor is also only expressed at low levels in normal vessels but is increased in arterial lesions (33). Understanding the regulation of growth factors and their receptors will help determine their individual roles in attraction and proliferation of cells in lesion formation. *In vitro* studies have enabled us to determine many of the growth mediators made by cells present in arterial lesions.

TABLE 1. *Growth factors and cytokines that may be delivered by infiltrating leukocytes or activation of arterial wall cells*

Growth factor or cytokine	Abbreviation	Cellular sources
Epidermal growth factor	EGF	P
Basic fibroblast growth factor	bFGF	EC, M, SMC
Granulocyte-macrophage colony stimulating factor	GM-CSF	EC, M, SMC, T
Insulin-growth factor I	IGF-I	EC, M, P, SMC
Interferon-γ	IFN-γ	T
Interleukin-1	IL-1	EC, M, SMC, T
Interleukin-2	IL-2	T
Monocyte-colony stimulating factor	M-CSF	EC, M, SMC
Monocyte chemotactic protein	MCP-1	EC, M, SMC
Platelet-derived growth factor	PDGF	EC, M, P, SMC
Platelet-derived endothelial growth factor	PDEGF	P
Transforming growth factor-α	TGF-α	M
Transforming growth factor-β	TGF-8,3	EC, M, P, SMC, T
Tumor necrosis factor-α	TNF-α	EC, M, SMC, T
Tumor necrosis factor-β (lymphotoxin)	TNF-β	T
Vascular endothelial cell growth factor	VEGF/VPF	M, SMC

EC, endothelial cell; M, monocyte/macrophage; P, platelet; SMC, smooth muscle cell; T, T cell.

The cellular events described above in experimentally induced hypercholesterolemia have led to the formulation of a hypothesis that has been modified and refined during the past 15 years, the Response to Injury Hypothesis of Atherosclerosis. This hypothesis suggests that some form of "injury" to the endothelial lining of the artery results in a sequence of events that leads to the development of the advanced lesions of atherosclerosis (29,30). The injury to the endothelium does not necessarily result in denudation, but it may induce subtle changes in function (endothelial dysfunction), such as the adherence of leukocytes described above. In addition to chronic hypercholesterolemia, factors that may lead to similar injury include altered shear stress, which may occur at branch points or bifurcations in arteries in hypertension, and dysfunction induced by toxins, viral infection, or other injurious agents. The Response to Injury Hypothesis also suggests a major role for the monocyte/macrophage in the initiation and evolution of lesions. A multitude of *in vitro* data further suggest that a number of different arterial cells may serve as local sources of growth factors, chemoattractants, and further endothelial injury. According to this hypothesis, if the injury to the endothelium were a self-limited event and endothelial function were restored, the proliferative lesions might be capable of regressing. However, if the injury at focal sites in the artery wall is either long-standing or chronic, the lesions could continue to progress and lead to advanced lesions, occlusion, and the resultant clinical sequelae.

THE ROLES OF DIFFERENT CELLS IN LESION FORMATION

The cells involved in lesion formation include arterial endothelium, monocyte-derived macrophages, T cells, SMC, and platelets. To understand the pathogenesis of atherosclerosis, it is necessary to understand the functional roles of each cell in both lesion induction and progression and the nature of the cellular interactions associated with an increased incidence of atherosclerosis. Table 2 summarizes the potential contribution of each cell type to major factors involved in development of lesions of atherosclerosis: lipid accumulation and metabolism, endothelial injury, release of chemoattractants, smooth muscle proliferation, immune modulation, formation of vasoactive agents, and matrix formation. Particular features of each of the cell types and major questions regarding their potential roles in lesion initiation and development will be discussed below.

The endothelium plays a critical role in providing a selective permeability barrier, regulating vascular tone, and in maintaining hemostasis and a nonthrombogenic lining to the artery wall. Removal of this barrier results in interactions between platelets and underlying connective tissue and exposes the underlying arterial cells to material released from platelets and to all plasma constituents. Such platelet-vessel wall interactions have been shown to occur in homocysteinemia (12); and it is likely that such interactions play a major role in lesion development at perianastomotic sites of coronary bypass grafts, following percutaneous transluminal coronary angioplasty, and in other traumatic vascular lesions. However, "nondenuding injury" (27) and endothelial activation (9,14,24) can alter endothelial cell function. Following activation, the endothelial cell is capable of expressing specific leukocytes adhesion molecules, actively participate in immune regulation and the release of growth factors, and is altered metabolically and structurally (9,22,24,37,39,40). Neovascularization associated with advanced lesions may also play an important role in lesion progression. Understanding the nature of endothelial cell activation in response to different risk factors is clearly central to understanding the pathogenesis of lesion formation.

The development of monoclonal antibodies has facilitated the identification of the monocytes/macrophage as the ubiquitous foam cell in both fatty streaks and advanced lesions of atherosclerosis. As detailed above, studies in experimental animals have also demonstrated the early attachment of monocytes to endothelium, followed by subendothelial migration. Once localized subendothelially, the monocyte-derived macrophage has the capacity to further modulate endothelial injury, metabolize and store lipid, secrete a number of different smooth muscle and leukocyte chemoattractants, induce smooth muscle proliferation, and actively participate in an immune reaction (see Table 2). It is clear that macrophages within lesions accumulate lipid. However, it is important to determine at what stages of lesion development the other multiple capacities of the macrophage are involved. Although the list of macrophage products and the ubiquitous presence of the macrophage at all stages of lesion development has

TABLE 2. *Possible role of different cells in development of lesions of atherosclerosis*

Possible role	Endothelium	Monocyte/macrophage	Platelets	Smooth muscle	T cells
Mediation of endothelial "injury" or dysfunction	Results in: Alteration of leukocyte adhesion; Altered pinocytosis; Procoagulant activity; Secretion of chemoattractant activity; Secretion of growth regulatory molecules	Able to secrete: Direct mediators proteases oxygen metabolites; Indirect mediators lipoprotein lipase; Cytokines IL-1 and TNF-α, which enhance leukocyte adhesion		Oxidized lipids	
Lipid accumulation metabolism	Peroxidation of LDL; Altered endothelial function allowing infiltration of plasma lipids; Transport of lipids	Accumulate large amounts of lipoprotein and cholesterol; Peroxidation of LDL; Principal fatty-streak foam cell	Enhance: ApoE production by macrophages; Cholesterol accumulation in macrophages and SMC	Internalize and store lipids; Can become foam cells; Peroxidation of LDL	Activated T cells inhibit SMC; Intracellular accumulation of cholesterol ester
Smooth muscle proliferation	Endothelial heparin (−); PDGF (++); bFGF (++); IGF-1 (+); IL-1 (indirect +); TGF-β (indirect +/−); Thrombospondin (+); TNF-α (indirect +)	bFGF (++); PDGF (++); TGF-α (+); IGF-1 (+); TGF-β (indirect +/−); IL-1 (indirect +); Thrombospondin (+); TNF-α (indirect +)	PDGF (++); EGF (+); TGF-β (indirect +/−); Thrombospondin (+); IGF-1 (+)	PDGF (++); IGF-1 (+); IL-1 (indirect +); TGF-β (indirect +/−); Heparan sulfate (−); bFGF (+); Thrombospondin (+)	IFN-γ (−); TGF-β (indirect +/−); TNF-α (indirect +); IL-1 (indirect +)
Monocyte/macrophage survival and proliferation	GM-CSF; M-CSF	GM-CSF; M-CSF		GM-CSF; M-CSF	GM-CSF

Function					
Smooth muscle chemoattractants	PDGF TGF-β bFGF	PDGF TGF-β 12-HETE bFGF	PDGF TGF-β Platelet-factor 4 β-thromboglobulin	PDGF TGF-β	TGF-β
Leukocyte chemoattractants	GM-CSF TGF-β Oxidatively modified LDL MCP-1	GM-CSF TGF-β C5a Leukotriene-B4 TNF-α IL-1 MCP-1	GM-CSF TGF-β Platelet-factor 4	GM-CSF MCP-1 TGF-β TNF-α Leukotriene-B4 Oxidatively modified LDL	GM-CSF IFN-γ (T cells) TGF-β TNF-α
Immune modulation	IFN-γ induces MHC class II expression Antigen presentation IL-1 enhances T-cell response	MHC class II expression Antigen presentation Cytolysis IL-1 enhances T-cell response	TGF-β inactivates macrophages	IFN-γ induces MHC class II expression Antigen presentation IL-1 enhances T-cell response	Cell-mediated immunity Antigen recognition Cytolysis IL-2, IL-2 receptor expression amplify response to antigen
Matrix formation	Macromolecules that form the basal lamina, including collagens, fibronectin, laminin, and proteoglycans			Responsible for the bulk of arterial connective tissue including collagen, elastic tissue, and proteoglycans	
Formation of vasoactive agents	Major source of PGI$_2$ (vasodilator) Endothelial-derived relaxing factor Endothelins (vasoconstrictors) Platelet-activating factor	Platelet-activating factor	Vasoconstrictor, thromboxane A$_2$ β-thromboglobulin inhibits PGI$_2$ production Platelet-activating factor	Vasoconstrictive amines PGI$_2$ (vasodilator) Platelet-activating factor	
Induction of angiogenesis	bFGF TGF-β TNF-α	bFGF TGF-β TGF-α TNF-α VEGF	TGF-β PDEGF	TGF-β TNF-α VEGF	TGF-β TNF-α

focused a great deal of attention on the macrophage as a possible mediator of lesion progression, an alternative role for the macrophage could be a protective one, and a failure of that protective role could be in part responsible for lesion progression. In most inflammatory situations, the macrophage contributes to the resolution by scavenging debris from the interstitial tissue and then migrating from the site of injury, thereby removing tissue debris. Is lesion progression due in part to a loss of effectiveness by the local macrophages to clear the area of excess lipid and altered lipids? Evaluation of the issues of macrophage activation and maturation at the molecular level is critical to our understanding of their potential role in developing lesions.

Platelets are a rich source of growth factors and chemoattractants (Tables 1 and 2) and thus are excellent candidates for the initiation of lesion formation. Platelet adhesion to subendothelial connective tissue and release of platelet products, including multiple growth factors, may be particularly important in denuding injury to the endothelium, such as that seen in homocystinemia (12), after bypass surgery or angioplasty. Inhibition of platelet function (5,6,12,13,21) or an inhibitor of thrombin (11) has prevented lesion formation in models of denuding injury. The importance of platelet adherence and release in lesion progression in nondenuding injury and at sites of altered endothelium (as seen in experimental models of atherosclerosis, described above) is less clear and remains to be determined.

Smooth muscle proliferation and connective tissue deposition are important in lesion progression and in the manifestation of clinical sequelae. SMC are capable of synthesizing a number of both positive and negative regulators of their own growth (Tables 1 and 2). They can also accumulate lipid or become foam cells. Furthermore, if autoimmunity is important in some forms of atherosclerosis, they can actively participate in the immune response (15,25). Because of the critical role of smooth muscle proliferation in lesion progression, it is particularly important to understand whether autocrine expression of growth factors is involved in lesion formation and whether inhibitors of smooth muscle growth are altered. In addition, it is necessary to determine what regulates expression of the receptors for these growth-regulatory factors.

The presence of T cells in developing lesions of atherosclerosis has recently been appreciated with the use of cell-specific monoclonal antibodies (2,10,16,23,38). Along with macrophages, T cells are a source of multiple leukocyte chemoattractants and, in particular, represent an effector of cell-mediated immunity (Table 2). What role, if any, do these cells play in lesion development and progression? Are they directed against specific antigens within the artery wall? These are issues that clearly need to be evaluated. Studies in experimental models of atherosclerosis and the use of monoclonal antibodies have facilitated definition of the cells involved in lesion development. *In vitro* studies of these cells have delineated their possible multiple capabilities in the initiation and progression of lesions of atherosclerosis. Further understanding of their relative contributions *in vivo* and of their interactive roles with neighboring cells are critical to the future design of antagonists, prevention, and therapy.

ACKNOWLEDGMENT

This research was supported in part by grants from the National Heart, Lung, and Blood Institute of the National Institutes of Health, grants HL-18645 and HL-03174 to R.R. and E.W.R., and NIH grant RR-00166 to the Northwest Regional Primate Center.

REFERENCES

1. Chobanian, A., Forney-Prescott, M., and Haudenschild, C. (1984): *Exp. Mol. Pathol.*, 41:153–169.
2. Emeson, E. E., and Robertson, A. A. (1988): *Am. J. Pathol.*, 130:369–376.
3. Faggiotto, A., and Ross, R. (1984): *Arteriosclerosis*, 4:341–356.
4. Faggiotto, A., Ross, R., and Harker, L. (1984): *Arteriosclerosis*, 4:323–340.
5. Fingerle, J., Johnson, R., Clowes, A. W., Majesky, M. W., and Reidy, M. A. (1989): *Proc. Natl. Acad. Sci. USA*, 86:8412–8416.
6. Friedman, R. J., Stemerman, M. B., Wenz, B., et al. (1977): *J. Clin. Invest.*, 60:1191–1201.
7. Gerrity, R. G. (1981a): *Am. J. Pathol.*, 103:181–190.
8. Gerrity, R. G. (1981b): *Am. J. Pathol.*, 103:191–200.
9. Gimbrone, M. A. (1980): In: Gotto, A. M. Jr., Smith, L. C., and Allen, B., eds. *Atherosclerosis V*. New York: Springer-Verlag, pp. 415–425.
10. Gown, A. M., Tsukada, T., and Ross, R. (1986): *Am. J. Pathol.*, 125:191–207.
11. Hanson, S. R., and Harker, L. A. (1988): *Proc. Natl. Acad. Sci. USA*, 85:3184–3188.
12. Harker, L. A., Harlan, J. M., and Ross, R. (1983): *Circ. Res.*, 53:731–739.
13. Harker, L. A., Ross, R., Slichter, S. J., and Scott, C. R. (1976): *J. Clin. Invest.*, 58:731–741.
14. Jaffe, E. (1987): *Hum. Pathol.*, 18:234–239.
15. Jonasson, L., Holm, J., and Hansson, G. K. (1988): *Lab. Invest.*, 58:310–315.
16. Jonasson, L., Holm, J., Skalli, O., Bondjers, G., and Hansson, G. K. (1986): *Arteriosclerosis*, 6: 131–138.
17. Kowala, M. C., Cuenoud, H. F., Joris, I., and Majno, G. (1986): *Exp. Mol. Pathol.*, 45:323–335.
18. McGill, H. C., Jr. (1984): *Arteriosclerosis*, 4:443–451.
19. Masuda, J., and Ross, R. (1990a): *Arteriosclerosis*, 10:164–177.
20. Masuda, J., and Ross, R. (1990b): *Arteriosclerosis*, 10:178–187.
21. Moore, S., Friedman, R. J., Singal, D. P., Gauldie, M. A., Blajchman, M. A., and Roberts, R. S. (1976): *Thromb. Haemost.*, 35:70–81.
22. Munro, J. M., and Cotran, R. S. (1988): *Lab. Invest.*, 58:249–261.
23. Munro, J. M., van der Walt, J. D., Munro, C. S., Chalmers, J. A., and Cox, E. L. (1987): *Hum. Pathol.*, 18:375–380.
24. Pober, J. S. (1988): *Am. J. Pathol.*, 133:426–433.
25. Pober, J., Collins, T., Gimbrone, M. A. Jr., Libby, P., and Reiss, C. S. (1986): *Transplantation*, 41:141–146.
26. Raines, E. W., Bowen-Pope, D. F., and Ross, R. (1990): In: Sporn, M. B., and Roberts, A. B., eds. *Handbook of experimental pharmacology: peptide growth factors and their receptors*, Vol. 95I. New York: Springer-Verlag, pp. 173–262.
27. Reidy, M. A., and Schwartz, S. M. (1984): *Exp. Mol. Pathol.*, 41:419–434.
28. Rosenfeld, M. E., and Ross, R. (1990): *Arteriosclerosis*, 10:680–687.
29. Ross, R. (1986): *N. Engl. J. Med.*, 314:488–500.
30. Ross, R., and Glomset, J. A. (1973): *Science*, 180:1332–1339.
31. Ross, R., Masuda, J., Raines, E. W., et al. (1990): *Science*, 248:1009–1012.
32. Ross, R., Raines, E. W., and Bowen-Pope, D. F. (1986): *Cell*, 46:155–169.
33. Rubin, K., Hansson, G. K., Ronnstrand, L., et al. (1988): *Lancet*, 1:1353–1356.
34. Schwenke, D. C., and Carew, T. C. (1989): *Arteriosclerosis*, 9:908–918.
35. Sporn, M. B., and Roberts, A. B. (1990): *Handbook of experimental pharmacology: peptide growth factors and their receptors*, Vol. 95I. New York: Springer-Verlag, pp. 3–15.

36. Sporn, M. B., and Roberts A. B. (1990): *Handbook of experimental pharmacology: peptide growth factors and their receptors,* Vol. 95I and 95II. New York: Springer-Verlag.
37. Springer, T. A. (1990): *Nature,* 346:425–434.
38. van der Wal, A. C., Das, P. K., van de Berg, D. B., van der Loos, C. M., and Becker, A. E. (1989): *Lab. Invest.,* 61:166–170.
39. Vane, J. R., Anggard, E. E., and Botting, R. M. (1990): *N. Engl. J. Med.,* 323:27–36.
40. Wallis, W. J., and Harlan, J. M. (1986): *Pathol. Immunopathol. Res.,* 5:73–103.

Atherosclerosis Reviews, Volume 23,
edited by P. C. Weber and A. Leaf.
Raven Press, Ltd., New York © 1991.

Interactions of Human Aortic Wall Cells in Co-Culture

Mahamad Navab, Lori A. Ross, Susan Hama, Feng Liao,
Gregory P. Hough, *Davis C. Drinkwater, *Hillel Laks,
and Alan M. Fogelman

*Division of Cardiology, Department of Medicine and *Division of Cardiothoracic
Surgery, Department of Surgery, School of Medicine, University of California,
Los Angeles, California 90024-1679*17

Under physiological conditions, there are a limited number of smooth muscle cells (SMC) and monocytes in the subendothelial space (SES) of large arteries, but in the course of atherogenesis, there is a marked migration of monocytes and SMC into the SES (38,46). The presence of monocytes, endothelial cells (EC), and SMC in such a confined space can be expected to lead to extensive cellular interactions. Accumulating evidence indicates that substantial direct physical contact and interaction occur between EC and SMC *in vitro* (1,7,16,18,29,39) and *in vivo* (3,7,17,43,48). The coculture of EC and SMC has been reported to result in the alteration of the amount and the composition of the extracellular matrix (ECM) (29). The interaction of EC and SMC in culture has been shown to produce increased lysosomal cholesteryl ester activity (16), reduced rate of SMC proliferation (15), and increased low-density lipoprotein (LDL) receptor activity (8). More recently, EC and perycytes (1) or EC and SMC (39) in mixed cultures were reported to produce active transforming growth factor beta (TGF-β). We have used an *in vitro* model of the artery wall to study the interaction of human aortic EC (HAEC), human aortic SMC (HASMC) and monocytes in co-culture. Our findings show that the interaction of HAEC, HASMC, and monocytes results in marked increases in the levels of several biologically important molecules.

GROWTH FACTORS

Co-cultures of HAEC and HASMC produced markedly higher levels of macrophage colony stimulating factor (M-CSF), granulocyte macrophage-CSF (GM-CSF), and TGF-β compared to those from the HAEC and HASMC cultured separately. M-CSF can support the growth and survival of monocytes/macrophages *in vitro* even in the absence of serum growth factors (31). High levels of M-CSF mRNA are present in the atherosclerotic lesions of both Watanabe Heritable Hyperlipidemic and cholesterol-fed rabbits (37). Presumably, many of the monocytes/macrophages observed in the SES in autopsy specimens of human coronary arteries would have died unless their survival had been supported by growth factors (46). M-CSF produced by the interaction of EC and SMC could potentially act as one such factor. GM-CSF could be another factor. GM-CSF has been shown to prolong the survival, differentiation, proliferation, and development of responsive cells *in vitro* and *in vivo* (19,31). In our studies, the co-cultures of HAEC and HASMC, which were in the form of a confluent EC monolayer on top of a confluent layer of SMC with ECM components in between them (35), also produced markedly higher levels of latent TGF-β. However, when EC and SMC co-cultures were grown not as multilayers but as mixed cultures, significant quantities of active TGF-β were produced (36).

The almost universal ability of cells to respond to TGF-β and the diversity of the effects of this multifunctional growth factor makes this peptide unique in terms of its role in regulating both normal and pathologic physiology (45). TGF-β has been shown to (a) activate gene transcription and increase synthesis and secretion of matrix proteins, (b) decrease synthesis of proteolytic enzymes that degrade matrix proteins while increasing the synthesis of protease inhibitors that block the activity of these enzymes and, (c) increase the transcription, translation, and processing of cellular receptors for matrix proteins (44). In addition, TGF-β is a potent regulator of myogenesis in *in vitro* models (44,45) and has been implicated in the maintenance and repair of cardiac myocytes (49). Since, however, all the cultured cells examined secreted TGF-β in a latent (inactive) form, the relevance of this factor as a growth modulator appears to lie in its activation. The *in vivo* mechanisms of this activation, however, are not fully understood. Possible mechanisms include perturbation of the carbohydrate structure of latent TGF-β (32,33) or proteolysis (25,40).

Sato and colleagues (40) reported that the activation of TGF-β appears to require cell-to-cell contact or very close apposition of the two different cell types. The activation reaction also required a plasmin-like enzyme; their work showed that inclusion of plasmin inhibitors in the heterotypic culture medium blocked the activation of TGF-β. In accordance with our findings, there was no significant increase in TGF-β mRNA levels in heterotypic cultures (36). Approximately 1% to 10% of the latent TGF-β was converted to active form in co-cultures (40). The active TGF-β induced the synthesis of plasminogen activator inhibitor 1 (PAI-1). PAI-1 blocks the subsequent conversion of plasminogen to plasmin, thereby suppressing further activation of latent TGF-β (40).

However, McCaffery and colleagues (26) have identified an interaction between heparin and TGF-β in which heparin potentiates the biological actions of TGF-β. Heparin appeared to free TGF-β from its complex with α_2-macroglobulin. Thus, heparin-like agents such as heparan sulfate proteoglycans may be important regulators of TGF-β biological activity. Danielpour and Sporn (6) postulated that α_2-macroglobulin may be involved in the regulation of activation of latent TGF-β. This binding protein is secreted by a variety of cell types. Most cell types studied express the receptor for this protein; through its presence in extracellular matrix it may act as an important regulator of the activity of TGF-β (6). In our studies, the addition to co-cultures of neutralizing antibody to TGF-β clearly altered the levels of ECM components. Therefore, it appears that TGF-β was activated in a microenvironment in the matrix produced by the interaction of the aortic wall cells.

MATRIX COMPONENTS

Co-cultures of EC and SMC were reported by Merrilees and Scott (29) to result in increased production of hyaluronic acid and glycosaminoglycans as compared with the separate cultures of the two cell types. The changes in ECM components were later demonstrated by the authors to be due to the presence of active TGF-β in the co-cultures (30). In our laboratory, the cocultures of the human aortic cells produced type I collagen levels that were significantly higher than those from separate cultures. Addition of neutralizing antibody to TGF-β significantly reduced the collagen levels in the co-culture medium and cell layers (36). The presence of a membrane filter between the HAEC and HASMC, which permitted access of the media but prevented direct EC-SMC contact, markedly reduced the collagen levels.

There was also a marked increase in the levels of another ECM component—fibronectin in the co-culture medium and cell layers (36). Addition of neutralizing TGF-β antibody to the co-cultures resulted in a significant decrease in the fibronectin levels. When HAEC and HASMC were separated by a filter in the same chamber and medium, permitting access of media but preventing EC-SMC contact, there was a marked decrease in fibronectin levels in the media and in the cell layers.

The results of these experiments indicated that the direct interaction of aortic wall cells can produce elevated levels of matrix components and that TGF-β is involved in this interaction. Because increased monocyte adhesion to the endothelium and transmigration to the SES is one of the early events in atherogenesis, we subsequently studied the effect of the interaction of human peripheral blood monocytes with the aortic wall cells. Addition of monocytes to the cocultures produced a dramatic increase (up to 22-fold) in the fibronectin levels in the culture media (36). The increase in collagen produced by the interaction of monocytes/macrophages and the cells of the artery wall was less pronounced (36). Both collagen and fibronectin have been implicated in atherogenesis (28). Increases in collagen have been shown in several experimental models of atherosclerosis (27). Additionally, atherosclerotic lesions of human intima are known to have an increased collagen content (23), and collagen type I was reported to be the prominent form in the diseased vessels (42). Substantial levels of fibronectin were observed in the ECM of fatty streaks and in some areas of fibrous plaque containing large numbers of subendothelial cells in human arteries (41). Moreover, increased fibronectin levels were seen in rabbit aorta 4 weeks after cholesterol feeding (50).

GAP JUNCTION PROTEIN

Both EC and SMC have been shown to express message for connexin43, a member of the family of related gap junction proteins (21,22). These junctions are membrane structures involved in intercellular communication. They have been implicated in buffering of cytoplasmic ions (4,22), synchronization of cellular behavior such as contraction of myocardial cells (2), growth control and differentiation (24), and suppression of deleterious effects of somatic cell mutations in a variety of enzymes (47). The induction of connexin43 as a result of the interaction of EC, SMC, and monocytes in co-culture has not been previously reported. In our studies, the interaction of HAEC and HASMC resulted in levels of mRNA for the gap junction protein connexin43 that were significantly higher than those from the components. There was no detectable signal for mRNA for connexin32. Interaction of human monocytes with HAEC produced markedly higher levels of connexin43 transcripts (36). Addition of monocytes to the co-cultures resulted in further increases in the induction of message for connexin43. Eghbali and colleagues (10) have demonstrated that stable transfection of gap junction–incompetent cells resulted in the expression of message for connexin paralleled by a dramatic increase in the gap junction formation and intercellular cytoplasmic transfer.

Lash and co-workers (22) have shown that microinjection of SMC connexin43 mRNA was sufficient to induce intercellular coupling in previously uncoupled blastomers (22). Dahl and colleagues (5) observed a concentration-dependent induction of cell-to-cell channels in response to an *in vitro* transcribed gap junction messenger RNA. The significant increase in connexin43 mRNA demonstrated in co-cultures of human aortic wall cells is, therefore, highly likely to be followed by heterotypic gap junction assembly and intercellular cytoplasmic transfer contributing to further cellular interactions.

INTERLEUKINS 1 AND 6

On activation, monocytes demonstrate markedly increased activities for numerous factors, including interleukin 1 (IL-1) (9). We have observed that during the process of monocyte transmigration into the subendothelial space of the co-cultures, the cells acquire the typical appearance of spread monocytes, suggesting the activation of these cells. Injection of IL-1 into rats has been reported to produce elevated serum levels of fibronectin (13). Leukocyte interleukins have also been reported to induce cultured EC to produce a highly organized pericellular matrix (34). IL-1 induces IL-6 in certain cell types (11). Monocytes stimulated by IL-1 were shown to produce increased levels of IL-6; that in turn resulted in elevated levels of fibronectin in cultured hepatocytes (14).

Lancer and Brown (20) recently showed that IL-6 is responsible for the increased fibronectin production by rat hepatocytes exposed to conditioned medium from stimulated monocytes. In studies employing the co-culture of human aortic cells, addition of neutralizing antibody to IL-1 or neutralizing antibody to IL-6 during the interaction of monocytes with the co-cultures resulted in marked reductions in the levels of fibronectin in the culture media (36). Presence of antibody to IL-1 together with antibody to IL-6 did not increase the blocking effect of anti–IL-6 antibody alone. Neutralizing antibodies to M-CSF and GM-CSF did not produce any significant changes in the increased levels of fibronectin. Therefore, it is likely that the exposure of monocytes to the co-cultures resulted in the activation of monocytes producing IL-1, which presumably induced IL-6 in the EC, which in turn resulted in increased levels of fibronectin.

CONCLUSION

The interaction between human aortic wall cells in co-culture produced a significant increase in the levels of M-CSF, GM-CSF, and TGF-β. The co-culture of HAEC and HASMC clearly led to an increase in the production of both fibronectin and collagen that depended on close physical approximation of the two cell types. This increase appeared to be mediated by TGF-β. The increased induction of the gap junction protein connexin43 in co-cultures of EC and SMC indicates the possibility of increased junctional communication and interaction between the EC and SMC in these co-cultures. Addition of human monocytes to the co-cultures amplified the production of the extracellular matrix molecules. This was paralleled by a marked induction of connexin43, raising the possibility of increased direct heterotypic cellular communications. The significant inhibition of monocyte-induced increase in fibronectin levels in co-cultures of artery wall cells by neutralizing antibodies to IL-1 and to IL-6 strongly suggests that these cytokines are involved in the monocyte–artery wall cell interactions. These findings, therefore, indicate that the migration of SMC and monocytes into the SES of the early atherosclerotic lesion may lead to cell-cell interactions that result in the production of several biologically important molecules that may amplify lesion development.

ACKNOWLEDGMENT

We thank Drs. Denise C. Polacek, Peter F. Davies, and David L. Paul for providing us with cDNA probes for connexins; Drs. Matt Ashby and Judith Berliner for valuable discussions; Dr. Phillip Koeffler for assistance obtaining human bone marrow cells; Farah Elahi for her excellent technical assistance; and the members of the UCLA Heart Transplant Team for collecting the aortic specimens.

This work was supported in part by U.S. Public Health Services grants HL 30568, IT 32 HL 07412, and RR 865; by the Laubisch Fund; and by the M. K. Grey Fund.

REFERENCES

1. Antonelli-Orlidge, A., Sunders, K. B., Smith, S. R., and D'Amore, P. A. (1989): An activated form of transforming growth factor beta is produced by cocultures of endothelial cells and pericytes. *Proc. Natl. Acad. Sci. USA,* 86:4544–4548.
2. Barr, L., Dewey, M. M., and Berger, W. (1965): Propagation of action potential and the structure of the nexus in cardiac muscle. *J. Gen. Physiol.,* 48:797–823.
3. Bruns, R. R., and Palade, G. E. (1968): Studies on blood capillaries. I. General organization of blood capillaries in muscle. *J. Cell Biol.,* 37:244–276.
4. Corsaro, C. M., and Migeon, B. R. (1977): Contact mediated communication of oubain resistance in mammalian cells in culture. *Nature (Lond.),* 268:737–739.
5. Dahl, G., Miller, T., Paul, D., Voellmy, R., and Werner, R. (1987): Expression of functional cell-cell channels from cloned rat liver gap junction complementary DNA. *Science,* 236:1290–1293.
6. Danielpour, D., and Sporn, M. B. (1990): Differential inhibition of transforming growth factor-$\beta 1$ and $\beta 2$ activity by alpha2-macroglobulin. *J. Biol. Chem.,* 265:6973–6977.
7. Davies, P. F., Olesen, S. P., Clapham, D. E., Morrel, C. M., and Shoen, D. J. (1988): Endothelial communication. State of the art lecture. *Hypertension,* 11:583–582.
8. Davies, P. F., Truskey, G. A., Warren, H. B., O'Connor, S. E., and Eisenhaure, B. H. (1985): Metabolic cooperation between vascular endothelial cells and smooth muscle cells in co-culture: Changes in low density lipoprotein metabolism. *J. Cell Biol.,* 101:871–879.
9. Dayer, J. M., de Rochemonteix, B., Burrus, B., Demczuk, S., and Dinarello, C. A. (1986): Human recombinant interleukin 1 stimulates collagenase and prostaglandin E2 production by human synovial cells. *J. Clin. Invest.,* 77:645–648.
10. Eghbali, B., Kessler, J. A., Spray, D. C. (1990): Expression of gap junction channels in communication-incompetent cells after stable transfection with cDNA encoding connexin 32. *Proc. Natl. Acad. Sci. USA,* 87:1328–1331.
11. Elias, J. A., and Lentz, V. (1990): IL-1 and tumor necrosis factor synergistically stimulate fibroblast IL-6 production and stabilize IL-6 messenger RNA. *J. Immunol.,* 145:161–166.
12. Fogelman, A. M., Elahi, F., Sykes, K., Van Lenten, B. J., Territo, M. C., and Berliner, J. A. (1988): Modification of the Recalde method for the isolation of human monocytes. *J. Lipid Res.,* 29:1243–1247.
13. Hagiwara, T., Kono, I., Nemoto, K., Kashiwagi, H., and Onozaki, K. (1989): Recombinant interleukin-1 triggers the increase of circulating fibronectin levels in rats. *Int. Arch. Allergy Appl. Immunol.,* 89:376–380.
14. Hagiwara, T., Suzuki, H., Kono, I., Kashiwagi, H., Akiyama, Y., and Onozaki, K. (1990): Regulation of fibronectin synthesis by interleukin-1 and interleukin-6 in rat hepatocytes. *Am. J. Pathol.,* 136:39–47.
15. Hajjar, D. P., Falcone, D. J., Amberson, J. B., and Heffon, J. M. (1985): Interaction of arterial cells. I. Endothelial cells alter cholesterol metabolism in co-cultured smooth muscle cells. *J. Lipid Res.,* 26:1212–1223.
16. Hajjar, D. P., Marcus, A. J., and Hajjar, K. A. (1987): Interactions of arterial cells. Studies on the mechanisms of endothelial cell modulation of cholesterol metabolism in co-cultured smooth muscle cells. *J. Biol. Chem.,* 262:6976–6981.
17. Huttner, I., Boutet, M., More, R. H. (1973): Gap junctions in arterial endothelium. *J. Cell Biol.,* 57:247–252.
18. Jones, P. (1979): Construction of an artificial blood vessel wall from cultured endothelial and smooth muscle cells. *Proc. Natl. Acad. Sci. USA,* 76:1882–1886.
19. Lang, R. A., Metcalf, D., Cuthbertson, R. A., et al. (1987): Transgenic mice expressing a hematopoietic growth factor gene (GM-CSF) develop accumulation of macrophages, blindness, and a fatal syndrome of tissue damage. *Cell,* 51:875–886.
20. Lanser, M. E., and Brown, G. E. (1989): Stimulation of rat hepatocyte fibronectin production by monocyte condition medium is due to interleukin 6. *J. Exp. Med.,* 170:1781–1786.
21. Larson, M., Haudenschild, C. C., and Beyer, E. C. (1990): Gap junction messenger RNA expression by vascular wall cells. *Circ. Res.,* 66:1074–1080.
22. Lash, J. A., Critser, E. S., and Pressler, M. L. (1990): Cloning of a gap junctional protein from

vascular smooth muscle and expression in two cell mouse embryos. *J. Biol. Chem.,* 265:13113–13117.

23. Levene, C. I., Poole, J. C. F. (1962): The collagen content of the normal and atherosclerotic human aortic intima. *Br. J. Exp. Pathol.,* 43:469–471.

24. Loewenstein, W. R. (1966): Permeability of membrane junctions. *Ann. NY Acad. Sci.,* 137:441–472.

25. Lyons, R., Gentry, L. E., Purchio, A. F., and Moses, H. L. (1990): Mechanism of activation of latent recombinant transforming growth factor β1 by plasmin. *J. Cell Biol.,* 110:1361–1367.

26. McCaffery, T. A., Falcone, D. J., Brayton, C. F., Agarwal, L. A., Welt, F. G. P., and Weksler, B. B. (1989): Transforming growth factor-β activity is potentiated by heparin via dissociation of the transforming growth factor-β/alpha2-macroglobulin inactive complex. *J. Cell Biol.,* 109:441–448.

27. Mayne, R. (1986): Collagenous proteins of blood vessels. *Arteriosclerosis,* 6:585–593.

28. Mecham, R. P., Whitehouse, L. A., Wrenn, D. S., et al. (1987): Smooth-muscle mediated connective tissue remodeling in pulmonary hypertension. *Science,* 237:423–426.

29. Merrilees, M. J., and Scott, L. (1981): Interaction of aortic endothelial and smooth muscle cells in culture. Effect on glycosaminoglycan levels. *Atherosclerosis,* 39:147–161.

30. Merrilees, M. J., and Scott, L. (1990): Endothelial cell stimulation of smooth muscle glycosaminoglycan synthesis can be accounted for by transforming growth factor beta activity. *Atherosclerosis,* 81:255–265.

31. Metcalf, D. (1989): The molecular control of cell division, differentiation commitment and maturation in haemopoietic cells. *Nature (Lond.),* 339:27–30.

32. Miyazono, K., and Heldin, C.-H. (1989): Role for carbohydrate structure in TGF-β1 latency. *Nature,* 338:158–160.

33. Miyazono, K., Hellman, U., Wernstedt, C., and Heldin, C.-H. (1988): Latent high molecular weight complex of transforming growth factor β1. *J. Biol. Chem.,* 263:6407–6415.

34. Montesano, R., Mossaz, A., Ryser, J.-E., Orci, L., and Vassalli, P. (1984): Leukocyte interleukins induce cultured endothelial cells to produce a highly organized glycosaminoglycan rich pericellular matrix. *J. Cell Biol.,* 99:1706–1715.

35. Navab, M., Hough, G. P., Stevenson, L. W., Drinkwater, D. C., Laks, H., and Fogelman, A. M. (1988): Monocyte migration into the subendothelial space of a coculture of adult human aortic endothelial and smooth muscle cells. *J. Clin. Invest.,* 82:1853–1863.

36. Navab, M., Liao, F., Hough, G. P., et al. (1991): Interaction of monocytes with coculture of human aortic wall cells involves interleukins 1 and 6 with marked increases in connexin43 message. *J. Clin. Invest.,* 87:1763–1772.

37. Rajavashisth, T. B., Andalibi, A., Territo, M. C., Berliner, J. A., Navab, M., Fogelman, A. M., and Lusis, A. J. (1990): Modified low density lipoproteins induce endothelial cell expression of granulocyte and macrophage colony stimulating factors. *Nature (Lond.),* 344:254–257.

38. Ross, R. (1986): The pathogenesis of atherosclerosis. An update. *N. Engl. J. Med.,* 314:488–500.

39. Sato, Y., and Rifkin, D. B. (1989): Inhibition of endothelial cell movement by pericytes and smooth muscle cells: activation of a latent transforming growth factor beta 1–like molecule by plasmin during coculture. *J. Cell. Biol.,* 109:309–315.

40. Sato, Y., Tsuboi, R., Lyons, R., Moses, H., and Rifkin, D. B. (1990): Characterization of the activation of latent TGF-β by cocultures of endothelial cells and pericytes or smooth muscle cells: a self-regulating system. *J. Cell Biol.,* 111:757–763.

41. Shekhonin, B. V., Domogatsky, S. P., Idelson, G. L., Koteliansky, V. E., and Rukosuev, V. S. (1987): Relative distribution of fibronectin and type I, III, IV, V collagens in normal and atherosclerotic intima of human arteries. *Atherosclerosis,* 67:9–16.

42. Smith, E. B. (1965): The influence of age and atherosclerosis on the chemistry of aortic intima. *J. Atheroscler. Res.,* 5:241–248.

43. Spagnoli, L. G., Villaschi, S., Neri, L., and Palmieri, G. (1982): Gap junctions in myo-endothelial bridges of rabbit carotid arteries. *Experientia,* 38:124–125.

44. Czech, M. P., Clairmont, K. B., Yagaloff, and Corvera, S. (1990): Properties and regulation of receptors for growth factors. In: Sporn, M. B., and Roberts, A. B., eds. *Handbook of experimental pharmacology; Peptide growth factors and their receptors.* Heidelberg: Springer-Verlag, pp. 37–65.

45. Sporn, M. B., and Roberts, A. B. (1988): Peptide growth factors are multifunctional. *Nature (Lond.),* 332:217–219.
46. Stary, H. (1989): Evolution and progression of atherosclerotic lesions in coronary arteries of children and young adults. *Arteriosclerosis,* 9(suppl.):I 19–32.
47. Subak-Share, H., Burk, R. R., and Pitts, J. D. (1969): Metabolic cooperation between biochemically marked mammalian cells in tissue culture. *J. Cell Science,* 4:353–367.
48. Thoma, R. (1921): Uber Die Intima der Arterien. *Virchows Arch.* [A], 230:1–45.
49. Thompson, N. L., Bazoberry, F., Speir, E. H., et al. (1988): Transforming growth factor beta-1 in myocardial infarction in rats. *Growth Factors,* 1:91–99.
50. Uematsu, M., Tanouchi, J., Ishihara, K., et al. (1989): Hypercholesterolemia without mechanical interventions induces early accumulation of fibronectin during fatty streak formation [Abstract]. *Arteriosclerosis,* 9:769a.

Atherosclerosis Reviews, Volume 23,
edited by P. C. Weber and A. Leaf.
Raven Press, Ltd., New York © 1991.

Interleukin-1 and Cytokine Antagonism

Charles A. Dinarello

Department of Medicine, Tufts University School of Medicine and New England Medical Center, Boston, Massachusetts 02111

Interleukin-1 (IL-1) is a polypeptide produced as a result of infection, toxic injury, trauma, or antigenic challenge (16). Although the macrophage/monocyte is a primary source of IL-1, B lymphocytes, endothelial, epithelial, mesangial, and smooth muscle cells (SMC), and fibroblasts also synthesize IL-1. Two distinct IL-1 cDNAs were cloned in 1984. They represent two separate gene products; IL-1β (2) codes for a neutral polypeptide, whereas IL-1α (32) is an acidic protein. At the mRNA level, IL-1β is more abundant than IL-1α (15). Neither IL-1α nor IL-1β contains a signal peptide; therefore, a considerable amount of IL-1 remains cell-associated. As much as 90% of IL-1α produced by human monocytes stimulated with bacterial endotoxin is found intracellularly, whereas 70% of IL-1β synthesized by these same cells is secreted (20,33). The secreted form of IL-1 is a 17,000-kDa polypeptide cleaved from 31-kDa precursor. It is unclear how the precursor of IL-1 is cleaved or secreted, but specific proteases (serine) appear to be involved. Biologically active "cell surface membrane" IL-1α has been described by a number of investigators (5,8,28). Fibroblast growth factors (α and β) are other examples of proteins without signal peptides. Fibroblast growth factor α shares 31% amino acid homology with IL-1β.

BIOLOGICAL PROPERTIES OF IL-1

IL-1 has both beneficial as well as detrimental activities. In recent clinical trials in patients, low doses of IL-1 stimulated bone marrow stem cells leading to increased neutrophil and platelet production, but high doses caused hyperpyrexia, general malaise, gastrointestinal disturbances, and hypotension. Other biological properties of IL-1 are clearly beneficial. There is justification for the use of IL-1 in the treatment of certain diseases, such as depressed bone marrow, protection from radiation, and increases in nonspecific resistance to infection. However, in this paper, only anti–IL-1 strategies will be discussed.

IL-1 AS A PROTOTYPE INFLAMMATORY CYTOKINE

IL-1 is a potent inflammatory molecule. IL-1 and tumor necrosis factor (TNF) share many biological properties (16); they are highly synergistic in both animal and *in vitro* experiments. IL-1 induces fever; in fact, IL-1 was likely the first endogenous pyrogen described and purified (17). In addition to triggering events in the central nervous system leading to fever, IL-1 also causes the release of a variety of neuropeptides, most importantly ACTH, corticotropin releasing factor, and somatostatin. IL-1 is an appetite suppressant (23). IL-1 also induces sleep via rapid increases in slow wave sleep, even before the onset of fever (50). The somogenic property of IL-1 is not, like fever or appetite suppression, blocked by inhibition of cyclooxygenase.

Within minutes of exposing cells to IL-1, there is an increase in new mRNA coding for cyclooxygenase and phospholipase A_2. In isolated tissues perfused with IL-1, PGE_2 increases in the perfusate and continues to rise for several hours after cessation of the IL-1 perfusion. The increased synthesis of lipid metabolites, such as the prostaglandins, and also of platelet activating factor by IL-1 contribute to the shock syndrome (14). The induction of hypotension, neutropenia, thrombocytopenia, lactic acidosis, and decreased systemic vascular resistance follows an intravenous injection of IL-1 (36); however, this is dramatically potentiated by co-injection with TNF. IL-1 and combinations of IL-1 plus TNF enhance endothelial procoagulant activity, the expression of leukocyte adhesion molecules, and synthesis of a plasminogen activator inhibitor.

IL-1 induces smooth muscle, fibroblast, and mesangial cell proliferation and is thought to be one of the macrophage products that play a role in the proliferative lesion of atherosclerosis (29). Recent evidence suggests that IL-1 is a growth factor, because it induces the synthesis of platelet-derived growth factor (PDGF)

TABLE 1. *IL-1–induced gene expression or gene suppression*

Increased gene expression	Suppression of gene expression
IL-1, IL-2, IL-3, IL-4	Albumin
IL-5, IL-6, IL-7, IL-8	Cytochrome P450
TNFα, TNFβ, INFβ-1	Lipoprotein lipase
GM-CSF, G-CSF, M-CSF	Aromatase
IL-2R (Tac antigen)	Aldosterone
Metallothionein; ceruloplasmin	Thyroglobulin
Complement; C2; Factor B	Thyroid peroxidase
Manganese superoxide dismutase	Prepro-insulin
Cyclooxygenase, phospholipase A_2	
Platelet-derived growth factor (AA)	IL-1Rtl
Adhesion molecules	
Oncogenes (c-fos; c-myc; c-jun)	
G protein α-i-2 subunit	
Interferon regulatory factor	
Tissue and urinary plasminogen activator	
Plasminogen activator inhibitor	
Preproendothelin-1	
Corticotropin releasing factor and pro-opiomelanocortin	
Amyloid A and amyloid beta proteins	
Collagenases and stromelysin	

(7,37). Smooth muscle proliferation by IL-1 *in vitro* is observed when the suppressive effect of prostaglandins is blocked by cyclooxygenase inhibitors (31). There is also evidence that PDGF up-regulates the expression of the IL-1 receptor type I, adding to the autocrine loop of growth factor production (9). This has been shown in synovial cells where both IL-1 and PDGF affect the inflammation tissue remodeling processes (27).

The most consistent biological property of IL-1 is its ability to up-regulate cellular metabolism and increase the expression of several genes. IL-1 predominantly activates transcription of several genes but also stabilizes mRNA for others, such as GM-CSF. On the other hand, the expression of household genes are reduced by IL-1—for example, those for albumin, lipoprotein lipase, cytochrome P450, and aromatase. Table 1 lists the effects of IL-1 on gene expression and suppression.

EXPRESSION OF THE IL-1 GENE

The tissue macrophage and blood monocyte are the major sources of IL-1 in a variety of inflammatory diseases, such as the inflamed joint, meninges, lung, intestinal tract, and likely the arterial wall. One approach to anti-inflammatory therapies has been the use of agents that block the induction of the IL-1 gene. The transcriptional activation of IL-1 by agents such as endotoxin begins within 15 min, and mRNA for IL-1β reaches peak concentrations 3 hr to 4 hr later (22,42). Using IL-1 as a stimulant of its own gene expression, mRNA levels remain elevated in human blood monocytes for over 30 hr (43). It appears that microbial agents trigger the synthesis of a transcriptional repressor or alternatively activate enzymes that break down IL-1 mRNA. What is most interesting for chronic inflammatory diseases is that IL-1 gene expression seems to escape its usual rapid reduction in steady-state mRNA levels.

CORTICOSTEROIDS AS INHIBITORS OF IL-1 GENE EXPRESSION

When added just prior to stimulation, corticosteroids block the transcriptional activation of IL-1 by a variety of exogenous stimulants (25). Other agents, including some lipoxygenase inhibitors, also reduce IL-1 at the transcriptional level. Because IL-1 stimulates gene expression for other cytokines (IL-2–IL-9, including TNF), reduction of IL-1 synthesis may provide an important approach to anti-inflammatory or immunosuppressive therapy.

INTERFERONS AS SUPPRESSORS OF IL-1 GENE EXPRESSION

Using IL-1 itself as a stimulator of IL-1 synthesis, both IFNγ and IFNα *reduce* IL-1 production by suppressing its transcription (43). The decrease in transcription of IL-1 by interferons is not due to increased degradation of IL-1 mRNA.

IL-1 is a growth factor for SMC. There may be an IL-1 autocrine effect in which IL-1-induction of IL-1 contributes to the proliferation of SMC and fibroblasts. Because IL-1 induces the genes for PDGF in fibroblasts and SMC (7,37), the efficacy of IFNα in Kaposi's sarcoma or in patients with angiogenic pulmonary fibrosis may be due to IFNα suppression of IL-1–induced genes in these cases. In an experimental setting, IFNγ suppresses gene expression for PDGF and IL-1β in cultured endothelial cells (47).

PREVENTING THE SYNTHESIS OF IL-1

During cell activation by a variety of IL-1–inducing agents, arachidonic acid (AA) is liberated. Formation of leukotrienes (LT) appears to provide a positive signal for cytokine synthesis. LTB$_4$ has been shown to stimulate IL-1 gene expression and synthesis. In addition, agents that inhibit the lipoxygenase pathway can also inhibit cytokine synthesis. The lipoxygenase product 13-hydroxyocta-decadienoic acid (13-HODD) has been identified as a likely lipoxygenase metabolite for TNF synthesis (41). To evaluate the effect of reduced LT formation on cytokine synthesis, the *ex vivo* production of IL-1α, IL-1β, and TNF was measured before, after and during two washout phases in human volunteers taking eicosapentaenoic acid supplements. A 50% to 60% decrease in total cytokine synthesis in nine volunteers was reported (21). We have also observed similar decreases in *ex vivo* cytokine production in women after 2 and 3 months of taking 1.5 g/day of EPA supplements (34). The effect of EPA supplements has also been observed in clinical studies (26).

The suppressive effect of PGE$_2$ and PGI$_2$ on cytokine synthesis appears to be due to increased cAMP formation (24). The methylxanthine drug pentoxifylline, which like PGE$_2$ increases cAMP formation, also reduces TNF synthesis (46). We recently observed similar suppression of cytokine synthesis using theophylline, which blocks the cyclic nucleotide hydrolyzing enzyme, phosphodiesterase; the addition of histamine—also an inducer of cAMP via the H$_2$ receptor—similarly reduces cytokine synthesis (48). Thus, in addition to changes in lipoxygenase products, one can also reduce cytokine synthesis employing agents that increase cAMP levels in cells. It should be interesting to observe the effect of drugs such as pentoxifylline or the H$_2$ receptor blockers on *in vivo* and *ex vivo* cytokine production.

IL-1 RECEPTORS

There are at least two IL-1R, and each is a separate gene product (6,10). A p80 glycoprotein (termed "IL-1RtI"), a member of the immunoglobulin superfamily, is found on macrophages, T cells, fibroblasts, endothelial cells, keratinocytes, and hepatocytes, whereas a p68 IL-1R (termed "IL-1RtII") is found on B cells and neutrophils. The p80 IL-1RtI contains an extracellular, a single transmembrane, and an intracellular portion; the intracellular portion has no intrinsic tyrosine kinase activity, although it resembles substrates for protein kinase C.

The IL-1RtII is a 68-kDa glycoprotein related structurally to the type I receptor in that it is also a member of the immunoglobulin superfamily. The extracellular portion of the type II receptor shares the same three Ig domains with the type I receptor and 28% amino acid homology. However, unlike the type I receptor, the type II receptor has a truncated cytosolic segment. In addition to the IL-1RtII on B cells, there is a 30-kDa binding protein observed on T cells, macrophages, and mesangial cells; but it is unclear whether this is a receptor or an associated protein (40). One hypothesis to explain the action of IL-1R is that, similar to other cytokine receptors, it is a heterocomplex of different polypeptide chains. However, a complete signal transduction event following exposure of cells to IL-1 leading to gene expression appears to be linked to the IL-1RtI in some cells; whereas in other cells apparently lacking the p80 IL-1R chain, IL-1 itself causes only phospholipid (phosphatidylcholine) hydrolysis (39) without evidence of new gene expression. In those cells, a second signal is required for full IL-1 activity.

THE IL-1 RECEPTOR ANTAGONIST

The IL-1 receptor antagonist (IL-1ra) molecule, originally called the IL-1 inhibitor, was isolated and purified from the urine of patients with myelomonocytic leukemia (44,45). A similar IL-1 inhibitory activity was found in the urine of patients with fever (30) and in the circulation of human subjects injected intravenously with endotoxin (18). In these reports, the biological characteristic of the IL-1 inhibitory activity was its ability to block IL-1 but not IL-2 or mitogen-induced T-cell proliferation. The "IL-1 inhibitor" purified from the urine had a molecular weight of 23 to 25 kDa. It blocked the binding of IL-1 to receptors on T cells but did not block the binding of TNF or IL-2 (4,44,45). Thus, the IL-1 inhibitor was a competitive inhibitor of IL-1/IL-1R interaction.

Using the IL-1 inhibitor purified from adherent monocytes (1), N-terminal sequence was obtained, and the molecule was cloned (19). The cDNA sequence codes for a polypeptide of approximately 17 kDa, whereas the 25 kDa molecular weight is due to glycosylation. The amino acid sequence deduced from the cDNA revealed 40% homology conserved amino acid to IL-1β and 39% to IL-1α. The recombinant IL-1 inhibitor competes with the binding of IL-1 to its cell surface receptors. Renamed the IL-1 receptor antagonist (IL-1ra), it blocks IL-1 activity *in vitro* and *in vivo*.

BIOLOGICAL EFFECTS OF IL-1ra

The IL-1ra blocks IL-1 effects in a variety of models, including IL-1–induced fever, corticosterone response, hypoglycemia, and neutrophilia. Rabbits given recombinant IL-1 develop hypotension, which can be reversed by prior administration of the IL-1ra (35). *E. coli* injected into rabbits produced several parameters of the septic shock syndrome—namely, hypotension, leukopenia, thrombocytopenia, and tissue damage. When rabbits were pretreated with the IL-1ra, only a transient hypotensive episode and a decrease in the leukopenia were observed (49). There were also reduced numbers of tissue infiltrating neutrophils. In these studies, the circulating levels of TNF and IL-1β (as determined by specific radioimmunoassay) were unchanged.

In a rabbit model of colitis, the degree of inflammation, edema, and necrosis in colonic tissue correlates with the tissue levels of IL-1 in these tissues (12). When rabbits were pretreated with the IL-1ra, a marked decrease in tissue inflammatory cell infiltration, edema, and necrosis was observed (12). In addition, decreased PGE_2 was measured in the rectal lumen, despite the fact that IL-1 tissue levels were unchanged (11). Together, these data demonstrate that blockade of IL-1 prevents the onset and development of the inflammatory lesion in this model of immune complex-induced colitis.

Several studies have reported that IL-1 induces colony stimulating factors from fibroblasts, endothelial cells, lymphocytes, and blood monocytes. Moreover, antibodies to human IL-1β completely reduced the spontaneous proliferation and colony stimulating activity of granulocytic and myelogenous leukemia cells (3,13). Therefore, it was hypothesized that growth factor production is under the control of IL-1 in these cells. Recent studies have shown that the IL-1ra blocks the spontaneous proliferation as well as spontaneous production of GM-CSF, IL-1, and IL-6 colony stimulating production in peripheral blood myelogenous leukemia cells *in vitro* (38). These studies suggest that IL-1 is controlling the production of GM-CSF in these cells and that treatment with IL-1ra would be highly effective in reducing the proliferation of these leukemia cells.

PRODUCTION OF IL-1 AND IL-1ra IN VARIOUS DISEASE STATES

It is clear that the IL-1ra is a copy of IL-1β and that it represents the third IL-1 form. It appears that expression of the IL-1ra gene is linked to the same types of stimuli that trigger gene expression for IL-1β and IL-1α. However, there may be distinct differences that can be exploited—i.e., preparations of IgG are potent stimulators of IL-1ra synthesis, but IgG is a poor stimulator of IL-1 production. This may account for some of the beneficial effects of intravenous IgG administration in some diseases. Moreover, it is possible that during some disease processes, more IL-1 and less IL-1ra are released. Alternatively, a situation where there was more IL-1ra and less IL-1 production would attenuate inflammation.

ACKNOWLEDGMENT

These studies were supported by NIH grant AI15614.

REFERENCES

1. Arend, W. P., Joslin, F. G., Thompson, R. C., and Hannum, C. H. (1989): *J. Immunol.*, 143: 1851–1858.
2. Auron, P. E., Webb, A. C., Rosenwasser, L. J., et al. (1984): *Proc. Natl. Acad. Sci. USA*, 81: 7907–7911.
3. Bagby, G. C. J., Dinarello, C. A., Neerhout, R. C., Ridgway, D., and McCall, E. (1988): *J. Clin. Invest.*, 82:1430–1436.
4. Balavoine, J. F., De, R. B., Williamson, K., Seckinger, P., Cruchaud, A., and Dayer, J. M. (1986): *J. Clin. Invest.* 78:1120–1124.
5. Beuscher, H. U., and Colten, H. R. (1988): *Mol. Immunol.*, 25:1189.
6. Bomsztyk, K., Sims, J. E., Stanton, T. H., et al. (1989): *Proc. Natl. Acad. Sci. USA*, 86:8034– 8038.
7. Bonin, P. D., Fici, G. J., and Singh, J. P. (1989): *Exp. Cell Res.*, 181:475–82.
8. Brody, D. T., and Durum, S. K. (1989): *J. Immunol.*, 143:1183.
9. Chiou, W. J., Bonin, P. D., Harris, P. K., Carter, D. B., and Singh, J. P. (1989): *J. Biol. Chem.*, 264:21442–21445.
10. Chizzonite, R., Truitt, T., Kilian, P. L., et al. (1989): *Proc. Natl. Acad. Sci. USA*, 86:8029–8033.
11. Cominelli, F., Llerena, F., Clark, B. D., Nast, C. C., Thompson, R. C., and Dinarello, C. A. (1990): *Lymphokine Res.*, 9:597.
12. Cominelli, F., Nast, C. C., Clark, B. D., et al. (1990): *J. Clin. Invest.*, (in press).
13. Cozzolino, F., Rubartelli, A., Aldinucci, D., et al. (1989): *Proc. Natl. Acad. Sci. USA*, 86:2369– 2373.
14. Dejana, E., Breviario, F., and Erroi, A., et al. (1987): *Blood*, 69:695–699.
15. Demczuk, S., Baumberger, C., Mach, B., and Dayer, J. M. (1987): *J. Mol. Cell Immunol.* X: 255–265.
16. Dinarello, C. A. (1989): *Adv. Immunol.*, 44:153–205.
17. Dinarello, C. A., Cannon, J. G., and Wolff, S. M. (1988): *Rev. Infect. Dis.*, 10:168–189.
18. Dinarello, C. A., Rosenwasser, L. J., and Wolff, S. M. (1981): *J. Immunol.*, 127:2517–2519.
19. Eisenberg, S. P., Evans, R. J., Arend, W. P., et al. (1990): *Nature*, 343:341–346.
20. Endres, S., Cannon, J. G., Ghorbani, R., et al. (1989): *Eur. J. Immunol.*, 19:2327–2333.
21. Endres, S., Ghorbani, R., Kelley, V. E., et al. (1989): *N. Engl. J. Med.*, 320:265–271.
22. Fenton, M. J., Clark, B. D., Collins, K. L., Webb, A. C., Rich, A., and Auron, P. E. (1987): *J. Immunol.*, 138:3972–3979.
23. Hellerstein, M. K., Meydani, S. N., Meydani, M., Wu, K., and Dinarello, C. A. (1989): *J. Clin. Invest.*, 84:228–235.
24. Knudsen, P. J., Dinarello, C. A., and Strom, T. B. (1986): *J. Immunol.*, 137:3189–3194.
25. Knudsen, P. J., Dinarello, C. A., and Strom, T. B. (1987): *J. Immunol.*, 139:4129–4134.
26. Kremer, J. M., Lawrence, D. A., Jubiz, W., et al. (1990): *Arthritis Rheum.*, 33:810–820.
27. Kumkumian, G. K., Lafyatis, R., Remmers, E. F., Case, J. P., Kim, S. J., and Wilder, R. L. (1989): *J. Immunol.*, 143:833–837.
28. Kurt-Jones, E. A., Beller, D. I., Mizel, S. B., and Unanue, E. R. (1985): *Proc. Natl. Acad. Sci. USA*, 82:1204.
29. Leaf, A. (1990): *Circulation*, 82:624–628.
30. Liao, Z., Grimshaw, R. S., and Rosenstreich, D. L. (1984): *J. Exp. Med.*, 159:125–136.
31. Libby, P., Warner, S. J., and Friedman, G. B. (1988): *J. Clin. Invest.*, 81:487–498.
32. Lomedico, P. T., Gubler, R., Hellmann, C. P., et al. (1984): *Nature*, 312:458–462.
33. Lonnemann, G., Endres, S., van der Meer, J. W., Cannon, J. G., Koch, K. M., and Dinarello, C. A. (1989): *Eur. J. Immunol.*, 19:1531–1536.
34. Meydani, S. N., Endres, S., Woods, M. M., et al. (1990): *J. Nutr.*, (in press).
35. Ohlsson, K., Bjork, P., and Bergenfeldt, M. et al. (1989): *Cytokine*, 1:131a.
36. Okusawa, S., Gelfand, J. A., Ikejima, T., Connolly, R. J., and Dinarello, C. A. (1988): *J. Clin. Invest.*, 81:1162–1172.
37. Raines, E. W., Dower, S. K., and Ross, R. (1989): *Science*, 243:393–396.
38. Rambaldi, A., Torcia, M., Bettoni, S., et al. (1990): *Blood*, (in press).
39. Rosoff, P. M., Savage, N., and Dinarello, C. A. (1988): *Cell*, 54:73–81.
40. Savage, N., Puren, A. J., Orencole, S. F., Ikejima, T., Clark, B. D., and Dinarello, C. A. (1989): *Cytokine*, 1:23–25.

41. Schade, U. F., Burmeister, I., and Engel, R. (1987): *Biochem. Biophys. Res. Comm.,* 147:695–700.
42. Schindler, R., Clark, B. D., and Dinarello, C. A. (1990): *J. Biol. Chem.* 265:10232–10237.
43. Schindler, R., Ghezzi, P., and Dinarello, C. A. (1990): *J. Immunol.,* 144:2216–2222.
44. Seckinger, P., and Dayer, J. M. (1987): *Ann. Inst. Pasteur Immunol.,* 138:461–516.
45. Seckinger, P., Lowenthal, J. W., Williamson, K., Dayer, J. M., and MacDonald, H. R. (1987): *J. Immunol.,* 139:1546–1549.
46. Streiter, R. M., Remick, P. A., Ward, P. A., et al. (1988): *Biochem. Biophys. Res. Comm.,* 155:1230–1236.
47. Suzuki, H., Shibano, K., Okane, M., et al. (1989): *Am. J. Pathol.,* 134:35–43.
48. Vannier, E., Miller, L. C., Schindler, R., Terlain, B., and Dinarello, C. A. (1989): *Cytokine,* 1:123.
49. Wakabayashi, G., Gelfand, J. A., Burke, J. F., Thompson, R. C., and Dinarello, C. A. (1990): *FASEB J.,* (in press).
50. Walter, J., Davenne, D., Shoham, S., Dinarello, C. A., and Krueger, J. M. (1986): *Am. J. Physiol.,* 86:R96–R103.

Atherosclerosis Reviews, Volume 23,
edited by P. C. Weber and A. Leaf.
Raven Press, Ltd., New York © 1991.

Immune Mechanisms in Plaque Formation

Göran K. Hansson

Cell Biology Research Laboratory, Department of Clinical Chemistry, Gothenburg University, Sahlgren's Hospital, S-413 45 Gothenburg, Sweden

Leukocytes interact with the cells of the vasculature both during the physiological inflammatory response and in many pathological conditions. In inflammation, vascular endothelial cells express cell surface proteins that serve as ligands for leukocytes equipped with the appropriate receptors. For example, the endothelial leukocyte adhesion molecule-1 (ELAM-1) promotes the adhesion of granulocytes and monocytes (2), and the VCAM-1 molecule is a receptor for the binding of lymphocytes to the endothelial surface (26). The addressins of the high endothelium of venules (HEV) in specialized regions of the vasculature serve as ligands for homing receptors of subsets of lymphocytes destined for homing to lymph nodes or inflammatory lesions (3).

Adherent leukocytes penetrate the endothelial lining through intercellular junctions and may accumulate in the subendothelial tissue during inflammatory conditions (5). Both cell culture studies and analysis of tissue specimens show that such leukocytes are often in an activated state and secrete bioactive substances that regulate gene expression in surrounding mesenchymal cells (5,15,23,27). Cytokines are proteins that are released by such activated leukocytes and exert hormone-like effects on surrounding cells. Local production of cytokines in vascular lesions is demonstrated both directly by *in situ* hybridization and indirectly by the detection of cytokine-inducible gene expression in target cells (6,20).

Several vascular diseases are characterized by inflammatory responses. The most obvious examples are found among the vasculitides. In giant cell arteritis, the arterial intima and media are filled with macrophages that fuse to giant cells and with CD4+ T lymphocytes (1). Similarly, the vasculitic lesion of systemic lupus erythematodes is characterized by mononuclear cell infiltrates (29).

INFLAMMATORY CELLS IN ATHEROSCLEROSIS

In atherosclerosis, classical histopathological studies have demonstrated the presence of lipid-laden macrophages (9). Immunohistochemical phenotypic analyses strongly suggest that these foam cells are derived from blood monocytes (10,19,30,34). Such immunohistochemical studies have also revealed the presence of substantial amounts of T lymphocytes in atherosclerotic plaques (19,20). T lymphocytes were initially observed in advanced plaques, but they have subsequently been identified also in fatty streaks and fibrous plaques that probably represent earlier phases of the disease (8,14,24).

Two observations strongly suggest that the mononuclear cell infiltrate in the plaque represents an active inflammatory or immunologic process and not simply a trapping of leukocytes in the tissue. First, a substantial proportion of plaque T cells were found to express cell surface receptors that are present only on activated T cells (12). These include the histocompatibility protein, HLA-DR; the receptor for the autocrine growth factor, interleukin-2; and the integrin receptor, VLA-1. Second, a high proportion of smooth muscle cells (SMC) and macrophages of the plaque express cell surface proteins that are inducible by lymphokines that are in turn released from activated T cells. HLA-DR expression is found on two-thirds of all cells, including SMC and macrophages in advanced plaques (20). The expression of this histocompatibility protein is induced by γ-interferon, one of the major secretory products of activated T cells (28).

CLONAL COMPOSITION OF PLAQUE T LYMPHOCYTES

These observations show that there are three major cellular components that interact in the subendothelium during plaque development: macrophages, T lymphocytes, and SMC. The pattern of activation is, however, unclear. Do the lymphocytes, for instance, constitute a homogeneous population of cells that respond to a single antigen? Alternatively, they might represent an immunologically heterogeneous population that has been recruited to the plaque, e.g., due to their expression of adhesion receptors.

This raises the question of clonality of the T lymphocytes in the plaque. In an immune response to a single antigen, only a limited number of T cells respond. After activation, they proliferate to give rise to a small number of T cell clones, each of which is derived from one progenitor cell and capable of responding to one specific antigenic epitope (4). An inflammatory infiltrate, on the other hand, is usually composed of many different lymphocytes, with different immunologic specificities and hence of different clonal origins (4).

The degree of clonality of a T lymphocyte population can be determined by analysis of the genes for the T cell antigen receptor (TCR). These genes are present in germline cells as segments dispersed along the chromosome. During T-cell differentiation, the segments are rearranged to form a functional TCR gene, and interspersed DNA is deleted (4,7,22). The precise sequence of the rearranged gene is unique for each T lymphoblast and remains unchanged throughout the life not only of the lymphoblast but also of the mature T lymphocyte and all daughter cells derived from it. Therefore, clonal proliferation during an immune response results in a population of T cells with identical TCR genes. In contrast, a polyclonal T-cell population contains as many TCR gene patterns as there are cells (4,7,22).

The rearranged TCR gene can be distinguished from the germline gene by DNA hybridization. Each individual TCR rearrangement pattern is unique and can be identified by Southern blotting after cleavage of the gene with appropriate restriction enzymes (4,7,22).

The T lymphocytes of the atherosclerotic plaque could represent a local immune response to one (or a few) specific antigens and constitute an oligoclonal population with a limited number of TCR rearrangement patterns. Alternatively, they might form the polyclonal population of an inflammatory response, in which case there should be as many TCR patterns as cells (Fig. 1). We have used a combination of T-cell cloning and TCR gene analysis to determine the clonal properties of T cells in the plaque (33).

T cells were isolated from endarterectomy specimens and immediately cloned by the limiting dilution technique. Irradiated autologous peripheral mononuclear cells were used as feeder cells and both growth factor (interleukin-2) and a polyclonal mitogen (CD3 antibodies) were added to promote growth of the cultures. Thirty to fifty T-cell clones were raised from each plaque and expanded to sufficient amounts for DNA analysis. DNA was cleaved with the restriction enzymes EcoRI and HindIII, separated by electrophoresis and blotted to nitrocellulose. The membranes were hybridized with gene probes specific for the TCR β and γ genes.

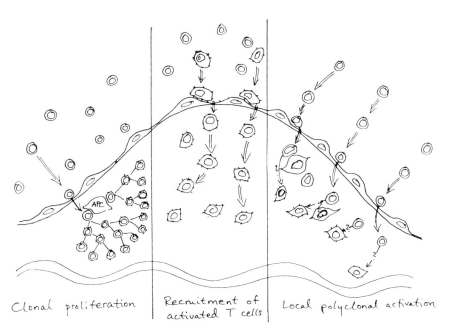

Clonal proliferation | Recruitment of activated T cells | Local polyclonal activation

FIG. 1. Three mechanisms that could lead to T lymphocyte accumulation in atherosclerotic plaques. Left: Clonal proliferation of antigen-specific T cells. Center: Recruitment of activated T cells that express adhesion receptors. Right: Polyclonal activation of T cells in the plaque.

Analysis of the TCR γ gene using a probe for its J (joining) segment showed heterogeneity between T-cell cultures. Only one-fifth of the clones showed identical rearrangement patterns and were reanalyzed using a probe for the C (constant) segment of the TCR β gene. In this way, all but two of the 250 clones could be separated into different TCR gene patterns. The last pair was reanalyzed after cleavage with a third restriction enzyme, KpnI, followed by TCR-J-γ hybridization. This analysis showed that also these two clones were different and thus not derived from any common progenitor T cell in the plaque (33).

In conclusion, the analysis indicated that the T-cell population of the atherosclerotic plaque is polyclonal (33). This argues against a local immune response to one or a few antigenic epitopes as a significant phenomenon in the mature atherosclerotic plaque. It cannot, however, be ruled out that such a response could take place earlier during the pathogenesis of the disease.

Our two findings—that (a) T cells of the plaque are in a state of activation, and that (b) they are polyclonal—suggest that there may be a preferential recruitment of activated T cells into the plaque (Fig. 1). The reason for this is unclear. One possibility is that the (endothelial or other) surface-forming cells of the plaque or in the vasa vasorum express receptors that bind to cell surface proteins specifically expressed on activated T lymphocytes. The other possibility would be a polyclonal activation of T cells in the plaque.

γ-INTERFERON REGULATES GENE EXPRESSION IN VASCULAR SMOOTH MUSCLE CELLS

The presence in the plaque of activated T lymphocytes, irrespective of their immunologic specificity, implies that lymphokines are secreted in the plaque. As mentioned above, both direct and indirect evidence show that this is the case. The finding of HLA-DR expression in the plaque strongly suggests that γ-interferon is released locally. We have therefore analyzed the effects of γ-interferon on vascular SMC and macrophages with regard to growth, differentiation, and lipid metabolism.

γ-Interferon induces expression of histocompatibility genes in SMC. Cultured human SMC do not normally express any class II histocompatibility genes but treatment with γ-interferon at ng/ml concentrations results in *de novo* gene expression of HLA-DR, DQ, and DP (32). In the rat, the equivalent histocompatibility genes RT1B and RT1D (also called I-A and I-E) are induced (13,18). However, treatment of the cells with γ-interferon not only induces histocompatibility genes but also inhibits growth of the cells (11,13). This is due to a block of growth factor–induced progression through the G_1 phase of the cell cycle and results in trapping of the cells in early G_1 and inhibition of DNA synthesis and proliferation (13).

Growth cessation is often associated with induction of differentiation. We

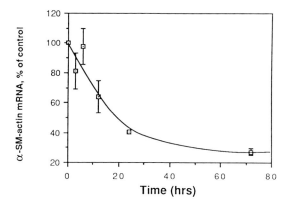

FIG. 2. γ-Interferon down-regulates αSM-actin mRNA in rat SMC cells. RNA was isolated from cells treated for different lengths of time with recombinant rat γ-interferon. α-SM-actin mRNA was quantitated by densitometry after hybridization with the cDNA probe, pRoαA-3'UT. (From ref. 15.)

therefore analyzed the effect of γ-interferon on expression of differentiation-specific α-smooth muscle actin (αSM-actin) (11). γ-Interferon–treated cells showed loss of αSM-actin containing stress fibers (11). This was due to an inhibition of expression of the gene for αSM-actin with a reduced steady-state level of αSM-actin mRNA (Fig. 2). There are two possible mechanisms for this regulation. γ-Interferon could either induce a transacting, negative regulatory factor for αSM-actin gene expression, or increase the degradation of αSM-actin mRNA. These possibilities are now being evaluated in our laboratory.

The *in vivo* relevance of the cell culture findings described above are not fully clear. It is possible that the down-regulation of αSM-actin expression results in a reduced contractility of the afflicted vascular segment; this action may explain the increased blood flow in inflammatory lesions.

More is known about the growth-inhibitory effect of γ-interferon. The histocompatibility genes, RT1B and RT1D, are expressed by SMC in the arterial response to injury *in vivo* (13,18). The response after balloon catheter injury therefore represents a good model for analysis of vascular responses to γ-interferon. RT1B+ SMC do not replicate their DNA, as indicated by their lack of [³H]thymidine uptake after *in vivo* injection in the rat (13). This implies that γ-interferon is an endogenous inhibitor of growth during the arterial response to injury. It also suggests that γ-interferon may be useful to block SMC proliferation—e.g., after angioplasty.

We recently tested the effect of parenteral recombinant γ-interferon on the arterial response to balloon catheter injury. Rats treated with γ-interferon developed significantly smaller lesions when compared to PBS-treated controls (15a). The effect was detectable two weeks after injury and persisted throughout the 10-week experimental period. This result leads us to conclude that γ-interferon could be useful as a drug to prevent arterial stenosis after angioplasty and vascular surgery.

γ-INTERFERON REGULATES MACROPHAGE LIPID METABOLISM

Finally, lymphokines are potent regulators of differentiation and activation in macrophages. The latter cell type develops into the cholesterol-laden foam cell that is characteristic of atherosclerosis, and we have therefore started to evaluate the effects of γ-interferon on lipid metabolism in the macrophage. We have concentrated on the enzyme, lipoprotein lipase (LPL), which is synthesized by macrophages and SMC (and adipocytes) and hydrolyzes triglycerides of very-low-density lipoproteins (VLDL), resulting in release of free fatty acids (FFA) and glycerol and the conversion of the lipoprotein into intermediate-density lipoproteins (IDL) (25).

First, we noted by immunofluorescence that there was an inverse correlation between cellular LPL and HLA-DR expression in the atherosclerotic plaque (16). This observation suggested to us that γ-interferon may regulate LPL expression in the cells. This possibility was tested in cultured human monocyte-derived macrophages.

LPL activity was analyzed in macrophage-conditioned culture medium (17). The activity was all but abolished in cells treated with recombinant γ-interferon

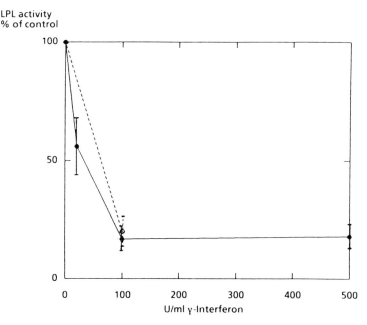

FIG. 3. γ-Interferon inhibits lipoprotein lipase activity in human monocyte-derived macrophages. Cells were treated for 2 days with different doses of recombinant γ-interferon (● — ●) or with T cell–conditioned medium in which the γ-interferon concentration was 100 U/ml (○ ---- ○). Lipoprotein lipase was released with heparin and assayed in the medium. (From ref. 17.)

(Fig. 3). Conditioned medium from activated T lymphocytes exerted a similar effect. Pretreatment of the medium with antibodies to γ-interferon eliminated the effect of such media on macrophage LPL, indicating that natural γ-interferon exerts the same effect as the recombinant protein and that γ-interferon is the only factor produced by T lymphocytes that inhibits LPL secretion.

The effect of γ-interferon on LPL synthesis was evaluated by metabolic labeling followed by immunoprecipitation (17). LPL synthesis was significantly reduced in γ-interferon–treated cells. This reduction was, however, not of the same magnitude as the reduction of LPL enzymatic activity secreted by the cells. It is therefore possible that γ-interferon may inhibit not only the synthesis but also the intracellular processing and transport of LPL (17).

Tumour necrosis factor (TNF) and interleukin-1 exert effects on LPL similar to γ-interferon (21,31). Because γ-interferon activates macrophages to release TNF and IL-1, several direct and indirect cytokine pathways may lead to an inhibition of lipolytic activity in inflammatory lesions and atherosclerotic plaques.

CONCLUSIONS

We have demonstrated the existence of inflammatory cells (macrophages and T lymphocytes) in atherosclerotic plaques and obtained evidence for a recruitment of activated, polyclonal T cells to the plaque. Cell culture studies show that cytokines released by these cells, particularly γ-interferon, exert important regulatory influences on growth and differentiation of these cells. The effects on contractile proteins and lipolytic enzymes are particularly interesting because they can influence basic functions involved in vascular disease.

ACKNOWLEDGMENT

The stimulating collaboration of my colleagues Jan Holm, Lena Jonasson, and Sten Stemme is gratefully acknowledged.

This work was supported by grants from the Swedish Medical Research Council (6816) and the Swedish Heart-Lung Foundation.

REFERENCES

1. Andersson, R., Hansson, G. K., Söderström, T., Jonsson, R., Bengtsson, B.-Å., and Nordborg, E. (1988): *Clin. Exp. Immunol.,* 73:82–87.
2. Bevilacqua, M. P., Stengelin, S., Gimbrone, M. A., and Seed, B. (1989): *Science,* 243:1160–1165.
3. Butcher, E. C. (1990): *Am. J. Pathol.,* 136:3–11.
4. Caccia, N., and Mak, T. W. (1989): *Transplant. Proc.,* 21:18–22.
5. Cotran, R. S. (1987): *Am. J. Pathol.,* 129:407–413.
6. Cotran, R. S., Gimbrone, M. A., Bevilacqua, M. P., Mendrick, D. L., and Pober, J. S. (1986): *J. Exp. Med.,* 164:661–666.
7. Davis, M. M. (1988): In: Hames, B. D., and Glover, D. M., eds. *Molecular Immunology.* Oxford: IRL Press, pp. 61–79.

8. Emeson, E., and Robertson, A. L. (1988): *Am. J. Pathol.,* 130:369–376.
9. Geer, J. C., McGill, H. C., and Strong, J. P. (1961): *Am. J. Pathol.,* 38:263–275.
10. Gown, A. M., Tsukada, T., and Ross, R. (1986): *Am. J. Pathol.,* 125:191–207.
11. Hansson, G. K., Hellstrand, M., Rymo, L., Rubbia, L., and Gabbiani, G. (1989): *J. Exp. Med.,* 170:1595–1608.
12. Hansson, G. K., Holm, J., and Jonasson, L. (1989): *Am. J. Pathol.,* 135:169–175.
13. Hansson, G. K., Jonasson, L., Holm, J., Clowes, M. M., and Clowes, A. W. (1988): *Circ. Res.,* 63:712–719.
14. Hansson, G. K., Jonasson, L., Lojsthed, B., Stemme, S., Kocher, O., and Gabbiani, G. (1988): *Atherosclerosis,* 72:135–141.
15. Hansson, G. K., Jonasson, L., Seifert, P. S., and Stemme, S. (1989): *Arteriosclerosis,* 9:567–578.
15a. Hansson, G. K., and Holm J. (1991): *Circulation* (in press).
16. Jonasson, L., Bondjers, G., and Hansson, G. K. (1987): *J. Lipid Res.,* 28:437–445.
17. Jonasson, L., Hansson, G. K., Bondjers, G., Noe, L., and Etienne, J. (1990): *Biochim. Biophys. Acta.,* 1053:43–48.
18. Jonasson, L., Holm, J., and Hansson, G. K. (1988): *Lab. Invest.,* 58:310–315.
19. Jonasson, L., Holm, J., Skalli, O., Bondjers, G., and Hansson, G. K. (1986): *Arteriosclerosis,* 6:131–138.
20. Jonasson, L., Holm, J., Skalli, O., Gabbiani, G., and Hansson, G. K. (1985): *J. Clin. Invest.,* 76:125–131.
21. Kawakami, M., Pekala, P. H., Lane, M. D., and Cerami, A. (1982): *Proc. Natl. Acad. Sci. USA,* 79:912–916.
22. Lefranc, M. P., and Rabbitts, T. H. (1989): *Trends Biochem. Sci.,* 14:214–218.
23. Libby, P., and Hansson, G. K. (1990): *Lab. Invest.*
24. Munro, J. M., van der Waly, J. D., Munro, C. S., Chalmers, J. A. C., and Cox, E. L. (1987): *Hum. Pathol.,* 18:375–380.
25. Nilsson-Ehle, P., Garfinkel, A. S., and Schotz, M. C. (1980): *Annu. Rev. Biochem.,* 49:667–693.
26. Osborn, L., Hession, C., Tizard, R., et al. (1989): *Cell,* 59:1203–1211.
27. Pober, J. S. (1988): *Am. J. Pathol.,* 133:426–433.
28. Revel, M., and Chebath, J. (1986): *Trends Biochem. Sci.,* 11:166–170.
29. Rothfield, N. (1985): *Clinical features of systemic lupus erythematosus.* 2nd ed. Philadelphia; W. B. Saunders, pp. 1070–1072.
30. Schaffner, T., Taylor, K., Bartucci, E. J., et al. (1980): *Am. J. Pathol.,* 100:57–80.
31. Semb, H., Peterson, J., Tavernier, J., and Olivecrona, T. (1987): *J. Biol. Chem.,* 262:8390–8394.
32. Stemme, S., Fager, G., and Hansson, G. K. (1990): *Immunology,* 69:243–249.
33. Stemme S., Rymo L., and Hansson, G. K. (1991): *Lab. Invest.* (in press).
34. Vedeler, C. A., Nyland, H., and Matre, R. (1984): *Acta Pathol. Microbiol. Immunol. Scand.,* 92C:133–137.

Atherosclerosis Reviews, Volume 23,
edited by P. C. Weber and A. Leaf.
Raven Press, Ltd., New York © 1991.

Determinants of Serum Cholesterol

D. M. Hegsted

*New England Regional Primate Research Center, Harvard Medical School,
Southboro, Massachusetts 01772*

The major determinants of individual serum cholesterol levels are the genetic makeup of the individual and his or her dietary habits. It is important to recognize that within most communities, the variation in serum cholesterol levels of individuals, even excluding those with marked hypercholesterolemia, greatly exceeds the variation caused by differences in diet.

GENETICS VERSUS DIET

The subjects of our study (9) were screened to remove those with exceptionally high or low serum cholesterol levels. We found that the serum cholesterol levels of the individuals differed by about 100 mg/dl (6) when all received the same diet. This group of men had a mean serum cholesterol level of about 225 mg/dl when consuming a diet similar to that of the average American. The maximum shift in the average cholesterol levels that we could achieve was a little more than 100 mg/dl, changing from a diet low in cholesterol with most fat in the form of safflower oil to a high-cholesterol diet with butterfat or coconut oil. This difference in dietary fat composition is much greater, of course, than will ever occur in ordinary diets.

The point is that we should not expect the diet of individuals to correlate very highly, if at all, with their serum cholesterol levels. Failure to find significant correlations between the diet of individuals and their cholesterol level has led some observers to conclude that diet plays an insignificant role. This conclusion is certainly wrong.

In addition, there is increasing evidence that all methods of collecting dietary data in the field have very serious problems. Because there is no foolproof way to determine the food intake of people under ordinary conditions, all investigators in the past have used evidence of reproducibility as evidence of validity (35). That is, if repeated measures of the diet, using the same or different methods, were significantly correlated, the data were assumed to be reasonably valid. Evidence to the contrary is now available.

The double-labeled water technique (33) provides an independent method of measuring energy expenditure. Energy expenditure must equal energy intake in individuals with stable body weight and physical activity. Thus, the measured energy expenditure can be used to validate energy intakes based on food records or other methods. Livingstone et al. (20), for example, found that although individuals examined twice with 7-day weighed food records reported similar intakes on the two occasions ($r = 0.79$)—i.e., the data appeared to be reproducible, but the correlation between the reported energy intake and the energy expenditure was very poor. Most of the subjects seriously underestimated their intake, some by as much as 50%. A summary (33) of the few studies that have compared energy expenditure with reported energy intake indicates that unless one is working with small, well-trained groups, the dietary data appear to be seriously biased and generally yield substantial underestimates of intake.

Attempts to relate the dietary practices of individuals to their health status are likely to yield incorrect conclusions (14,30,36). What is even worse, if food intake cannot be accurately monitored, field trials to test the effects of dietary modification must be suspect, especially large field trials. There is also reason to believe that participants in studies who know what they are supposed to eat are likely to produce dietary records that are especially suspect (3).

Comparisons of mean intakes of populations appear more reliable, especially if there are considerable differences in food habits. When applied to a large group, even crude measures yield a reasonable estimate of the mean intake of the group, and the biases in dietary data are similar when the same method is applied to different groups. The results of immigrant studies suggest that the genetic differences in susceptibility are not large in different populations. Hence, the comparison of disease incidence, biochemical markers like serum cholesterol, or mortality in groups with average diets of such groups is meaningful and worthwhile. Nevertheless, the reliability of dietary information, however it is gathered, is going to be under serious scrutiny in the coming years, and the outlook is rather discouraging.

DIETARY FAT AND SERUM CHOLESTEROL

An increasing number of reports indicate that a variety of food constituents—plant sterols, dietary fiber, tocotrienols, saponins, and unidentified materials—may affect serum lipid levels and atherosclerosis. Data on the effects of such materials in human subjects are very limited so far, but attention will have to be paid to these kinds of materials in the immediate future. It is likely that variations in these components in experimental diets used to investigate the effects of dietary fats and cholesterol may explain—at least in part—some of inconsistencies that have been reported.

Although dietary fat and cholesterol were implicated early in the search for factors affecting serum cholesterol levels, it was the work of Keys et al. (18), as well as our own laboratory (9), that provided the principal basis for the general recommendations of the American Heart Association. These studies showed that saturated fats increased serum cholesterol and were the primary determinant of serum cholesterol levels, that polyunsaturated fatty acids decreased serum cholesterol, and that monounsaturated fatty acids had no specific effect. In the 30 years since these publications appeared, there have been numerous studies in which dietary fats were varied and the change in serum cholesterol measured. In the last few years, the conclusion of Keys et al. and Hegsted et al. that monounsaturated fatty acids have no specific effect on serum cholesterol has been challenged (25,27).

In a preliminary report (7) made 2 years ago, we attempted an analysis of the literature on the effects of dietary fats upon serum cholesterol in humans. At that time, we were able to identify some 210 dietary comparisons that had been published. Regression analysis of these combined data confirmed the principal conclusions of Keys and Hegsted. The best predictive equation for the combined data obtained in what we called "metabolic studies," where the diets were prepared and fed to groups of human subjects, was:

$$\Delta SC = 2.22\Delta S - 0.98\Delta P + 0.066\Delta C \qquad r = 0.92$$

where ΔS represents change in intake of saturated fatty acids, ΔP represents change in intake of polyunsaturated fatty acids expressed as percentage of calories, and ΔC represents change in intake of cholesterol expressed as mg/1,000 calories.

No improvement in predictability was obtained when the monounsaturated fatty acids were included in the equation, which then became:

$$\Delta SC = 2.22\Delta S - 0.96\Delta P + 0.065\Delta C + 0.16\Delta M \qquad r = 0.92$$

In these equations the coefficients for ΔS, ΔP, and ΔC are highly significant ($p = 0.001$); that of ΔM is not.

Since that report, we have identified additional literature, including several published within the last year. The total number of dietary comparisons now available appears to be about 250. An analysis of these data is now being prepared. We are certain, however, that the previous conclusions will not be greatly modified. We simply cannot find an independent effect of the monounsaturated fatty acids, nor are they equivalent to the polyunsaturated fatty acids.

Although the regression equations developed by Keys or myself, or used in our analysis of the total data account for a large proportion of the variance, there is a considerable spread of the points around any of these regression lines. In the Keys data, for example, data points deviate by about 10 mg/dl. The deviation around the regression line in the Hegsted data (Fig. 1) is somewhat larger. Obviously, the general equations do not agree with many of the individual points, or one can easily select points in either data set that disagree with the results predicted by the general equations. The real merit of the Keys and Hegsted data is that a sufficient number of fats were studied to draw general conclusions. All studies conducted since that time have reported on only two or three different fats. It is not surprising that some of these studies agree and others disagree with the predictive equations.

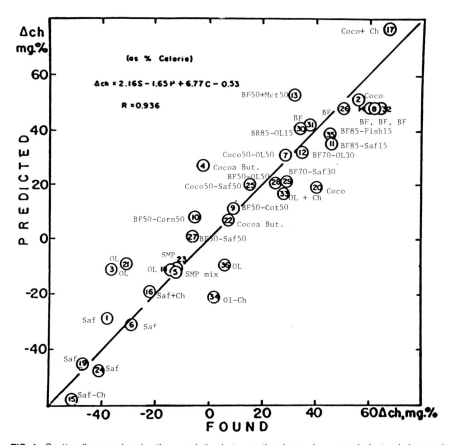

FIG. 1. Scatter diagram showing the correlation between the change in serum cholesterol observed and that predicted by the regression equation. Note that although the regression equation accounts for 88% of the total variance, there is considerable spread around the regression line. Modified from Hegsted et al. (9).

We do not know why the outcomes of studies of this kind are as variable as they are. There may be inadequate description or monitoring of the diets, inadequate definition of the scrum cholesterol levels, variability in the responsiveness of the subjects studied, other factors that affect serum cholesterol, etc. Unfortunately, there appear to be no data available to estimate the reproducibility of such findings. Katan et al. (16) have concluded that when the same individuals are retested, the serum cholesterol response is not reproducible. If this is true, the reproducibility of data from small groups is also likely to be variable.

This field suffers from what has recently been labeled the "oat bran syndrome" (24). Each new article, especially if it appears in the *New England Journal of Medicine, Science,* or *Lancet,* is publicized as though it were the final answer. It is exploited by those with commercial or scientific interests, even though the results may disagree with much other data. In discussing "uncertainty" recently,

Moore (28) commented that we should "learn to look for overall patterns and not attempt a causal explanation for each outcome." It seems obvious that there is considerable uncertainty in small dietary trials, even those that appear well controlled. The overall pattern of serum cholesterol response to dietary fatty acids is now established. Isolated findings cannot and do not modify this pattern.

MONOUNSATURATED VERSUS POLYUNSATURATED FATTY ACIDS

Putting aside the general question of whether we can generalize from small studies, which I believe is dangerous, it is important to note that Mattson and Grundy (25) utilized "formula diets" in their studies. We (10) have examined all of the relevant papers in which formula diets have been used, starting with the classic paper of Ahrens et al. (1). The data obtained with formula diets over the years show two important effects that differ from results obtained with ordinary diets. First, formula diets markedly lower serum cholesterol even when they contain saturated fats. Second, all such studies find equivalent effects of oils high in mono- and polyunsaturated fats on serum cholesterol. Hence, these studies simply confirm what Ahrens et al. (1) reported in 1957.

We are forced to conclude that, for reasons unknown but perhaps because the diets are free of cholesterol, formula diets attenuate the effects of fats upon serum cholesterol and specifically fail to distinguish between oils high in mono- and

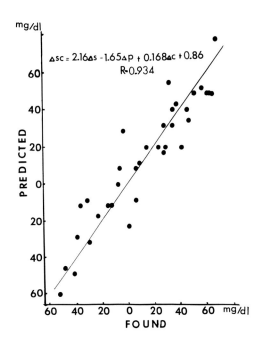

FIG. 2. The data of Hegsted et al. (9), as in Fig. 1, recalculated with change in diet expressed as mg/1,000 kcal.

polyunsaturated fatty acids. This finding is contrary to most of the data obtained with diets composed of ordinary foods. Hence, we believe that such data cannot be extrapolated to other conditions until it has been specifically shown that similar results are obtained with ordinary diets. Such comparative data have not been produced.

Obviously this criticism does not apply to the work of Mensink and Katan (27), who used ordinary diets. However, there appears to be a widespread misconception about the discriminatory capacity of studies of this kind. Figure 2 shows the original data of Hegsted recalculated with dietary cholesterol expressed as mg/1,000 kcals. Figure 3 shows the same calculation with the data of Mensink and Katan included. It would seem clear that inclusion of these data does not significantly modify the general conclusions based upon the original data. Similarly, if these data are included with the original Keys data, they do not significantly change the original conclusions. Therefore, these isolated comparisons of a few diets cannot seriously challenge the overall conclusions now based on >250 dietary comparisons. If further progress is to be made in defining the role of dietary fats upon serum cholesterol, new designs and approaches are needed. In particular, investigators must demonstrate that their results are reproducible.

The most complete comparison of an oil high in monounsaturates (olive oil) and one high in polyunsaturates (safflower oil) was published in 1965 (9) (Fig. 4). Three oils were fed with three levels of dietary cholesterol (in the form of eggs). Olive oil caused almost no change in serum cholesterol from the baseline levels, whereas safflower oil clearly lowered serum cholesterol levels. The first

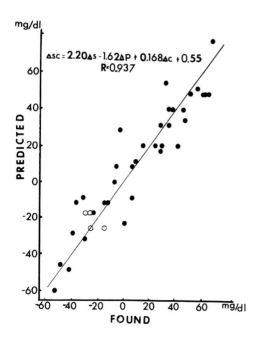

FIG. 3. The regression equation calculated from the combined data of Hegsted et al. (9) and those of Mensink and Katan (27) (open circles). Note that the addition of the latter data results in a minimal change when compared to Fig. 2.

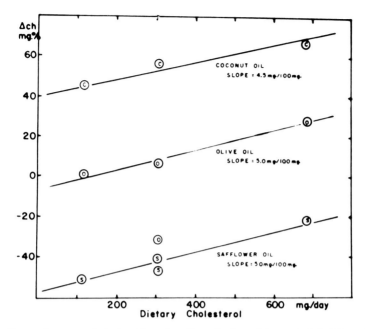

FIG. 4. Change in serum cholesterol from baseline with three fats, each fed at three levels of dietary cholesterol (egg). Olive oil caused essentially no change from baseline.

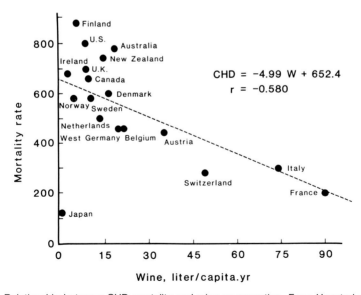

FIG. 5. Relationship between CHD mortality and wine consumption. From Hegsted and Ausman (8).

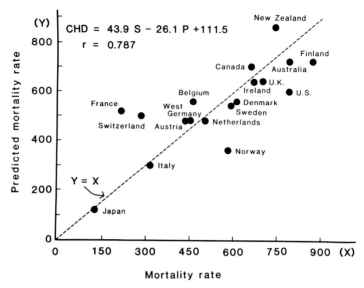

FIG. 6. CHD mortality predicted by saturated (S) and polyunsaturated (P) fatty acids in the food supply versus observed mortality (8).

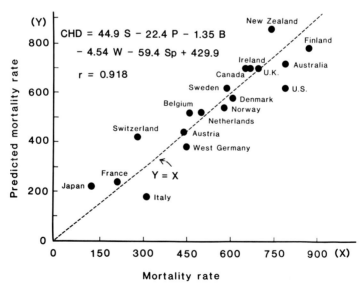

FIG. 7. CHD mortality predicted by saturated (S) and polyunsaturated (P) fatty acids in the food supply and alcohol consumption. Wine (W), beer (B), and spirits (Sp) all have negative regression coefficients suggesting that all sources of alcohol provide some protection (8).

time we fed olive oil, the change in serum cholesterol approximated that obtained with safflower oil and seemed aberrant compared to the other data. When the feeding was repeated, it fell to about the level expected. Aberrant data are sometimes obtained for unknown reasons.

We are all aware, of course, that the fabled "Mediterranean diet" is always offered up as the final evidence of the value of a diet high in monounsaturated fatty acids. However, as Keys has noted (17), the low level of saturated fatty acids in the diet would suffice to explain the reduced levels of serum cholesterol in these populations. We (8) believe that wine consumption is also important. Figure 5 shows the relationship between wine consumption alone and coronary heart disease (CHD) mortality. Figure 6 shows that consumption of saturated and polyunsaturated fatty acids explains a good deal of the variance, but a much better fit is obtained when alcohol as well as fat consumption is considered. All of the sources of alcohol—wine, beer, and spirits—yield negative regression coefficients, indicating protection against death from coronary disease (Fig. 7).

Overall, the evidence shows that, to the degree that they replace saturated fats, monounsaturated fatty acids lower serum cholesterol. The data do not support the conclusion that they have any ability to lower serum cholesterol levels, as do the polyunsaturated fatty acids.

SERUM LIPOPROTEINS

It is obvious, of course, that changes in serum cholesterol are no longer sufficient; we are interested in the changes in the lipoproteins. There are many fewer data on fat-induced changes of low-density (LDL) and high-density lipoproteins (HDL) than of total cholesterol, and the lipoproteins are more difficult to quantitate. However, as one would expect, it appears that changes in LDL cholesterol are similar to the changes in total cholesterol discussed above. This would be expected because LDL carries most of the serum cholesterol. There are even fewer data available on dietary effects on HDL. The studies showing substantial drops in HDL when polyunsaturated fatty acids have been fed were based on diets containing excessive amounts of polyunsaturated fatty acids—diets that no one eats. It is not at all clear that the drops in HDL are of concern when any reasonable level of linoleic acid is provided. Several authors have concluded that low-fat diets lower HDL and are therefore presumably undesirable. I would only emphasize that there appear to be abundant epidemiologic data showing that low-fat diets protect against CHD. This, after all, is our primary concern, regardless of serum lipoprotein levels. Similarly, diets high in polyunsaturated fatty acids prevent atherosclerosis in animals.

Just as small, limited studies often yield erroneous results on the effects of diet on total serum cholesterol, this is doubly true of effects upon lipoproteins. Generalizations must be based on an adequate body of data rather than the most recent publication. There are not sufficient data on the effects of various fatty acids on lipoprotein levels to draw general conclusions at this time; nor are there sufficient data to relate these changes to atherosclerosis and CHD.

SATURATED AND TRANS FATTY ACIDS

Another issue that has yet to be settled is the relative potency of the various saturated fatty acids. There is considerable evidence to show that stearic acid is less hypercholesterolemic than some of the others (2,5,9) but almost no data on the relative potency of the other saturated fatty acids. Yet I would emphasize that in the transesterified fats we studied (23), we could not demonstrate that laurate, myristate, palmitate, and stearate had different potencies. If stearate is usually less hypercholesterolemic than other saturated fatty acids, the only apparent explanation would seem to be that the position of the fatty acids in the trigryceride molecule is significant. Again, the data are very limited, so it is too early to draw definitive conclusions about the specific effects of any of the saturated fatty acids.

The trans fatty acids have physical properties that are similar to the saturated fatty acids. Despite limited data (4), there has been reason to believe that they might have effects on serum cholesterol more like saturated fatty acids. The recent articles of Mensink and Katan (27) provides the most convincing evidence that this is true. These studies need confirmation, but it is likely that such data will have an important effect upon the formulation of margarines and other hydrogenated products.

FISH OILS

As the importance of the n-3 fatty acids began to be appreciated, including their effect on many parameters related to cardiovascular disease (19), it has also become apparent that the effects of dietary fat cannot be considered only in terms of their effect on serum lipids. The n-6 polyunsaturated fatty acids may also affect functions other than the serum lipids. As Hetzel et al. (11) have emphasized, the principal dietary change in the United States and Australia in recent years has been the substantial increase in the consumption of linoleic acid. This consumption has been associated with a marked fall in CHD mortality, especially sudden death, which appears to be greater than can be explained by the modest fall in serum cholesterol levels. The decrease in mortality is consistent with the experimental finding that increased intake of either n-3 or n-6 polyunsaturated fatty acids decreases susceptibility to arrhythmias in experimental animals (21,22). Limited studies on the fatty acid composition of adipose and other tissues indicate that low levels of linoleic acid are associated with CHD (15,31,34,37). Changes in the fatty acid content of tissue membranes may affect many functions (13,29,38).

It seems likely that the role of serum lipids has been somewhat overemphasized, and other functions of fatty acids will become increasingly important. There is a serious need for data indicating the appropriate balance between n-3 and n-6 fatty acids and the levels of each in the diet. It is dangerous to extrapolate from data that compare extreme situations, such as diets that contain only fish oil or corn oil.

Although I believe that serum lipids will receive less emphasis in the future than they have in the past, there is some danger that the pendulum might swing too far. The important causal role of elevated serum cholesterol levels in atherosclerosis and the benefits achieved by reducing them by dietary or pharmacologic means is now very well established. And we still have relatively little quantitative information on the n-3 fatty acids and their relationship to other fatty acids in the diet.

The largest deliberate dietary experiment ever done has been the change in the diet fat in the United States and a few other countries, with apparently beneficial effects. The goal has been to increase the consumption of linoleic acid. We must not be so enthusiastic about the monounsaturated fatty acids, stearic acid, the n-3 fatty acids, oxidized LDL, etc., that we reverse the favorable trends in cardiovascular disease for inadequate reasons.

CONCLUSIONS

We now have a massive body of data on the effect of dietary fats on serum cholesterol and, to a lesser extent, the serum lipoproteins. These data support the general conclusions of Keys et al. (18) and Hegsted et al. (9) that saturated fatty acids elevate and polyunsaturated fatty acids lower serum cholesterol, whereas the monounsaturated fatty acids have no specific effect. The absolute quantitative effects of the fatty acids and dietary cholesterol are probably not definable, because it is likely that they depend to some degree upon interactions between the fatty acids, cholesterol, and perhaps other dietary constituents.

What is discouraging is the conclusion that simple comparisons of two or three different diets, regardless of what they show, cannot refute the overall findings of 30 years of research. If these issues are to be further refined, they require new approaches and experimental designs. In the future, all investigators should provide clear evidence that their data are reproducible, preferably in more than one group of subjects.

Defining the effects of dietary fats upon total serum cholesterol levels is a relatively straightforward problem, but 30 years of extensive study leave many unanswered questions. Determining the effects of fats upon the various lipoproteins and many other functions will be, no doubt, substantially more difficult. If we are not to spend another 30 years on these issues, serious thought should be given to developing more effective and efficient research designs than we are using now.

Finally, it is important to remember that national dietary policies cannot be determined by the effects of diet on heart disease alone.

ACKNOWLEDGMENT

This work was supported in part by the National Institutes of Health grant RR00158 from the Division of Research Resources.

REFERENCES

1. Ahrens, E. H., Hirsch, J., Insull, W., Tsaltas, T. T., Blomstrand, R., and Peterson, M. L. (1957): *Lancet,* 1:943–953.
2. Bonanome, A., and Grundy, S. M. (1988): *N. Engl. J. Med.,* 318:1244–1248.
3. Gorbach, S. L., Morrill-LaBrode, A., and Woods, M. N., et al. (1990): *J. Am. Diet. Assoc.,* 90: 802–809.
4. Gottenbos, J. J. (1983): In: Visek, W. J., ed. *Dietary fats and health.* American Oil Chemists Society, Champaign, IL: pp. 375–390.
5. Grande, F., Anderson, J. T., and Keys, A. (1970): *Am. J. Clin. Nutr.,* 23:1184–1193.
6. Hegsted, D. M. (1985): *Nutr. Rev.,* 42:357–367.
7. Hegsted, D. M. (1989): In: *Proceedings of the Scientific Conference on Effects of Fatty Acids on Serum Lipoproteins and Hemostasis.* Washington, D.C.: American Heart Association, pp. 103–114.
8. Hegsted, D. M., and Ausman, L. M. (1989): *J. Nutr.,* 118:1184–1189.
9. Hegsted, D. M., McGandy, R. B., Myers, M. L., and Stare, F. J. (1965): *Am. J. Clin. Nutr.,* 17: 281–295.
10. Hegsted, D. M., and Nicolosi, R. J. (1990): *J. Vasc. Med. Biol.,* 2:68–73.
11. Hetzel, B. S., Charnock, J. S., Dwyer, T., and McLennan, P. L. (1989): *J. Clin. Epidemiol.,* 42: 885–893.
13. Hwang, T.-C., Guggino, S. E., and Guggino, W. B. (1990): *Proc. Natl. Acad. Sci. U.S.A.,* 87: 5706–5709.
14. Jones, D. Y., Schatzkin, A., and Green, S. B. (1978): *J. Natl. Cancer Inst.,* 79:465–471.
15. Katan, M. B., and Beynen, A. C. (1981): *Lancet,* 2:371.
16. Katan, M. B., van Gastel, A. C., de Rover, C. M., van Montfort, M. A. J., and Knuiman, J. T. (1988): *Eur. J. Clin. Invest.,* 18:644–647.
17. Keys, A. (1990): *J. Am. College Nutr.,* 9:288–291.
18. Keys, A., Anderson, J. T., and Grande, F. (1957): *Lancet,* 2:959–966.
19. Leaf, A. (1990): *Circulation,* 82:624–628.
20. Livingstone, M. B. E., Prentice, A. M., Strain, J. J., et al. (1990): *Br. Med. J.,* 300:708–712.
21. McLennan, P. L., Abeywardena, M. Y., and Charnock, J. S. (1989): *Aust. N. Z. J. Med.,* 19:1–5.
22. McLennan, P. L., Abeywardena, M. Y., and Charnock, J. S. (1990): *Am. J. Clin. Nutr.,* 51:53–58.
23. McGandy, R. B., Hegsted, D. M., and Myers, M. L. (1970): *Am. J. Clin. Nutr.,* 23:1288–1298.
24. Mann, C. (1990): *Science,* 249:476–480.
25. Mattson, F. H., and Grundy, S. M. (1985): *J. Lipid Res.,* 26:194–202.
26. Mensink, R. P., and Katan, M. B. (1989): *N. Engl. J. Med.,* 321:436–441.
27. Mensink, R. P., and Katan, M. B. (1990): *N. Engl. J. Med.,* 323:439–445.
28. Moore, D. S. (1990): In: Steen, L. A., ed. *On the shoulders of giants; new approaches to numeracy.* Washington, D.C.: National Academy Press, pp. 95–137.
29. Nicolosi, R. J., Stucchi, A. F., Kowala, M. C., Hennessy, L. K., Hegsted, D. M., and Schaefer, E. J. (1990): *Arteriosclerosis,* 10:119–128.
30. Nichols, A. B., Rosencroft, C., Lamphiear, D. E., and Ostrander, L. D. (1976): *Am. J. Clin. Nutr.,* 29:1384–1392.
31. Riemersma, R. A., Wood, D. A., Butler, S., et al. (1986): *Br. Med. J.,* 292:1423–1427.
32. Rossouw, J. E., Lewis, B., and Rifkind, B. M. (1990): *N. Engl. J. Med.,* 323:1112–1119.
33. Schoeller, D. A. (1990): *Nutr. Rev.,* 48:373–379.

34. Simpson, H. C. R., Barker, K., Carter, R. D., Cassels, E., and Mann, J. I. (1982): *Brit. Med. J.,* 285:683–684.
35. Willett, W. C., Sampson, L., Stampfer, M. J., et al. (1985): *Am. J. Epidemiol.,* 122:51–65.
36. Willett, W. C., Stampfer, M. J., Colditz, G. A., Rósner, B. A., Hennekens, C. H., and Speizer, F. E. (1987): *N. Engl. J. Med.,* 316:22–28.
37. Wood, D. A., Riemersma, R. A., Butler, S., et al. (1987): *Lancet,* 1:177–183.
38. Woollett, L. A., Spady, D. K., and Dietschy, J. M. (1989): *J. Clin. Invest.,* 84:119–128.

Atherosclerosis Reviews, Volume 23,
edited by P. C. Weber and A. Leaf.
Raven Press, Ltd., New York © 1991.

N-3 Fatty Acids: Effects on the Plasma Lipids and Lipoproteins and on Neural Development

William E. Connor

Division of Endocrinology, Metabolism and Clinical Nutrition, Department of Medicine, Oregon Health Sciences University, Portland, Oregon 97201-3098

The past 15 years have seen a veritable explosion of knowledge about the biological role of the n-3 fatty acids, especially eicosapentaenoic (EPA) and docosahexaenoic (DHA), which are derived only from marine organisms (3,4,11, 15,17,21,23,24,35,51,52). These fatty acids have diverse biological actions, which include:

1. Prostaglandin and leukotriene precursors (and inhibitors)
2. Anti–platelet aggregation; anti-thrombotic
3. Inhibit the synthesis of triglycerides (TG), very-low-density lipoproteins (VLDL), and low-density lipoproteins (LDL)
4. Hypolipidemic action
5. Anti-atherosclerotic (promotes endothelial-derived relaxing factor and inhibits cellular growth factors)
6. Immunologic effects; anti-cancer?
7. Essential fatty acids, especially for the brain, retina, and spermatozoa

Several of these actions can affect the atherosclerosis process (16,19,34,45,48); others are important in infancy. Among their most important actions are their effects on the plasma lipids and lipoproteins and their function in the development of the brain and retina in the newborn infant.

EFFECTS OF N-3 FATTY ACIDS UPON THE PLASMA LIPIDS AND LIPOPROTEINS

It has been known for more than two decades that fish oils, which contain the highly polyunsaturated n-3 fatty acids, have a hypolipidemic effect (21). However, until recently, their hypolipidemic action was considered similar to the plasma lipid-lowering caused by polyunsaturated vegetable oils rich in n-6 linoleic acid. No distinction was made between these two types of edible oils even though fish oils contain little of the n-6 linoleic acid that is so abundant in vegetable oils but instead are rich in the n-3 fatty acids, EPA (20:5) and DHA (22:6). The hypolipidemic action of polyunsaturated fat generally is related to its high amount of unsaturation rather than its content of linoleic acid.

Therefore, we set out to compare the hypotriglyceridemic actions of fish oil to polyunsaturated vegetable oils. We particularly wanted to study the metabolic differences between these two groups of polyunsaturated fats and to determine their mechanisms of action.

Hypolipidemic Effects in Normal Subjects and Hyperlipidemia Patients

We first tested the hypolipidemic actions of n-3 fatty acids supplied as salmon and salmon oil first to 12 normal adults (six men and six women) (28) and later to hyperlipidemic patients. Three diets that differed only in fatty acid composition were fed in random order for 4 weeks each: (a) a "saturated" control diet, (b) a salmon oil diet containing considerable amounts of ω-3 fatty acids, and (c) a vegetable oil diet high in ω-6 fatty acids. Each diet provided 40% of the calories as fat, 15% as protein, and 45% as carbohydrate (CHO); it also supplied about 500 mg/day of cholesterol. The control diet, designed to simulate the fatty acid composition of a typical American diet, contained cocoa butter and peanut oil. The vegetable oil diet was identical to the control diet, except that a mixture of safflower and corn oils provided the dietary fat. The salmon diet contained salmon fillets and salmon oil. Salmon was chosen as the source of ω-3 fatty acids because of its ready accessibility in the Pacific Northwest, its exceptionally good taste, and its high fat content (approximately 15%). Salmon also contains relatively high amounts of ω-3 fatty acids.

For subjects fed the salmon oil diet versus the control diet, plasma levels of cholesterol fell from 188 mg/dl to 162 mg/dl ($p < 0.001$). In similar fashion, VLDL cholesterol levels fell from 13 mg/dl to 8 mg/dl ($p < 0.001$), while LDL decreased from 128 mg/dl to 108 mg/dl ($p < 0.005$). HDL cholesterol levels were not affected by the salmon oil diet. The changes in plasma TG were most striking: from 76 mg/dl to 50 mg/dl. The polyunsaturated vegetable oils decreased the plasma cholesterol similarly but did not affect VLDL and TG levels.

The most striking finding of this study was the ability of salmon oil to lower plasma TG and VLDL levels, as well as plasma cholesterol and LDL levels, in normolipidemic subjects. Although the hypocholesterolemic effect of marine oils was a consistent finding in studies of the 1950s, its hypotriglyceridemic action was not appreciated (2,9,33,37). In more recent studies, fish oil feeding has invariably led to lower TG levels (8,50).

Our finding that, of the three fats tested, only salmon oil was hypotriglyceridemic indicates that its polyunsaturated ω-3 fatty acids have metabolic effects different than from ω-6 fatty acids. This encouraged us to begin a series of studies in hypertriglyceridemic patients (44). (The terms "n-3" and "ω-3" or "n-6" and "ω-6" are used interchangeably.) Because the depression of plasma TG and VLDL appeared to be a unique effect of ω-3 fatty acids from fish oil, we selected two groups of patients characterized by hypertriglyceridemia. Overproduction of VLDL has been a characteristic feature of most patients with hypertriglyceridemia (22).

Twenty hypertriglyceridemic patients (8 men and 12 women) volunteered for the study (44). Ten of the patients presented with increased levels of both VLDL and LDL, consistent with the type IIb phenotype, according to established criteria (20). Their mean plasma lipid levels at time of entry were 337 mg/dl for cholesterol and 355 mg/dl for TG. Clinically, many of these patients had familial combined hyperlipidemia, a disorder characterized by a strong disposition to the development of coronary heart disease (CHD) and by overproduction of lipoproteins, particularly VLDL (20).

The other 10 patients had apparent type V hyperlipidemia, as characterized by increased chylomicrons (CYM) and greatly increased VLDL levels in the fasting state. Their mean plasma lipid levels at entry were 514 mg/dl for cholesterol and 2,874 mg/dl for TG. The type V phenotype is characterized by both overproduction of VLDL and impaired clearance of the remnants of CYM and VLDL metabolism. Some type V patients belong to families with familial combined hyperlipidemia. Clinically, type V patients are characterized by episodes of abdominal pain from enlargement of abdominal viscera (hepatomegaly and splenomegaly) and by episodes of acute pancreatitis. These patients also suffer from eruptive xanthomata, neuropathy, and lipemia retinalis. Although LDL levels are low in type V patients, the presence of the atherogenic remnant particles predisposes them to the development of atherosclerotic complications, including CHD.

Two different control diets were used for the two groups of hypertriglyceridemic patients, depending on the phenotype of hyperlipidemia. Type IIb patients received their usual low-cholesterol (100 mg), low-fat (20 to 30% of total calories) diet. Subsequent dietary periods for type IIb patients consisted of a fish oil diet for 4 weeks, followed, in some patients, by a 4-week period of a diet high in a vegetable oil containing a predominance of ω-6 fatty acids. Both of these diets were balanced for cholesterol content ($\sim$250 mg/day) and contained 30% of calories as fat. The diets in all periods were eucaloric, such that the subjects neither gained nor lost weight.

For type V patients, the control diet consisted of a very-low-fat diet (5%) to lower plasma TG levels maximally (12). The next dietary interval contained fish oil at 20% or 30% of total calories. Finally, a polyunsaturated vegetable oil diet was also provided. This diet contained 20% to 30% of total calories as fat, and 200 mg to 300 mg of cholesterol. Both the fish oil and the vegetable oil diets were initially used cautiously in the type V patients in order to minimize the risk of hepatosplenomegaly, abdominal pain, and acute pancreatitis.

The salmon oil diet provided about 20 g/day of ω-3 fatty acids for an intake of 2,600 kcal, with 30% of total calories as fat. The commercial fish oil preparation supplied 30 g of ω-3 fatty acids under similar circumstances. On the other hand, the vegetable oil diet provided about 47 g of the ω-6 polyunsaturated fatty acid,

TABLE 1. *Plasma lipid and lipoprotein levels in patients with the type IIb phenotype after a diet rich in fish oil[a]*

| | Cholesterol (mg/dl) | | | | | | | |
| | Total | | VLDL | | LDL | | HDL | |
Patient no.	Control	Fish	Control	Fish	Control	Fish	Control	Fish
1	286	201	92	21	162	153	32	22
2	280	184	107	24	140	142	31	33
3	296	196	75	20	180	141	38	38
4	279	214	47	7	208	188	41	37
5	241	175	32	8	188	147	33	33
6	394	308	47	11	256	288	48	26
7	402	321	92	30	277	268	33	15
8	347	301	26	24	261	224	68	55
9	447	287	55	16	343	236	38	44
10	263	182	47	13	182	148	47	34
Mean ± S.D.	324 ± 69	236 ± 60	62 ± 28	17 ± 8	220 ± 63	194 ± 56	41 ± 11	34 ± 11
Change	−88		−45		−26		−7	
p value	<0.001		<0.001		<0.05		<0.05	

NS, not significant.

[a] To convert cholesterol and triglyceride values from milligrams per deciliter to millimoles per liter, multiply by 0.026 and 0.0113, respectively.

linoleic acid. Thus, the fish oil diets actually provided 43% to 64% less total polyunsaturated fatty acids than the vegetable oil diet, gram for gram.

The fish oil diet decreased the plasma cholesterol levels in type IIb patients by 27% (Table 1). Of individual lipoprotein cholesterol changes, the decline of VLDL cholesterol was most striking, but LDL and HDL cholesterol also de-

TABLE 2. *Plasma lipid and lipoprotein levels in patients with the type IIb phenotype after a diet rich in fish oil[a]*

| | Triglyceride (mg/dl) | | | | | |
| | Total | | VLDL | | LDL | |
Patient no.	Control	Fish	Control	Fish	Control	Fish
1	393	157	352	78	70	73
2	462	130	399	71	44	63
3	420	156	314	91	41	47
4	333	103	149	34	80	73
5	185	99	114	99	64	69
6	293	104	142	42	106	63
7	458	137	—	—	—	—
8	169	112	102	27	50	50
9	319	79	180	20	200	77
10	314	100	207	35	107	54
Mean ± S.D.	334 ± 102	118 ± 26	216 ± 112	55 ± 30	85 ± 50	63 ± 11
Change	−206		−161		−22	
p value	<0.001		<0.005		NS	

NS, not significant.

[a] To convert cholesterol and triglyceride values from milligrams per deciliter to millimoles per liter, multiply by 0.026 and 0.0113, respectively.

creased. The plasma TG changes were even greater than the cholesterol changes with the fish oil diet (−64%). This occurred largely because of the change in VLDL TG, which was lowered from 216 mg/dl to 55 mg/dl (Table 2).

The highly polyunsaturated vegetable oil diet led to less marked plasma cholesterol and TG lowering in type IIb patients, in contrast to the effects of fish oil, because the vegetable oil diet had much less effect upon VLDL cholesterol and TG. LDL values were similar; but in contrast, HDL cholesterol was higher after the vegetable oil diet. Plasma apolipoprotein changes reflected the lipoprotein lipid changes. In the type IIb patients, there were significant reductions in apoB and apoC-III levels in the fish oil period, which paralleled the declines in LDL and VLDL levels.

In the type V patients, the effects of the fish oil diet were even more striking (Figs. 1 and 2; Table 3). In subjects fed the very-low-fat control diet, initial

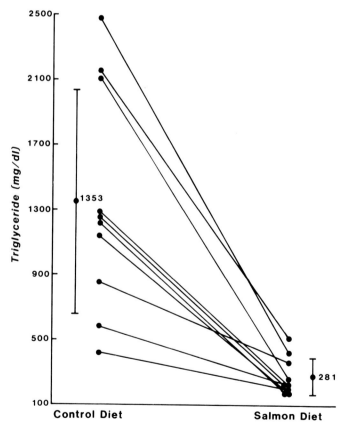

FIG. 1. The changes in plasma triglyceride levels in the 10 type V patients: control diet versus fish oil diet (Δ = −1,072 mg/dl, $p < 0.001$). (To convert triglyceride from milligrams per deciliter to millimoles per liter, multiply by 0.0113.)

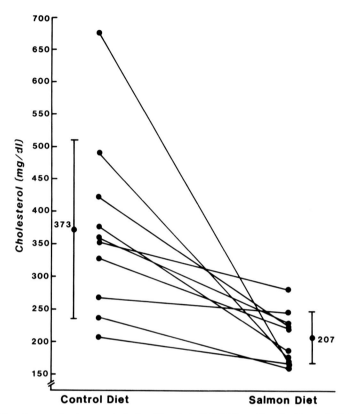

FIG. 2. The changes in plasma cholesterol levels in the 10 type V patients: control diet versus fish oil diet ($\Delta = -166$ mg/dl, $p < 0.01$). (To convert cholesterol from milligrams per deciliter to millimoles per liter, multiply by 0.026.)

plasma lipid levels declined considerably but still remained greatly elevated. Many of these patients still had milky-appearing plasma, and CYM were present in the fasting state. The first change to occur after introduction of the fish oil diet was the virtual disappearance of fasting chylomicronemia, which had been present in five of the patients. TG content of these CYM fractions declined from a mean value of 443 ± 210 to 22 ± 31 mg/dl. During the fish oil diet, total plasma TG decreased from a control value of 1,353 mg/dl to 281 mg/dl, a drop of 79% (Fig. 1). VLDL TG decreased similarly, from 1,087 mg/dl to 167 mg/ dl. Plasma cholesterol levels declined into the normal range after the fish diet, from 373 mg/dl to 207 mg/dl (Fig. 2). Most of this total plasma cholesterol decrease occurred as the result of marked changes in the amount of VLDL cholesterol, which decreased from 270 mg/dl to 70 mg/dl. Of interest was the 48% concomitant rise of LDL cholesterol, from the low value of 84 mg/dl to 125 mg/dl. Apolipoprotein levels changed to reflect the altered lipoprotein lipid levels. ApoA-1 levels did not change, whereas apoB, apoC-III, and apoE all decreased significantly.

TABLE 3. *Plasma lipid changes in eight patients with the type V phenotype after the control, vegetable-oil and fish oil diets[a]*

Plamsa lipids (mg/dl)	Control	Fish oil	Vegetable oil	p value Control vs. fish oil	p value Fish vs. vegetable oil
Total cholesterol	377 ± 155	195 ± 31	264 ± 97	<0.01	NS
Total triglyceride	1,432 ± 750	282 ± 120	841 ± 514	<0.01	<0.05
VLDL cholesterol	251 ± 148	74 ± 67	216 ± 219	<0.05	<0.05
VLDL triglyceride	1,249 ± 681	171 ± 119	550 ± 360	<0.01	NS
LDL cholesterol	77 ± 55	110 ± 34	79 ± 30	<0.05	<0.05
LDL triglyceride	70 ± 34	65 ± 18	71 ± 31	NS	NS
HDL cholesterol	31 ± 7	35 ± 12	31 ± 11	NS	NS

NS, not significant

[a] Values are means ± S.D. To convert cholesterol and triglyceride values from milligrams per deciliter to millimoles per liter, multiply by 0.026 and 0.0113, repsectively. There were no significant differences between the control and vegetable oil diets.

When the ω-6-rich vegetable oil replaced the fish oil in the diets of eight type V patients, all of them showed increases in plasma TG levels within 3 to 4 days (Table 3). After 10 to 14 days of the vegetable oil feeding, the mean plasma TG values rose 198%, and VLDL triglyceride increased from 171 mg/dl to 550 mg/dl. Plasma cholesterol also increased, from 195 mg/dl to 264 mg/dl. LDL levels, on the contrary, were decreased 28% by the vegetable oil diet—another indication that the metabolic abnormality of the type V phenotype was worsening. Because of enhanced hypertriglyceridemia and the risk of development of abdominal pain typical of this type V disorder, the vegetable oil feeding period was discontinued prematurely in all type V patients.

The disappearance of CYM after the fish oil feeding in the type V patients was also remarkable. Studies of this CYM effect have been performed in normal individuals given a fatty meal for breakfast with different background diets. When the background diet consisted of ω-3 fatty acids, the usual fat tolerance curve—with TG increases at 4 hr to 6 hr of one to three times the fasting TG values—was not observed at all (25). When the background diet consisted of the typical American, more saturated fat diet or one containing the ω-6 vegetable oils, the usual fat tolerance curve was inscribed. These data suggested either that CYM were not formed as usual, perhaps because of a disturbance of fat absorption, or else were removed much more rapidly. The absorption of ω-3 fatty acids from fish oil was, however, complete, as indicated by stool fat balance studies. Therefore, our hypothesis that smaller CYM were synthesized by the intestinal mucosa and were, in turn, removed more rapidly.

Mechanism of the Hypolipidemic Effects of Fish Oil

Two further experiments have determined how ω-3 fatty acids decrease the levels of plasma TG and cholesterol. One focused on the inhibition by fish oil of the usual hypertriglyceridemia that inevitably results when a high-CHO diet is suddenly fed to humans (25); the other examined the effects of fish oil on VLDL and LDL production and turnover.

The well-known phenomenon of CHO-induced hypertriglyceridemia is a physiologic response. In this model, VLDL triglyceride synthesis is stimulated as dietary CHO intake abruptly increases. The increased VLDL synthesis leads to hypertriglyceridemia, which may persist for many weeks (1,38,47,54). If ω-3 fatty acids do inhibit VLDL synthesis, then the usual CHO-induced hyper-triglyceridemia should not occur when fish oil is incorporated into the high-CHO diet.

Seven mildly hypertriglyceridemic but otherwise healthy subjects (ages, 22 to 54 years) were fed three different experimental diets (25). Each was composed of a liquid formula plus three bran muffins per day to supply fiber. The baseline diet contained 45% from CHO. The two high-CHO diets (control and fish oil) contained 15%, 10%, and 75% of calories as fat, protein, and CHO, respectively. In the baseline and high-CHO control diets, a blend of peanut oil and cocoa butter provided the fat, which was replaced by fish oil, in the form of a com-mercially available marine lipid concentrate, in the high-CHO fish oil diet. The total amount of fish oil consumed per day was 50 g (in a 3,000-kcal diet), equiv-alent to approximately 3.5 tablespoons of oil. This amount provided 8.5 g of EPA (C20:5 ω-3) and 5.5 g of DHA (22:6 ω-3).

The three experimental diets were fed in three different sequences at our Clinical Research Center (Fig. 3). In the first sequence, the high-CHO control diet preceded the high-CHO fish oil diet (Fig. 3A). In the second sequence, the high-CHO diet was given for 20 days instead of 10 days to demonstrate that the hypertriglyceridemia did not spontaneously resolve after the first 10 days. It was then followed by the fish oil diet (Fig. 3B). In the third sequence, the fish oil was fed first with the high-CHO diet for 25 days and then removed to permit the effects of the high CHO to be manifest for the next 15 days (Fig. 3C). Three subjects were studied with the first sequence, and two subjects each were studied with the second and third sequences.

In all seven subjects, the high-CHO control diet increased the plasma TG levels over the baseline diet: from 105 mg/dl to 194 mg/dl (data not shown). The magnitude of the CHO-induced hypertriglyceridemia correlated significantly with each individual's baseline TG levels. The rise in plasma TG levels was complete by day 5 and resulted almost entirely from an increase in the VLDL triglyceride fraction, which more than doubled during the control diet: from 69 mg/dl to 156 mg/dl (Fig. 4). Although the total plasma cholesterol levels did not change, VLDL cholesterol levels approximately doubled from 18 mg/dl to 34 mg/dl. LDL fell from 125 mg/dl to 106 mg/dl and HDL cholesterol was reduced from 49 mg/dl to 41 mg/dl.

When the fat of the high-CHO control diet was replaced isocalorically with fish oil, the elevated plasma TG concentration was reduced from 194 mg/dl to 75 mg/dl, a decrease of 61%. This decrease usually occurred within 3 days (Fig. 3A). Once again, changes in VLDL triglyceride levels were largely responsible

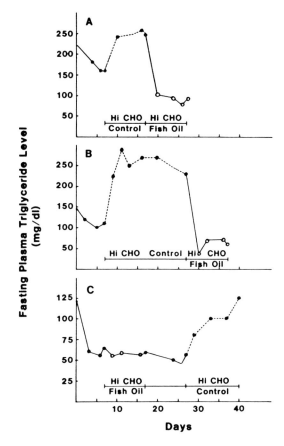

FIG. 3. Effects of the baseline diet and the control and fish oil diets on plasma triglyceride levels in three subjects. We see the reversal of carbohydrate-induced hypertriglyceridemia by dietary fish oil (**A**), the persistence of the hypertriglyceridemia (throughout 20 days) and the subsequent reversal by fish oil (**B**), and the prevention of carbohydrate-induced hypertriglyceridemia by fish oil (**C**).

for this effect (156 mg/dl to 34 mg/dl). Total cholesterol levels decreased insignificantly during the high-CHO fish oil diet—from 172 mg/dl to 153 mg/dl—primarily because of the drop in VLDL cholesterol levels (34 mg/dl to 12 mg/dl).

When the period of CHO induction was prolonged from 10 to 20 days, the hypertriglyceridemia persisted and did not significantly decrease until the high-CHO fish oil diet began (Fig. 3B). When the high-CHO fish oil diet followed the baseline diet, the plasma TG level did not rise, but the level increased when the high-CHO control diet was fed subsequently (Fig. 3C). The high-CHO control diet decreased the levels of apoB and increased apoC-III concentrations; apoA-1 and apoE levels did not change. The high-CHO fish oil diet decreased apoA-1 and apoC-III levels; apoB and apoE concentrations did not change.

The incorporation of corn oil in place of fish oil into the high-CHO regimen did not affect the induced hypertriglyceridemia. For the three subjects who participated in this corn oil study, TG levels were measured in milligrams per deciliter: baseline, 93 ± 23; high-CHO control, 196 ± 58; high-CHO corn oil,

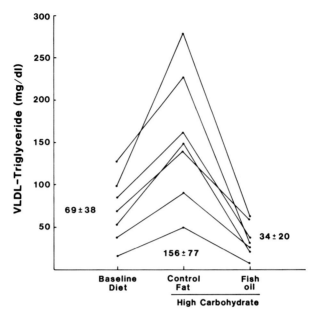

FIG. 4. The effects of the high carbohydrate control and fish oil diets upon the plasma VLDL triglyceride levels in the seven subjects.

215 ± 90; and high-CHO fish oil, 86 ± 10. In this study, dietary fish oil not only prevented but also rapidly reversed the dietary, CHO-induced elevations in plasma TG and VLDL levels, whereas the ω-6 fatty acid rich corn oil had no effect at all. Because the primary difference between corn oil and the commercial fish oil preparation is the *type* of polyunsaturated fatty acids present (corn, 57% 18:2 ω-6; linoleic acid; the commercially available fish oil preparation, 32% ω-3 fatty acids), the difference was probably due to the ω-3 fatty acids in the fish oil. This finding suggests that ω-3 fatty acids inhibit hepatic VLDL production.

Dietary fish oil probably affects either the synthesis or the removal of VLDL. The hypothesis that ω-3 fatty acids reduces VLDL levels by inhibiting its synthesis was further supported by a study designed to elucidate the hypotriglyceridemic effect of ω-3 fatty acids (26). The rates of flux and turnover of VLDL TG were measured after injection of [³H]glycerol into subjects fed one of two diets. One contained fish oil; the other, fats typical of the American diet. This technique allowed us to calculate both the rate of synthesis and the rate of removal of VLDL.

We selected 10 male subjects with a wide range of fasting plasma TG concentrations (34 to 4,180 mg/dl) to test the hypothesis about the mechanism of action of dietary fish oils in subjects with greatly different pool sizes of plasma TG. Liquid formula diets containing 15% to 20% fat, 65% to 75% CHO, and 10% to 15% protein were fed during both the control and the fish oil dietary periods.

The two diets differed only in the type of fat they contained. In the control diet, a blend of cocoa butter and peanut oil (1:2) was incorporated into the formulas. In the fish oil period, the fish oil was taken in three doses daily rather than being mixed into the formulas. The principal difference was the higher content of linoleic acid (C18:2 ω-6) in the control diet and the presence of ω-3 fatty acids in the fish oil diet. The control contained virtually no ω-3 fatty acids, whereas the fish oil provided about 17 g/day of these highly polyunsaturated fatty acids.

The experimental diets were consumed for a period of 3 weeks to 5 weeks before the actual VLDL turnover procedure was conducted. This time was needed for the plasma TG levels to stabilize, particularly in the subjects whose TG levels were above normal. Seven subjects consumed the control diet first, followed by the fish oil diet; in the remaining three, the order was reversed. The order in which the diets were administered did not affect the results.

The isocaloric substitution of fish oil for the control vegetable fat produced the expected significant reductions in the total and lipoprotein lipid levels in all 10 subjects. The mean values for the normal and hypertriglyceridemic groups are given in Table 4. Total cholesterol levels for all 10 subjects fell from 195 mg/dl to 144 mg/dl, a reduction of 22% ($p < 0.025$). Decreases in VLDL levels accounted for most of the drop in plasma cholesterol (83 mg/dl to 21 mg/dl; $p < 0.005$). LDL cholesterol levels did not change significantly, whereas HDL cholesterol concentrations fell from 31 mg/dl to 24 mg/dl ($p < 0.005$). All of these changes were evident in both groups (Table 4).

After the administration of [^{3}H]glycerol and its incorporation into the TG of

TABLE 4. *The effects of fish oil[a] upon plasma lipid and lipoprotein levels (means ± SD in mg/dl)*

	Cholesterol				Triglyceride	
	Total	VLDL	LDL	HDL	Total	VLDL
Normal (n = 3)						
Control						
Commercial fish oil	151 ± 0.5	14 ± 6	106 ± 23	39 ± 7	102 ± 34	62 ± 34
preparation	129 ± 9	3 ± 2	90 ± 14	40 ± 9	48 ± 10	13 ± 3
Hyperlipidemic (n = 7)						
Control	213 ± 36[b]	113 ± 56[c]	79 ± 36	27 ± 5[c]	581 ± 255[c]	542 ± 257[c]
Commercial fish oil preparation	147 ± 42	29 ± 15	108 ± 59	16 ± 5	194 ± 74	118 ± 71
Total (n = 10)						
Control	195 ± 44[c]	83 ± 66[c]	87 ± 34	31 ± 8[c]	442 ± 314[b]	398 ± 317[c]
Commercial fish oil preparation	144 ± 40	21 ± 17	103 ± 50	24 ± 13	150 ± 93	87 ± 77

No symbol, not significant.
[a] Control fats and commercial fish oil preparation were fed at 15% to 20% of total calories.
[b] $p < 0.025$.
[c] $p < 0.005$.

TABLE 5. *Effects of dietary fish oil on VLDL metabolism*

Subject	Diet	VLDL Lipids		VLDL-TG pool size (g)	VLDL-triglyceride synthesis		VLDL-TG FCR (h^{-1})	Residence time of VLDL-TG in plasma (hr)	Fast/slow synthetic pathway (ratio)
		TG^a (mg/dl)	Chol/TG (ratio)		(mg/h)	(mg/kg IBW)			
Mean ± SD	Control	330 ± 282	0.18 ± 0.3	11.4 ± 10.2	1685 ± 1073	23.0 ± 14.3	0.23 ± 0.12	5.8 ± 3.4	2.3 ± 0.79
	Fish Oil	92 ± 67	0.25 ± 0.08	3.2 ± 2.5	918 ± 563	12.6 ± 7.5	0.38 ± 0.16	3.2 ± 1.6	2.4 ± 1.34
p value		<0.005	<0.05	<0.025	<0.005	<0.005	<0.005	<0.005	NS
Percent change		−72%	+39%	−72%	−46%	−45%	+65%	−45%	+3%
Normal values (n = 13)		113 ± 10	0.21 ± 0.01		806 ± 123	11.5 ± 1.8	0.19 ± 0.01	5.2 ± 0.38	2.7 ± 0.36

[a] Represents the average VLDL-TG concentration during the 48-hr turnover study.

VLDL, the kinetic decay curves were analyzed by a computer-model system, so that VLDL synthesis and turnover could be calculated (26). The incorporation of ω-3 fatty acids into the diet caused a 72% decrease in the VLDL triglyceride pool size (11.4 g to 3.2 g; $p < 0.025$) (Table 5). The decreased pool size was associated with a 45% reduction in the VLDL TG synthetic rate (23 mg/hr/IW to 12.6 mg/hr/IW; $p < 0.005$) and a 45% decrease in the prevalence time of VLDL TG in the plasma (5.8 hr to 3.2 hr; $p < 0.005$). The reciprocal of the prevalence time is the fractional catabolic rate (FCR), which was increased by 65% (0.23 hr^{-1} to 0.38 hr^{-1}; $p < 0.005$). There was a significant rise in the cholesterol/TG ratio in VLDL during the fish oil interval (0.18 to 0.25; $p < 0.05$). Finally, the ratio of the fast to the slow synthetic pathways did not change with fish oil feeding. The same trends were seen in both normal and hypertriglyceridemic patients. Similar results have also been found using a slightly different dietary plan with the addition of apoB labeling (39).

Direct evidence that the hepatic synthesis of TG and VLDL is suppressed by ω-3 fatty acids from fish oil has been supplied by three *in vitro* studies of the perfused rat liver and of liver cells from rats and rabbits in primary culture (5,55,56). In all studies, TG synthesis was reduced. In one, enhanced ketone body production resulted; in the others, there was a diversion of ω-3 fatty acids from TG synthesis into phospholipid synthesis. Taking the net results of all of these studies together, the evidence is very strong that suppression of VLDL and TG synthesis is a primary mechanism of ω-3 acids to explain their hypolipidemic effects.

Divergent or Conflicting Results

Many other studies throughout the world have confirmed the TG lowering action of fish oil even when it was administered as a supplement with little or no dietary control (23). However, in many of these experiments, LDL increased, particularly in type IV hyperlipidemia but also in a few patients with familial combined hyperlipidemia (18,23,29). ApoB concentrations were lowered in some of the metabolically controlled studies but increased somewhat in other studies (18,23,44).

Because of vastly different experimental conditions, it is difficult to interpret the effects of fish oil in various hyperlipidemic patients. In some studies, fish oil was simply added as a supplement to the usual diet in doses of 8 to 16/g day. In the control period, a placebo such as olive oil or safflower oil was not always utilized. Other studies employed a standard American diet supplemented with a placebo oil. Furthermore, various kinds of fish oil have been used, some containing a considerable amount of cholesterol and saturated fat. Newer fish oils are much less saturated; they contain higher concentrations of ω-3 fatty acids and have a very low cholesterol content. (See Table 6 for lipid analyses of various fish oils and fish.)

TABLE 6. *Fat and ω-3 fatty acid content of fish and fish oils[a]*
(100 g, edible portion, raw)

	Fat (gm)	ω-3 fatty acids[b] (gm)
Fish		
Anchovy, European	4.8	1.4
Bass, striped	2.3	0.8
Bluefish	6.5	1.2
Carp	5.6	0.3
Catfish, channel	4.3	0.3
Cod, Atlantic	0.7	0.3
Cod, Pacific	0.6	0.2
Flounder, unspecified	1.0	0.2
Haddock	0.7	0.2
Halibut, Pacific	2.3	0.4
Herring, Atlantic,	9.0	1.6
Herring, Pacific	13.9	1.7
Mackerel, Atlantic	13.9	2.5
Mullet, unspecified	4.4	1.1
Ocean perch	1.6	0.2
Pike, Walleye	1.2	0.3
Pompano, Florida	9.5	0.6
Sablefish	15.3	1.4
Salmon, Atlantic	5.4	1.2
Salmon, Chinook	10.4	1.4
Salmon, pink	3.4	1.0
Salmon, Sockeye	8.6	1.2
Sardines, in sardine oil	15.5	3.3
Shark	1.9	0.5
Snapper, red	1.2	0.2
Sole	1.2	0.1
Sturgeon	3.3	0.3
Swordfish	2.1	0.2
Trout, brook	2.7	0.4
Trout, lake	9.7	1.6
Trout, rainbow	3.4	0.5
Tuna	2.5	0.5
Crustaceans		
Crab, Alaska King	0.8	0.3
Crab, Dungeness	1.0	0.3
Crayfish, unspecified	1.4	0.1
Lobster, Northern	0.9	0.2
Shrimp, unspecified	1.1	0.3
Mollusks		
Abalone, New Zealand	1.0	tr
Clam, hardshell	0.6	tr
Clam, Littleneck	0.8	tr
Mussel, blue	2.2	0.5
Octopus, common	1.0	0.2
Oyster, Pacific	2.3	0.6
Scallop, unspecified	0.8	0.2
Squid, unspecified	1.1	0.3
Fish Oils		
Cod liver oil	100.0	18.5
Herring oil	100.0	11.4
MaxEPA[c]	100.0	29.4
Promega[d]	100.0	44.2
Salmon oil	100.0	19.9

[a] Data taken from Hepburn, F. N., Exler, J., Weihrauch, J. L. (1986): Provisional tables on the content of ω-3 fatty acids and other fat components of selected foods. *J. Am. Diet. Assoc.*, 86:788–793.

[b] 20:5 plus 22:6.

[c] Analysis by the Atherosclerosis Research Laboratory, 1987.

[d] Concentrated fish body oils.

Several conclusions have emerged from the wide variety of studies, most of which have not been metabolically controlled. Fish oil is most effective when administered at 6% to 30% of total calories and when the diet is metabolically controlled. In these studies, LDL was usually lowered. In addition, profound VLDL and TG lowering has been reported in normal subjects and in a wide variety of hyperlipidemic states. In our experience, this lowering of plasma cholesterol levels occurs in patients with types V, IIa, IIb, III, and IV hyperlipidemia; the most dramatic results occur in type V patients who do not tolerate any other kind of dietary fat (11,24,44). In our experience, which has generally been corroborated by other investigators, HDL levels are not greatly affected by fish oil. Clearly, the use of fish oil in hyperlipidemia must be individualized in terms of use and dosage.

At lower dosages, when fish oil was used as a supplement, TG lowering is usually observed. Paradoxically, in some studies, levels of cholesterol and LDL did not change after fish oil; whereas in other studies, some increases were seen in LDL and apoB. Why plasma LDL and apoB at times increase after fish oil when at the same time plasma VLDL and TG decrease is a challenging question (23). This effect may relate to fundamental aspects of VLDL-LDL metabolism. Normally, LDL is derived from two sources—conversion from VLDL and direct synthesis by the liver. The catabolism of VLDL is likewise in two directions through intermediate-density lipoprotein (IDL). IDL may be removed by the apoE receptor in the liver or converted to LDL.

The experiments of Huff and Telford suggest why in some instances fish oil might increase LDL (32). Turnover studies in the miniature pig revealed that fish oil feeding increased the proportion of VLDL being converted to LDL. Apparently, the ω-3 fatty acids of fish oil produce a smaller VLDL particle that is more likely to be converted to LDL. However, LDL concentrations did not increase because the reduction of the direct synthesis of LDL caused by the fish oil was greater than the increase in LDL from VLDL. Although these pig studies await confirmation in humans, they do explain why LDL may increase in some humans fed fish oil: More VLDL is converted to LDL and direct LDL synthesis does not decrease; the net result is more LDL.

Summary and Conclusions

In the experimental studies reported here, dietary ω-3 fatty acids from fish and fish oil had profound hypolipidemic effects in normal subjects and in hypertriglyceridemic patients with combined hyperlipidemia (type IIb) and type V hyperlipidemia. A study population of 68 adults participated in carefully controlled metabolic experiments. In all cases, there were marked reductions in plasma cholesterol and TG concentrations; TG lowering was especially great. There were also reductions in VLDL, CYM, remnants, LDL, apoB, and apoE. The HDL changes were inconstant and varied from subject to subject.

Whereas the mechanism of the hypolipidemic action of the ω-6–rich vegetable oils containing linoleic acid such as corn or safflower oil still remains obscure, the mechanism of action of the ω-3 fatty acids in fish oil has been well documented within a few years of their use as hypolipidemic agents. The synthesis of TG and VLDL in the liver is greatly reduced by ω-3 fatty acids. At the same time, the turnover of VLDL in plasma is greatly shortened, and LDL production is decreased.

Combined with other dietary manipulations, such as a reduction in saturated fat and dietary cholesterol, the use of ω-3 fatty acids to treat hyperlipidemic and especially hypertriglyceridemic patients would appear to have a well-supported rationale. Further studies are required to determine exact doses and precise indications for different types of hyperlipidemia and to differentiate the effects if any, of the two major ω-3 fatty acids in fish oil, EPA and DHA. Coupled with the known anti-thrombotic actions of ω-3 fatty acids from fish oil because of changes in prostaglandin secretion and platelet function, these hypolipidemic effects have an important potential role in the control of CHD and other atherosclerotic disorders.

EFFECTS OF N-3 FATTY ACIDS AS ESSENTIAL FATTY ACIDS FOR THE BRAIN AND RETINA

A diet deficient in n-3 fatty acids leads to a triad of signs in the rhesus monkey: visual impairment, abnormalities of the electroretinogram (ERG), and polydipsia (13,42,43,46). Profound biochemical changes in the fatty acid composition of the membranes of the retina, brain, and other organs accompany these other disturbances (36,42). Low concentrations of n-3 fatty acids occur at birth in the plasma, red blood cells, and neural tissues of infants born from mothers fed an n-3–deficient diet (43). Docosahexaenoic acid (DHA, 22:6 n-3), an n-3 fatty acid that is uniquely rich in neural membranes, is found in very low concentrations in these infant monkeys. These concentrations even become lower when the deficient diet is continued postnatally. By 4 weeks of age, visual impairment can be demonstrated; shortly after that, abnormalities of the ERG are seen (41–43). Polydipsia develops later in life (36).

DHA is the most prominent fatty acid of the retina, brain, and spermatozoa. It generally occupies the sn-2 position of the phospholipid membranes of these organs (36). It is especially concentrated in the outer segment membranes of the retinal rod and cone photoreceptors and in the synaptosomes of the cerebral cortex. Other functions of the n-3 fatty acids are currently being described, such as serving as precursors of prostaglandins and eicosanoids and perhaps also as inhibitors of the n-6 series of prostaglandins.

In contrast to the more obvious clinical stigmata of n-6 fatty acid deficiency, the findings of n-3 deficiency are far more subtle, as might be expected for a fatty acid class required for neural membranes. N-3 fatty acid–deficient rhesus

TABLE 7. *Characteristics of n-3 and n-6 essential fatty acids deficiencies*

	n-3	n-6
Clinical features	Normal skin, growth and reproduction Reduced learning Abnormal electroretinogram Impaired vision Polydipsia	Growth retardation Skin lesions Reproductive failure Fatty liver Polydipsia
Biochemical markers	Decreased 18:3 n-3 and 22:6 n-3 Increased 22:4 n-6 and 22:5 n-6 Increased 20:3 n-9 (only if n-6 also low)	Decreased 18:2 n-6 and 20:4 n-6 Increased 20:3 n-9 (only if n-3 also low)

monkeys appear grossly normal even after long-term depletion. The fur and the skin do not show the conspicuous dermatitis found in n-6 fatty acid deficiency. Fatty liver does not occur either. Table 7 illustrates the characteristic clinical and biochemical differences of the two essential fatty acid series, n-6 and n-3. Although n-6 fatty acid deficiency has often been described in both animals and humans (10,30), until recently, n-3 fatty acid deficiency, because it is less conspicuous in its symptomatology, has been less well categorized. At times, it has even been combined with n-6 fatty acid deficiency (6,7,31,53).

Methods

Rhesus monkeys were examined after a combination of maternal and postnatal deprivation of dietary n-3 fatty acids. Throughout pregnancy, the adult female monkeys were given a semipurified diet with safflower oil as the only fat source (43). Their infants were fed the same liquid diet from birth onward. Safflower oil is particularly low in n-3 fatty acids; less than 0.3% of its total fatty acids are in the form of linolenic acid (18:3 n-3). Safflower oil is especially high in n-6 fatty acids; the ratio of n-6 to n-3 fatty acids was about 250:1. Mothers and infants in the control group received similar diets except that the fat source was soybean oil, which provides 7.7% of total fatty acids as in the form of linolenic acid and has an n-6 to n-3 ratio of 7:1. The more highly polyunsaturated fatty acids of the n-3 series, such as EPA and DHA, were not present in these diets.

To test the reversibility of the deficiency, five of the deficient offspring were repleted with very long chain and highly polyunsaturated n-3 fatty acids from fish oil beginning at 10 to 24 months of age (14). In the repletion diet, fish oil replaced 80% of the safflower oil. The remaining safflower oil provided ample n-6 linoleic acid (4.5% of calories), and the fish oil supplied large amounts of n-3 fatty acids, including DHA (22:6) and EPA (20:5).

Plasma, erythrocytes, and tissue samples including whole retina and cerebral cortex were analyzed for fatty acid composition by capillary column gas-liquid chromatography after separation of total phospholipids or individual phospho-lipid classes by thin-layer chromatography (14). In the repletion study, the fatty acids of plasma and erythrocytes were determined. In addition, in order to follow the time course of the biochemical changes, serial biopsies of the frontal cortical gray matter were obtained for fatty acid analysis after craniotomy.

Visual acuity was measured by the preferential-looking method, as described previously (43). The specific physiological effects of n-3 fatty acid deficiency on the function of the retina were examined by the ERG (41).

Results

Fatty Acid Composition of Plasma and Tissues

Dietary deprivation of n-3 fatty acids resulted in low plasma and red blood cell concentrations of all n-3 fatty acids (Fig. 5). Especially notable was the low concentration of n-3 fatty acids even at birth in the deficient monkeys. The n-3 fatty acid concentrations in the plasma of their mothers was also <50% of controls. In the deficient animals, the n-3 fatty acids were barely detectable by 24 weeks of age in the phospholipids of plasma and erythrocytes; by contrast, there were appreciable concentrations in the control animals.

The brain and retina had also very low levels of n-3 fatty acids and, in particular, DHA. In deficient animals at or near birth, DHA concentrations in phosphati-dylethanolamine were reduced by 50% in the retina and 75% in the cerebral cortex compared to the control values (Fig. 6). The proportion of DHA in both tissues doubled between birth and 22 months of age in control monkeys but failed to increase in the deficient group; thus, by 22 months, DHA concentrations in deficient monkeys were reduced to 15% to 20% of control values. It is notable that n-6 fatty acids—22:5 particularly—compensatorily increased in response to the reduced DHA, so that polyunsaturation of the phospholipid membranes was preserved as much as possible. This n-6 fatty acid comprises <1% of total fatty acids in the tissue phospholipids of normal animals; but in 22-month-old deficient animals, it rose to ~20% in the phosphatidylethanolamine of the cerebral cortex and nearly 30% in the retina.

After dietary repletion with fish oil, these changes in fatty acid composition were rapidly reversed, as indicated by changes in plasma phospholipids, red blood cells, and biopsy specimens of frontal cortex (14) (Fig. 7). The changes in the fatty acid composition of the frontal cortex also occurred rapidly, as early as 1 week after fish oil supplementation. By 24–28 weeks, the DHA in phos-phatidylethanolamine increased from 4.2% to 29.3% of total fatty acids (Fig. 8) compared to the 22.3% in soybean oil–fed control animals. Of interest with regard to membrane function was the fact that EPA and 22:5 n-3 both increased from 0% to ~3% in the cerebral cortex. At the same time, the concentrations of 22:5 n-6 and other longer chain n-6 fatty acids decreased.

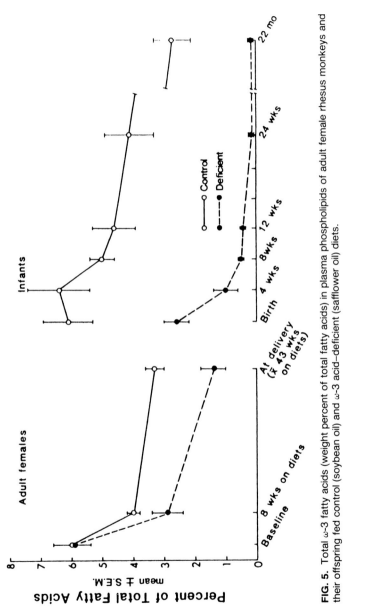

FIG. 5. Total ω-3 fatty acids (weight percent of total fatty acids) in plasma phospholipids of adult female rhesus monkeys and their offspring fed control (soybean oil) and ω-3 acid–deficient (safflower oil) diets.

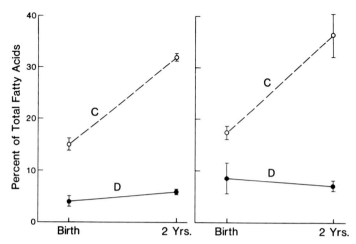

FIG. 6. The concentrations of docosahexaenoic acid (DHA) in the cerebral cortex (**left**) and retina (**right**) of control animals (C) and deficient animals (D) as provided by birth and at 2 years. Note that at birth both retina and cerebral cortex had much higher levels of DHA than deficient animals, but these disparities increase greatly after 2 years of development.

Visual Function and Electroretinograms

The visual acuity of n-3 fatty acid–deficient infants was reduced by half at 8 and 12 weeks of age (Fig. 9), as previously reported (43). Furthermore, deficient monkeys developed a number of abnormalities in the ERG (41). The timing of the ERG response was altered, with significant delays in the peak latency (time to the B-wave peak) of both cone and rod responses (Fig. 10). In contrast to previous studies in n-3 fatty acid deficient rats, differences in response amplitudes were not detected at 7 to 24 months of age. However, more recent recordings of younger infants at 3 to 4 months of age have demonstrated clear differences in the A-wave amplitudes of both rod and cone responses. The reason for the transient nature of this effect is unknown. Deficient animals also showed a specific abnormality in the rate of recovery of the ERG response after an initial bright flash. This effect was present at 3 months but increased in magnitude with age. With an interval of 3.2 sec between flashes, response amplitude in the deficient animals was reduced nearly twice as much as in controls, relative to the maximal amplitude seen to the first flash or to flashes presented at long (20-sec) intervals (Fig. 11). Thus, recovery of the capacity to generate a full ERG response was significantly slowed.

In deficient monkeys repleted with fish oil, ERG were recorded at 3, 6, and 9 months after the beginning of the repletion phase. Despite the increase in n-3 fatty acid levels in tissues, no improvement was seen in either peak latencies or in the ERG recovery function (14).

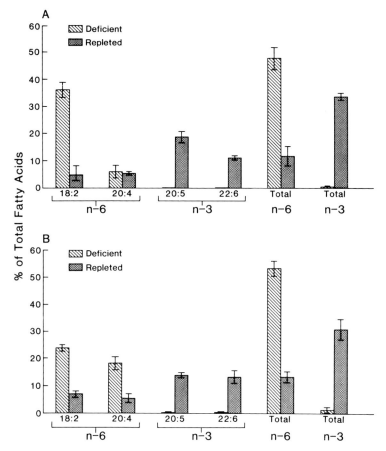

FIG. 7. The fatty acids of the plasma phospholipids (**A**) and erythrocyte phospholipids (**B**) in n-3 fatty acid–deficient monkeys as compared with monkeys replete with fish oil. Note the reciprocal relationships between the n-3 and n-6 fatty acids, with n-3 fatty acids increasing after the fish oil repletion diet and n-6 fatty acids diminishing greatly from the deficient state.

Polydipsia in Deficient Monkeys

Cage behavior in n-3 fatty acid deficient and control monkeys was monitored by videotaping. The deficient monkeys visited the water spouts of their cages much more often than did control monkeys, suggesting the possibility of greater water intake. A study of 24-hr water intakes was then carried out to confirm and quantify this difference (46). Figure 12 depicts the monkeys' mean water intake over 24 hr. The intake for deficient monkeys was almost four times that for control monkeys (264 g/kg versus 70 g/kg). The excretion or output was necessarily a combined output of feces and water because the urine was mixed with soft stools. The output was also more than double for deficient monkeys

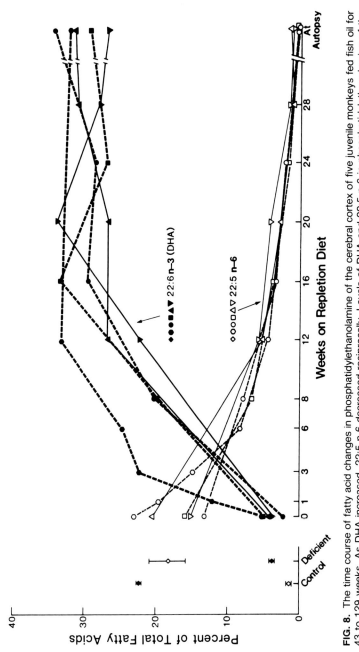

FIG. 8. The time course of fatty acid changes in phosphatidylethanolamine of the cerebral cortex of five juvenile monkeys fed fish oil for 43 to 129 weeks. As DHA increased, 22:5 n-6 decreased reciprocally. Levels of DHA and 22:5 n-6 in phosphatidylethanolamine of the frontal cortex of monkeys fed control (soybean oil) and deficient diets from a previous study (24) are given for comparison. DHA and 22:5 n-6 in control monkeys were 22.3 ± 0.3% and 21.4 ± 0.3% of total fatty acids, respectively. DHA and 22:5 n-6 in the deficient monkeys were 3.8 ± 0.4% and 18.3 ± 2.5%, respectively.

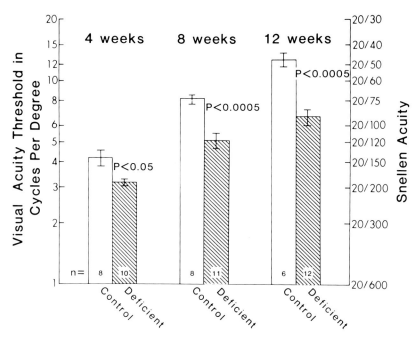

FIG. 9. Visual acuity thresholds (mean SEM) as determined by the preferential-looking method for control and ω-3 fatty acid–deficient infant monkeys. Thresholds are expressed in cycles per degree of visual angle and in the equivalent Snellen values. The *p* values for statistical significance were determined by Student's *t* test.

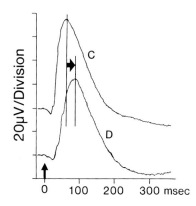

FIG. 10. Representative ERG waveforms from control and ω-3 fatty acid–deficient monkeys under conditions selectively stimulating the rod system. The vertical arrow indicates time of flash. B-wave peak latencies were delayed in the deficient group; vertical lines have been drawn through the peaks to aid comparison.

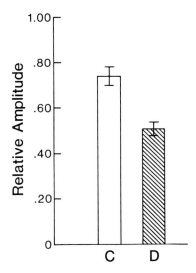

FIG. 11. Relative B-wave amplitude (mean SEM) of the ERG elicited by flashes at 3.2-sec intervals, as a percent of the maximal amplitude produced at intervals of 20 sec or more. Relative amplitude is significantly reduced in the deficient group ($p < 0.01$).

(268 g/kg versus 121 g/kg) (Fig. 12). These input and output studies were repeated on several different occasions with similar results in monkeys of varying ages (from 1.8 months to young adulthood).

Although the mechanism of the polydipsia is not yet understood, several possible explanations can be eliminated. The effect is probably not caused by an osmotic imbalance. Dietary electrolytes and serum electrolytes were similar in both control and deficient animals. Fasting glucose levels were normal, indicating that polydipsia did not result from fluid losses as a result as diabetes. The blood urine nitrogen and creatinine levels were also equal and normal, and there was no indication of renal insufficiency in either group.

Polydipsia does occur in ω-6 dietary deficiency because of increased skin permeability and the resulting loss of water by evaporation. However, the skin and fur of the deficient animals appeared completely normal. The amount of ω-6 fatty acids in the diet was actually 50% higher in deficient than in control monkeys. Increased fluid consumption could not have been activated by a diet deficient in calories because the deficient and control monkeys received the same amount of food. Investigations are now under way to describe possible hormonal and prostaglandin mechanisms of the polydipsia.

Discussion

This study has shown that dietary n-3 fatty acid deficiency leads to severe and progressive depletion of n-3 fatty acids from the plasma and from all tissues analyzed, including red blood cells, liver, skin, fat, cerebral cortex, and retina. In particular, the very long chain n-3 fatty acid, DHA, 22:6, was selectively depleted from neural and retinal phospholipids and was replaced by n-6 fatty

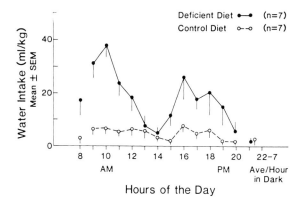

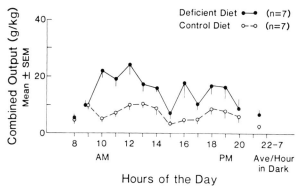

FIG. 12. The mean hourly water intake (ml/kg) over a 24-hr period and the hourly mean output of combined urine and feces (g/kg) over 24 hr. "Ave/Hour in Dark" refers to the measurement taken at the end of the 10-hr dark period divided by 10.

acids,—in particular, 22:5. Associated with these biochemical changes was a significant impairment in the development of visual acuity and abnormalities in the ERG.

In the initial experiments, linolenic acid (18:3) was the only dietary source of n-3 fatty acids. In the control animals, DHA was synthesized by successive and multiple steps of desaturation and elongation from linolenic acid. DHA then selectively accumulated in brain and retinal phospholipids, particularly in the phosphatidylethanolamine and phosphatidylserine fractions (13). The conversion of linolenic acid to DHA may occur in the liver, in the brain or retina, or in the placenta during fetal development. In the deficient monkeys, the dietary supply of linolenic acid was insufficient to support the synthesis of adequate levels of DHA; high levels of dietary linoleic acid may also have suppressed the synthesis of DHA from the available linolenic acid (49). However, during intrauterine life, our experimental monkeys probably received some DHA directly from their mothers via the placenta. Although deficient mothers had been receiving the n-3 fatty acid–deficient diet for at least 2 months before conception, their stores of DHA probably were depleted very slowly. The plasma of newborn deficient infants and their mothers revealed the presence of some DHA. The levels were consistently higher in the infants' plasma than in the mothers' plasma (selective biomagnification). However, plasma concentrations of DHA were much lower in the deficient infants than in controls. Once the infants were removed from any maternal sources of n-3 fatty acids, their plasma levels fell rapidly. They were permanently separated from their mothers at birth and therefore did not have access to maternal milk, a natural source of DHA.

DHA is the predominant fatty acid in phospholipids of the retina, particularly in the outer segment membranes of the photoreceptor cells. This fatty acid is thought to be responsible for the special biophysical properties of the outer segment membranes, which contain the visual pigment (41). Depletion of DHA from these membranes would be expected to alter their physical properties and therefore the efficiency of the visual process. It is also possible that DHA has a more specific biochemical function in the retina. In addition, DHA is a major fatty acid of brain gray matter and especially of synaptic membranes which, like photoreceptor membranes, are excitable and highly fluid. Thus, the change in membrane phospholipid composition produced by n-3 fatty acid deficiency might alter the transmission of information through the brain's visual pathways as well as affecting the photoreceptive process in the retina.

A few cases of n-3 fatty acid deficiency have been described in humans. Holman et al. reported a clinical case of peripheral neuropathy and blurred vision in a child receiving total parenteral nutrition (31). The symptoms were attributed to n-3 fatty acid deficiency because safflower oil, as in our study, was the sole fat source. Replacement of the safflower oil emulsion with linolenic acid–rich soybean oil was associated with recovery. However, it is difficult to be certain that the symptoms were due to n-3 fatty acid deficiency rather than to some other metabolic disturbance induced by long-term parenteral nutrition.

More recently, Bjerve et al. described 10 cases of so-called linolenic acid deficiency occurring in nursing home patients in Norway, some of whom were semicomatose, and had been fed by gastric tube over several years (6,7). Their diet was based on a commercially available powder supplement containing small amounts of corn oil (1.3 g/100 g) and mixed with skim milk. The authors reported that these patients developed very low plasma levels of n-3 fatty acids and a scaly dermatitis. Although corn oil contains very little n-3 linolenic acid (0.3%), if supplied in quantity, it would meet the patients' needs for n-6 essential fatty acids (i.e., linoleic 18:2). However, the diet furnished only 0.5% of energy as 18: 2 n-6; plasma 18:2 n-6 was low [9–15% of total plasma fatty acids versus 35% in healthy control subjects (53)]; and levels of eicosatrienoic acid (20:3 n-9) were substantially elevated. These observations suggest that the patients were also deficient in n-6 fatty acids and that the skin lesions were the result of the n-6 deficiency, since dermatitis has not been found in animals deficient in pure n-3 fatty acid (see Table 7). However, these 10 patients certainly did have an n-3 deficiency in addition to the n-6 deficiency—i.e., a combined essential fatty acid deficiency.

The findings of our study provide the first experimental evidence for a dietary requirement for n-3 fatty acids in primates and corroborate the extensive studies in rats emphasizing the need for linolenic acid (49). N-3 fatty acids are essential nutrients for retinal and brain function, especially during fetal and postnatal development. Both biochemical and functional stigmata are characteristic of the n-3 fatty acid–deficient state. A recent review details the experimental background of n-3 fatty acid deficiency in different species (40).

Summary and Implications

In summary, n-3 fatty acid deficiency in rhesus monkeys is characterized by a triad of problems: impaired vision, abnormal ERG, and polydipsia. Concomitant with the visual and ERG defects is the disturbed biochemistry of the retinal outer segment membranes: a great decrease in DHA (22:6 n-3) in the retinal phospholipids and a reciprocal increase of the n-6 fatty acids, particularly 22:5. In the absence of n-3 fatty acids, the body produces the most similar polyunsaturated fatty acids possible from precursors, so that the amount of polyunsaturation of the tissue membranes is largely maintained. The polydipsia may also be related to the altered biochemistry of the brain. Polydipsia does not appear to be mediated by abnormalities of the posterior pituitary hormones, renal disease, or osmotic regulation. However, the precise mechanism of this phenomenon has yet to be elucidated.

The diagnosis of n-3 fatty acid deficiency can be made at birth and later in life by fatty acid determinations of plasma and red cells of cord and peripheral venous blood. There will be low levels of the n-3 fatty acids 18:3 and 22:6 and high levels of the n-6 22:5, which is normally very low in both plasma and tissues of primates. The deficiency state at any age can be prevented by the provision of adequate amounts of n-3 fatty acids in the diet. It is not yet known whether several n-3 fatty acids are required for optimal development; i.e., linolenic acid and DHA, both of which are found in human milk. Once the deficiency state is well developed—by 10 months of age, for example,—biochemical correction in the tissues may not necessarily restore all the functional defects, especially the abnormal ERG.

The most critical periods of life for providing adequate n-3 fatty acids are during pregnancy, when fatty acids are transferred to the fetus via the placenta; in infancy, when n-3 fatty acids continue to accumulate in the brain and retina; and during lactation, when fatty acids are supplied postnatally via mother's milk. The diet of nursing mothers does affect the n-3 content of their milk (27). If formula feeding is used, its fats and oils should provide an adequate and balanced source of both n-3 and n-6 fatty acids. In all probability, n-3 fatty acids are also needed during childhood and even in adult life. The elderly and other patients may be at risk for n-3 fatty acid deficiency.

As dietary requirements for n-3 fatty acids, we suggest 0.5% to 1% of total calories. Ideally, these requirements would include both 18:3 and 22:6, as does human milk. The ratio of n-6 to n-3 fatty acids is important; it should range from about 4 to 12. Too high a ratio, like that found in the n-3 fatty acid–deficient safflower oil, might further exacerbate the deficiency. It is unfortunate that some infant formulas, particularly the dry powdered formulas containing corn and coconut oil, are marginal in their supply of n-3 fatty acids, which can be as low as 0.1%–0.2% of total calories. The ratio of n-6 to n-3 fatty acids is also high, at 75 (unpublished data).

These studies lend further credence to the recommendation that adequate amounts of both n-3 and n-6 fatty acids be included in the diet throughout life. They further show that their ratio is of great importance. This advice is particularly important for infants fed formulas whose fat sources include coconut oil, corn oil, or safflower oil. Some of these formulas do not provide adequate n-3 fatty acids yet include an excess of n-6 fatty acids. Ideally, the fat content and fatty acid composition of infant formulas should approximate that of human milk. This objective seems not only reasonable but also technologically feasible.

ACKNOWLEDGMENT

This work was supported by research grants from the National Institutes of Health (HL25687 and DK29930) and from the General Clinical Research Center (RR00334).

REFERENCES

1. Ahrens, E. H., Hirsch, J., Oette, K., Farquhar, J. W., and Stein, Y. (1961): Carbohydrate-induced and fat-induced lipemia. *Trans. Assoc. Am. Physicians,* 74:134.
2. Ahrens, E. H., Insull, W., and Hirsch, J., et al. (1959): The effect on human serum lipids of a dietary fat, highly unsaturated, but poor in essential fatty acids. *Lancet,* 1:115.
3. Bang, H. O., and Dyerberg, J. (1980): Lipid metabolism and ischemic heart disease in Greenland Eskimos. In: Draper HH, ed. *Advanced nutrition research;* vol 3. New York: Plenum, pp. 1–22.
4. Bang, H. O., Dyerberg, J., and Hyorne, N. (1973): The composition of food consumed by Greenlandic Eskimos. *Acta Med. Scand.,* 200:69–73.
5. Benner, K. G., Sasaki, A., Gowen, D. R., Weaver, A., and Connor, W. E. (1990): The differential effect of eicosapentaenoic acid and oleic acid on lipid synthesis and VLDL secretion in rabbit hepatocytes. *Lipids,* 25:534–540.
6. Bjerve, K. S., Fischer, S., and Alme, K. (1987): Alpha-linolenic acid deficiency in man: effect of ethyl linolenate on plasma and erythrocyte fatty acid composition and biosynthesis of prostanoids. *Am. J. Clin. Nutr.,* 46:570–576.
7. Bjerve, K. S., Mostad, I. L., and Thoresen, L. (1987): Alpha-linolenic acid deficiency in patients on long-term gastric tube feeding: estimation of linolenic acid and long-chain unsaturated n-3 fatty acid requirement in man. *Am. J. Clin. Nutr.,* 45:66–77.
8. Bronsgeest-Schoute, H. C., van Gent, C. M., Luten, J. B., and Ruiter, A. (1981): The effects of various intakes of omega-3 fatty acids on the blood lipid composition in healthy human subjects. *Am. J. Clin. Nutr.,* 34:1752.
9. Bronte-Stewart, B., Antonis, A., Eales, L., and Brock, J. F. (1956): Effects of feeding different fats on serum cholesterol levels. *Lancet,* 1:521.

10. Brown, W. R., Hansen, A. E., Burr, G. D., and McQuarrie, I. (1938): Effects of prolonged use of extremely low-fat diet on an adult human subject. *J. Nutr.,* 16:511–524.

11. Connor, W. E. (1986): Hypolipidemic effects of dietary omega-3 fatty acids in normal and hyperlipidemic humans: effectiveness and mechanisms. In: A. P. Simopoulos, ed. *Health effects of polyunsaturated fatty acids in seafoods.* New York: Academic Press, pp. 173–210.

12. Connor, W. E., and Connor, S. L. (1982): The dietary treatment of hyperlipidemia: rationale, technique and efficacy. *Med. Clin. North Am.,* 66:475.

13. Connor, W. E., Neuringer, M., Barstad, L., and Lin, D. S. (1984): Dietary deprivation of linolenic acid in rhesus monkeys: effects on plasma and tissue fatty acid composition and visual function. *Trans. Assoc. Am. Phys.* 97:1–9.

14. Connor, W. E., Neuringer, M., and Lin, D. S. (1990): Dietary effects upon brain fatty acid composition: the reversibility of n-3 fatty acid deficiency and turnover of docosahexaenoic acid in the brain, erythrocytes and plasma of rhesus monkeys. *J. Lipid Res.,* 31:237–248.

15. Davis, H. R., Bridenstine, R. T., Vesselinovitch, D., and Wissler, R. W. (1987): Fish oil inhibits development of atherosclerosis in Rhesus monkeys. *Arteriosclerosis,* 7:441–449.

16. Dehmer, G. J., Popma, J. J., and VandenBerg, E. K., et al. (1988): Reduction in the rate of early restenosis after coronary angioplasty by a diet supplemented with n-3 fatty acids. *N. Engl. J. Med.,* 319:733–740.

17. Dyerberg, J., and Bang, H. O. (1979): Hemostatic function and platelet polyunsaturated fatty acids in Eskimos. *Lancet,* 2:433–435.

18. Failor, R. A., Childs, M. T., and Bierman, E. L. (1988): The effects of omega-3 and omega-6 fatty acid-enriched diets on plasma lipoproteins and apoproteins in familial combined hyperlipidemia. *Metabolism,* 37:1021–1028.

19. Fox, P. L., and DiCorleto, P. E. (1988): Fish oils inhibit endothelial cell production of platelet-derived growth factor–like protein. *Science,* 214:453–456.

20. Fredrickson, D. S., and Levy, R. I. (1972): Familial hyperlipoproteinemia. In: Stanbury, J. B., Wyngaarden, J. B., Fredrickson, D. S., eds: *Metabolic basis of inherited disease.* 3rd ed. New York: McGraw-Hill, p. 545.

21. Goodnight, S. H. Jr., Harris, W. S., Connor, W. E., and Illingworth, D. R. (1982): Polyunsaturated fatty acids, hyperlipidemia and thrombosis. *Arteriosclerosis,* 2:87–113.

22. Grundy, S. M., Mok, Y. H. I., Zeck, L., Steinberg, O., and Berman, M. (1979): Transport of very low density lipoprotein triglycerides in varying degrees of obesity and hypertriglyceridemia. *J. Clin. Invest.* 63:1274.

23. Harris, W. S. (1989): Fish oils and plasma lipid and lipoprotein metabolism in humans: a critical review. *J. Lipid Res.,* 30:785–807.

24. Harris, W. S., and Connor, W. E. (1980): The effects of salmon oil upon plasma lipids, lipoprotein and triglyceride clearance. *Trans. Assoc. Am. Phys.,* 93:148–155.

25. Harris, W. S., Connor, W. E., Alam, N., and Illingworth, D. R. (1988): The reduction of postprandial triglyceride in humans by dietary n-3 fatty acids. *J. Lipid Res.,* 29:1451–1460.

26. Harris, W. S., Connor, W. E., and Illingworth, D. R. (1990): Effect of fish oil on VLDL triglyceride kinetics in man. *J. Lipid Res.,* 31:1549–1558.

27. Harris, W. S., Connor, W. E., and Lindsey, S. (1984): Will dietary omega-3 fatty acids change the composition of human milk? *Am. J. Clin. Nutr.,* 40:780–785.

28. Harris, W. S., Connor, W. E., and McMurry, M. P. (1983): The comparative reduction of the plasma lipids and lipoproteins by dietary polyunsaturated fats: salmon oil versus vegetable oils. *Metabolism,* 32:179.

29. Harris, W. S., Dujovne, C. A., Zucker, M. L., and Johnson, B. E. (1988): Effects of a low saturated fat, low cholesterol fish oil supplement in hypertriglyceridemic patients. *Ann. Int. Med.,* 109: 465–470.

30. Holman, R. T. (1970): Essential fatty acid deficiency. *Prog. Chem. Fats Other Lipids,* 9:275–339.

31. Holman, R. T., Johnson, S. B., and Hatch, T. F. (1982): A case of human linolenic acid deficiency involving neurological abnormalities. *Am. J. Clin. Nutr.,* 35:617–623.

32. Huff, M. W., and Telford, D. E. (1989): Dietary fish oil increases the conversion of very low density lipoprotein B, to low density lipoprotein. *Arteriosclerosis,* 9:58–66.

33. Keys, A., Anderson, J. T., and Grande, F. (1957): "Essential" fatty acids, degree of unsaturation and effects of corn (maize) oil on the serum cholesterol level in man. *Lancet,* 1:66.

34. Landymore, R. W., MacAulaym, M., Sheridan, B., and Cameron, C. (1986): Comparison of

cod-liver oil and aspirin-dipyridamole for the prevention of intimal hyperplasia in autologous vein grafts. *Ann. Thorac. Surg.,* 41:54–57.

35. Leaf, A., and Weber, P. C. (1988): Cardiovascular effects of n-3 fatty acids. *N. Engl. J. Med.,* 318:549–557.

36. Lin, D. S., Connor, W. E., Anderson, G. J., and Neuringer, M. (1990): The effects of dietary n-3 fatty acids upon the phospholipid molecular species of monkey brain. *J. Neurochem.,* 55:1200–1209.

37. Malmros, H., and Wigand, G. (1957): The effect on serum cholesterol of diets containing different fats. *Lancet,* 2:1.

38. Mancini, M., Mattock, M., Rabaya, E., Chait, A., and Lewis, B. (1973): Studies on the mechanisms of carbohydrate-induced lipemia in normal man. *Atherosclerosis,* 17:445.

39. Nestel, P. J., Connor, W. E., Reardon, M. R., and Connor, S. (1984): Suppression by diets rich in fish oil of very low density lipoprotein production in men. *J. Clin. Invest.,* 74:82.

40. Neuringer, M., Anderson, G. J., and Connor, W. E. (1988): The essentiality of n-3 fatty acids for the development and function of the retina and brain. *Ann. Rev. Nutr.,* 8:517–541.

41. Neuringer, M., and Connor, W. E. (1989): Omega-3 fatty acids in the retina. In: Galli, C., and Simopoulos, A. P., eds. *Dietary n-3 and n-6 fatty acids: biological effects and nutritional essentiality.* New York: Plenum, pp. 177–190.

42. Neuringer, M. D., Connor, W. E., Lin, D. S., Barstad, L., and Luck, S. (1986): Biochemical and functional effects of prenatal and postnatal omega-3 fatty acid deficiency on retina and brain in rhesus monkeys. *Proc. Natl. Acad. Sci. USA,* 83:4021–4025.

43. Neuringer, M., Connor, W. E., Van Petten, C., and Barstad, L. (1984): Dietary omega-3 fatty acid deficiency and visual loss in infant rhesus monkeys. *J. Clin. Invest.,* 73:272–276.

44. Phillipson, B. E., Rothrock, D. W., Connor, W. E., Harris, W. S., and Illingworth, D. R. (1985): The reduction of plasma lipids, lipoproteins, and apoproteins in hypertriglyceridemic patients by dietary fish oils. *N. Engl. J. Med.,* 312:1210.

45. Reis, G. J., Sipperly, M. E., and Boucher, T. M., et al. (1988): Results of a randomized, double-blind placebo-controlled trial of fish oil for prevention of restenosis after PTCA. *Circulation,* 78(suppl 11-291):1159A.

46. Reisbick, S., Neuringer, M., Hasnain, R., and Connor, W. E. (1990): Polydipsia in rhesus monkeys deficient in omega-3 fatty acids. *Physiol. Behav.,* 47:315–323.

47. Ruderman, N. B., Jones, A. L., Krauss, R. M., and Shafrir, E. (1971): A biochemical and morphologic study of very low density lipoproteins in carbohydrate-induced hypertriglyceridemia. *J. Clin. Invest.,* 50:1355.

48. Shimokawa, H., Lam, J. Y. T., Chesebro, J. H., Bowie, E. J. W., and Vanhoutte, P. M. (1987): Effects of dietary supplementation with cod-liver oil on endothelium-dependent response in porcine coronary arteries. *Circulation,* 76:898–905.

49. Tinoco, J. (1982): Dietary requirements and functions of α-linolenic acid in animals. *Prog. Lipid Res.,* 21:1–45.

50. von Lossonczy, T. O., Ruiter, A., and Bronsgeest-Schoute, H. C., et al. (1978): The effect of a fish diet on serum lipids in healthy human subjects. *Am. J. Clin. Nutr.,* 31:1340.

51. VonSchacky, C. (1988): Prophylaxis of atherosclerosis with marine omega-3 fatty acids: a comprehensive strategy. *Ann. Intern. Med.,* 107:890–899.

52. Weiner, B. H., Ockene, I. S., and Levine, P. H., et al. (1986): Inhibition of atherosclerosis by cod liver oil in a hyperlipidemic swine model. *N. Engl. J. Med.,* 315:841–846.

53. Wene, J. D., Connor, W. E., and DenBesten, L. (1975): The development of essential fatty acid deficiency in healthy men fed fat-free diets intravenously and orally. *J. Clin. Invest.,* 56:127–134.

54. Witztum, J. L., and Schonfeld, G. (1978): Carbohydrate diet-induced changes in very low density lipoprotein composition and structures. *Diabetes,* 27:1215.

55. Wong, S., Reardon, M., and Nestel, P. (1985): Reduced triglyceride formation from long chain polyenoic fatty acids in rat hepatocytes. *Metabolism,* 34:900–905.

56. Wong, S. H., Nestel, P. H., and Trimble, R. P. (1983): The adaptive effects of dietary fish and safflower oil on lipid and lipoprotein metabolism in perfused rat liver. *Biochem. Biophys. Acta,* 792:103.

Atherosclerosis Reviews, Volume 23,
edited by P. C. Weber and A. Leaf.
Raven Press, Ltd., New York © 1991.

A New Role for the Low-Density Lipoprotein Receptor Pathway: To Deliver Arachidonic Acid to Cells for Eicosanoid Formation

P. B. Salbach, U. Janßen-Timmen,
and A. J. R. Habenicht

*University of Heidelberg, Department of Medicine, Division of Endocrinology
and Metabolism, D-6900 Heidelberg, Germany*

It is well established that the low-density lipoprotein (LDL) pathway (1,4) functions to maintain a constant concentration of cellular cholesterol, but LDL effects that are unrelated to cholesterol metabolism have not been studied in great detail. We have suggested previously that the LDL pathway is directly linked to eicosanoid production in cells stimulated to divide by platelet-derived growth factor (PDGF), because low concentrations of LDL and very-low-density lipoproteins (VLDL) but not high-density-lipoproteins (HDL) stimulated prostaglandin (PG) E_2 formation in these cells, and because chloroquine, an inhibitor of lysosomal activity, prevented LDL-dependent PG synthesis (5). Herein, we report on studies designed to elucidate the molecular mechanism of the PG stimulatory activity of LDL. We provide evidence that LDL stimulate prostacyclin and PGE_2 synthesis in PDGF-stimulated cells through delivery of arachidonic acid (AA), that this delivery depends on the LDL receptor, and that LDL inhibit PGH synthase, the rate-limiting enzyme in PG and thromboxane formation. Taken together, our results suggest a new role for the LDL pathway and raise the possibility that LDL, and possibly other lipoprotein classes that are taken up through the LDL pathway, may be involved in the regulation of eicosanoid synthesis (2, 6–9).

LDL STIMULATE PG SYNTHESIS BY THE DELIVERY OF ARACHIDONIC ACID TO PDGF-STIMULATED FIBROBLASTS

We and others have observed stimulatory effects of plasma lipoproteins on the formation of prostacyclin and PGE_2 in cultured endothelial cells, smooth muscle cells, and fibroblasts (5,13). These preliminary results were of interest because prostacyclin and PGE_2 have potent biological activities, including anti-aggregatory effects toward platelets and inhibition of the early stages of macrophage and lymphocyte activation (12). However, the molecular mechanism underlying the PG stimulatory effect of the lipoproteins has remained uncertain (5).

To study the possibility that LDL stimulate PG synthesis through delivery of AA to fibroblasts, we reconstituted native human plasma LDL using the cholesteryl ester of ^{14}C-labeled AA [recLDL-(^{14}C-AA-CE)] according to Krieger (11). This approach allowed us to follow the metabolism of LDL-derived AA into different cell compartments and in particular into the pathways of the AA cascade. Furthermore, the use of recLDL-(^{14}C-AA-CE) was suitable to answer the question of whether the stimulatory effect of LDL depends on the classical LDL receptor pathway of Brown and Goldstein (1,4), because reconstituted LDL retains its ability to bind to the LDL receptor.

As shown in Fig. 1, normal quiescent fibroblasts (i.e., fibroblasts maintained in the absence of PDGF), when incubated with recLDL-(^{14}C-AA-CE), formed only small amounts of prostacyclin and PGE_2. In contrast, PDGF-stimulated normal fibroblasts formed significant amounts (Fig. 1B). This experiment demonstrated that LDL delivers AA to PDGF-stimulated but not quiescent cells for the formation of PGE_2 and prostacyclin.

To study whether stimulation of PG synthesis by recLDL-(^{14}C-AA-CE) depended on the LDL receptor, we first used fibroblasts of several patients afflicted with the LDL-receptor-negative phenotype of familial hypercholesterolemia (FH). Neither quiescent nor PDGF-stimulated FH cells were able to form significant amounts of eicosanoids from recLDL-(^{14}C-AA-CE) (Fig. 1A and B), whereas they formed normal rates of eicosanoids when unesterified ^{14}C-AA was used as the substrate. FH fibroblasts were also responsive to PDGF by doubling their cell number within 48 hr or less (not shown). This finding indicated that the inability of FH cells to produce eicosanoids in response to LDL depended on the receptor defect rather than on a deficiency in the enzymes of AA metabolism or an unresponsiveness to PDGF. Furthermore, anti-LDL receptor antibodies prevented the stimulatory effect of recLDL-(^{14}C-AA-CE) in normal fibroblasts, and chloroquine, an inhibitor of lysosomes, largely reduced the activity (Fig. 2A and B). When taken together, these results demonstrate that LDL stimulate PG synthesis through delivery of AA to cells; this activity depends on the LDL pathway of Brown and Goldstein.

LDL INHIBIT THE RATE-LIMITING ENZYME
OF PG SYNTHESIS, THE PGH SYNTHASE

The results presented in Figs. 1 and 2 raised another intriguing possibility. Previous studies by Smith and Lands (17) had shown that unesterified AA inhibits PGH synthase, presumably by the generation of endoperoxide intermediates.

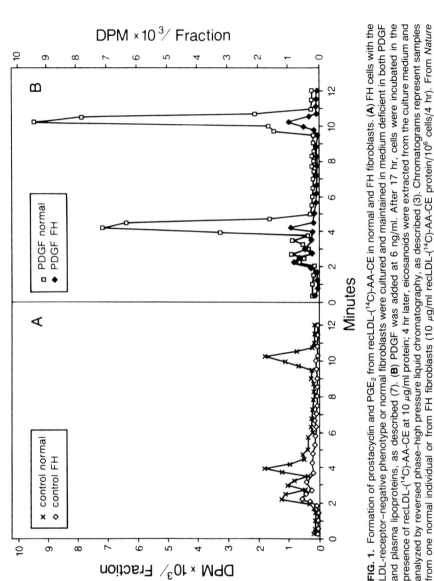

FIG. 1. Formation of prostacyclin and PGE$_2$ from recLDL-(^{14}C)-AA-CE in normal and FH fibroblasts. **(A)** FH cells with the LDL-receptor–negative phenotype or normal fibroblasts were cultured and maintained in medium deficient in both PDGF and plasma lipoproteins, as described (7). **(B)** PDGF was added at 6 ng/ml. After 17 hr, cells were incubated in the presence of recLDL-(^{14}C)-AA-CE at 10 μg/ml protein; 4 hr later, eicosanoids were extracted from the culture medium and analyzed by reversed phase–high pressure liquid chromatography, as described (3). Chromatograms represent samples from one normal individual or from FH fibroblasts (10 μg/ml recLDL-(^{14}C)-AA-CE protein/10^6 cells/4 hr). *From Nature* 1990;345:634–636, with permission of the publisher.

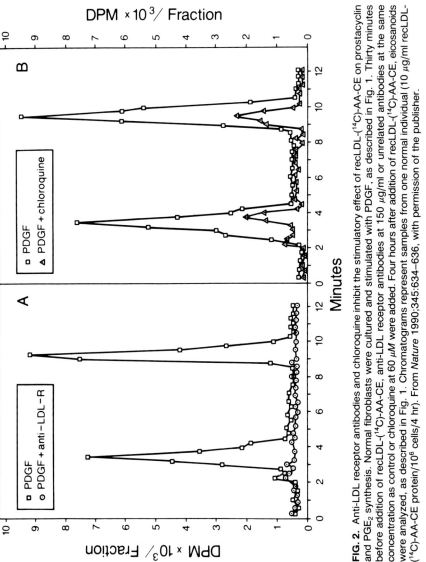

FIG. 2. Anti-LDL receptor antibodies and chloroquine inhibit the stimulatory effect of recLDL-(^{14}C)-AA-CE on prostacyclin and PGE$_2$ synthesis. Normal fibroblasts were cultured and stimulated with PDGF, as described in Fig. 1. Thirty minutes before addition of recLDL-(^{14}C)-AA-CE, anti-LDL receptor antibodies at 150 μg/ml or unrelated antibodies at the same concentration as control or chloroquine at 60 μM were added. Four hours after addition of recLDL-(^{14}C)-AA-CE, eicosanoids were analyzed, as described in Fig. 1. Chromatograms represent samples from one normal individual (10 μg/ml recLDL-(^{14}C)-AA-CE protein/10^6 cells/4 hr). From *Nature* 1990;345:634–636, with permission of the publisher.

We therefore tested the possibility that LDL inhibits PGH synthase in intact cell experiments. As shown in Fig. 3, LDL had a pronounced inhibitory effect on PGH synthase in a concentration-dependent and time-dependent way. Assays using microsomal preparations of cells that had been preincubated in the presence of LDL or unesterified AA showed that LDL and AA strongly reduced the maximal velocity of PGH synthase, whereas the apparent affinity for its substrate remained unchanged (10) (data not shown). This effect of LDL was reversed

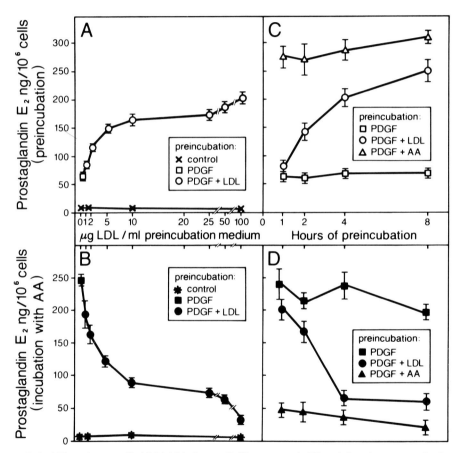

FIG. 3. LDL and unesterified AA inhibit the rate-limiting enzyme in PG and thromboxane synthesis, PGH synthase. Swiss 3T3 cells were cultured, as described for human skin fibroblasts in Fig. 1. Seventeen hours after addition of PDGF, parallel cultures were either incubated with increasing concentrations of native human plasma LDL (**A**) or with 10 μg/ml LDL protein for increasing periods of time or 10 μM unesterified AA dissolved in 10 μl ethanol (**C**). After this preincubation with LDL or AA, the culture medium was analyzed for the presence of PGE$_2$, as described (8). Identical cultures were then incubated in the presence of 10 μM AA to determine residual total cellular PGH synthase activity (**B, D**) (10). From *Nature* 1990;345:634–636, with permission of the publisher.

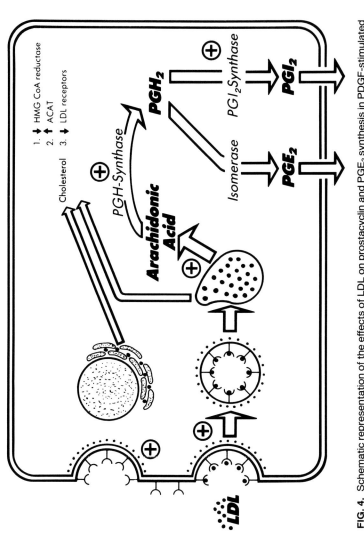

FIG. 4. Schematic representation of the effects of LDL on prostacyclin and PGE₂ synthesis in PDGF-stimulated fibroblasts. In this figure, + indicates a stimulatory effect of PDGF [see (3) and (8) for reference]. LDL is taken up through the classical LDL pathway of Brown and Goldstein (1,4), AA is released from the lysosomal compartment and subsequently converted into prostacyclin (PGI₂) and PGE₂ by the coupled action of PGH synthase and prostacyclin synthase or PGH₂/PGE₂ isomerase, respectively.

within 4 hr–6 hr after removal of the inhibitor. Reversal required *de novo* synthesis of protein, because it was completely prevented by cycloheximide (data not shown).

CONCLUSIONS

These results show that LDL delivers AA to PDGF-stimulated fibroblasts for prostacyclin and PGE$_2$ formation, that this effect depends on the classical LDL receptor pathway of Brown and Goldstein, and that LDL concomitantly inhibits the key enzyme of this pathway, the PGH synthase (Fig. 4). It is likely that cell types other than fibroblasts, including those of hematopoietic origin, also produce eicosanoids in response to LDL. Thus, we have shown, that human blood-derived monocytes/macrophages form products of the PGH synthase pathway including thromboxane and that they also form several products of the 5-lipoxygenase pathway, leukotrienes C$_4$, and leukotriene B$_4$ (15,16), in response to recLDL-(^{14}C-AA-CE) (Salbach, Glomset, and Habenicht, unpublished observations). It is now important to study the biological effects of the eicosanoids that are produced in response to LDL. PGE$_2$ has strong inhibitory effects on the early stages of activation of macrophages and lymphocytes—two cell types that are major cellular constituents of atherosclerotic lesions in patients afflicted with cardiovascular disease (14).

REFERENCES

1. Brown, M. S., and Goldstein, J. L. (1986): *Science,* 232:34–47.
2. Goerig, M., Habenicht, A. J. R., and Heitz, R., et al. (1987): *J. Clin. Invest.,* 75:1381–1387.
3. Goerig, M., Habenicht, A. J. R., and Zeh, W., et al. (1988): *J. Biol. Chem.,* 263:19384–19391.
4. Goldstein, J. L., and Brown, M. S. (1990): *Nature,* 343:425–430.
5. Habenicht, A. J. R., Dresel, H. A., and Goerig, M., et al. (1986): *Proc. Natl. Acad. Sci. USA,* 83: 1344–1348.
6. Habenicht, A. J. R., Glomset, J. A., King, W. C., Nist, C., Mitchell, C. D., and Ross, R. (1981): *J. Biol. Chem.,* 256:12329–12335.
7. Habenicht, A. J. R., Glomset, J. A., and Ross, R. (1980): *J. Biol. Chem.,* 255:5134–5140.
8. Habenicht, A. J. R., Goerig, M., and Grulich, J., et al. (1985): *J. Clin. Invest.,* 75:1381–1387.
9. Habenicht, A. J. R., Goerig, M., and Rothe, D. E. R., et al. (1989): *Proc. Natl. Acad. Sci. USA,* 86:921–924.
10. Habenicht, A. J. R., Salbach, P., and Goerig, M., et al. (1990): *Nature,* 345:634–636.
11. Krieger, M. (1986): *Methods Enzymol.,* 128:608–613.
12. Needleman, P., Turk, J., Jakschik, B. A., and Morrison, A. R. (1986): *Ann. Rev. Biochem.,* 55: 69–102.
13. Pomerantz, K. B., Tall, A. R., Feinmark, S. J., and Cannon, P. J. (1984): *Circ. Res.,* 54:554–565.
14. Ross, R. (1986): *N. Engl. J. Med.,* 314:488–500.
15. Samuelsson, B., Dahlen, D. A., Lindgren, C. A., Rouzer, C. A., and Serhan, C. N. (1987): *Science,* 237:1171–1176.
16. Samuelsson, B., and Funk, C. D. (1989): *J. Biol. Chem.,* 264:19469–19472.
17. Smith, W. L., and Lands, W. E. M. (1972): *Biochemistry,* 11:3283–3289.

Atherosclerosis Reviews, Volume 23,
edited by P. C. Weber and A. Leaf.
Raven Press, Ltd., New York © 1991.

Evidence for the Formation of Oxidized Lipoproteins in Cholesterol-Fed Rabbits

Michael E. Rosenfeld, Seppo Ylä-Herttuala,
Sampath Parthasarathy, John C. Khoo, and Thomas E. Carew

Division of Endocrinology and Metabolism, Department of Medicine, 0613D,
University of California–San Diego, La Jolla, California 92093

The oxidative modification hypothesis of atherogenesis suggests that lipoproteins entering the artery wall become oxidized, setting in motion a chain of events that leads to an influx of monocytes into the artery, the increased recognition and uptake of the oxidized lipoproteins by arterial macrophages, and the formation of macrophage-derived foam cells (24). Recently, we demonstrated that macrophages within atherosclerotic lesions of the Watanabe Heritable Hyperlipemic (WHHL) rabbit contain immunoreactive oxidation-specific lipid protein adducts (12,13,20). Such adducts are likely to have been derived in part from oxidized low-density lipoprotein (LDL), because LDL with all the properties of *in vitro* oxidized LDL can be extracted from the same lesions (12,29). Studies by Carew et al. (4) and Kita et al. (8) have further demonstrated that chronic administration of probucol, a potent antioxidant, to WHHL rabbits is effective in reducing atherosclerosis in the aorta (Table 1). In addition, recent data suggest that this may be due to a reduction in the formation of macrophage-derived foam cells (10,11).

The WHHL rabbit is a unique animal model of human familial hypercholesterolemia (FH) (26). The hypercholesterolemia that spontaneously occurs in these rabbits is primarily due to an increase in LDL (7). In contrast, in normal rabbits fed high levels of cholesterol, the resulting hypercholesterolemia is in large part due to an increase in beta–very-low-density lipoprotein (β-VLDL) (22). Although *in vitro*, β-VLDL can be oxidized both by cells and during incubation with copper ions and is chemotactic for monocytes (14), there are no data that demonstrate the presence of oxidized β-VLDL or other oxidized lipoproteins in cholesterol-fed rabbit arteries *in vivo*. Previous studies of the effects of probucol on the formation of atherosclerotic lesions in the cholesterol-fed rabbit have yielded conflicting results (5,9,23).

This article presents recent data on atherosclerotic lesions from cholesterol-fed rabbits and on macrophage-derived foam cells freshly isolated from ballooned, cholesterol-fed rabbits that suggest that oxidized lipoproteins are present in mac-

TABLE 1. *Effects of probucol on atherosclerotic lesions in the aorta of WHHL rabbits: extent of aortic lesions, percent of surface area involved*

Experimental group	Total aorta	Aortic arch	Descending thoracic	Abdominal
Untreated ($n = 6$)	40.6 ± 5.1	87.5 ± 3.5	37.7 ± 8.3	16.8 ± 3.2
Lovastatin ($n = 11$)	27.5 ± 4.6	65.0 ± 4.9	21.6 ± 6.2	14.3 ± 3.0
Probucol ($n = 11$)	14.3 ± 2.1	47.1 ± 5.3	6.6 ± 2.0	6.4 ± 1.0

Data are expressed as mean $\pm$ SEM. The statistical analysis was performed on log-transformed data. Differences between experimental groups in extent of lesions in the total aorta were compared by t tests: probucol group versus lovastatin group, $p < 0.01$; probucol group versus untreated group, $p < 0.0005$; lovastatin group versus untreated group, $p = 0.06$. Differences between groups in extent of lesions in the three aortic segments were compared by analysis of variance with a repeated measures design: probucol group versus lovastatin group, $p < 0.01$; probucol group versus untreated group, $p < 0.001$; lovastatin group versus untreated group, $p = 0.10$. (The data were originally published in the *Proc. Natl. Acad. Sci. USA*, 1987; 84:7725–7729, and are included with the permission of the authors.)

rophages within the artery, and that this animal model should be an appropriate model for analyzing the effects of antioxidants on atherogenesis.

METHODS

Isolation of Foam Cells

To increase the percentage of macrophage-derived foam cells (MFC) within atherosclerotic lesions of cholesterol-fed rabbits, the endothelial cells of the aorta and left iliac artery of New Zealand White rabbits (NZW) were removed with a Fogarty embolectomy catheter (4F). The animals were placed on a high-cholesterol diet (2%) for 13 weeks (1 week prior to the catheterization and 12 weeks following the denudation procedure) as described (19). Under a sterile hood and on ice, atherosclerotic lesion (intima) dissected from four to six animals was minced and the MFC were released from the tissue using the enzymatic digestion procedure of Berberian et al. (2). The cells were purified with a discontinuous density gradient of metrizamide (Sigma) (30% cushion, 10% top, centrifuged at $\times 1,200$ g in a swinging bucket rotor for 15 min at 10°C). The isolated cells were washed, plated, and maintained overnight in Opti-MEM I reduced-serum medium (Gibco) containing 0.5% fetal calf serum (FCS).

The purity of the foam cell preparations were assessed immunocytochemically with the monoclonal antibody RAM-11 (27), which is specific for rabbit macrophages, as well as monoclonal antibody HHF-35 (Enzo Biochemicals) (28), which recognizes smooth muscle actin. All immunostaining procedures were done with an avidin–biotin system conjugated with either horseradish peroxidase or alkaline phosphatase (Vector Labs). All experimental procedures with rabbits were conducted under a protocol approved by the Animal Care and Use Committee of the University of California–San Diego.

Detection of Oxidized Lipid-Protein Adducts

To determine whether the atherosclerotic lesions in the ballooned, cholesterol-fed rabbits, as well as the MFC isolated from the same lesions, contained oxidation-specific lipid-protein adducts, small segments of the abdominal aorta were immersion-fixed with formal-sucrose and immunostained with the following antibodies: guinea pig polyclonal antiserum MAL-2 and the mouse monoclonal antibody MDA-2, both generated against autologous malondialdehyde-conjugated LDL (MDA-LDL), as previously described (12,13,20).

Lipoprotein Degradation Assays

LDL (d = 1.019–1.063) and LPDS (d > 1.215) were isolated by preparative ultracentrifugation from fresh human plasma. The lipoproteins were dialyzed extensively against PBS containing 0.01% EDTA (pH, 7.4). β-VLDL (d < 1.006) was isolated by preparative ultracentrifugation from the plasma of cholesterol-fed rabbits. Lipoproteins were radio-iodinated with carrier-free sodium ^{125}I-iodide (Amersham/Searle) by the method of Salacinski et al. (21) using the solid-phase oxidizing agent, Iodogen (Pierce Chemical Co.). Acetyl-LDL was prepared according to the method of Basu et al. (1); and copper (Cu^{2+})-oxidized LDL was prepared as described by Steinbrecher et al. (25). The degradation of ^{125}I-LDL, ^{125}I-acetyl-LDL, ^{125}I-β-VLDL, ^{125}I-Cu^{2+}-oxidized LDL, and ^{125}I-oxidized β-VLDL was determined as described by Goldstein et al. (6).

Induction of Lipoprotein Oxidation

After an overnight incubation of all cells, the medium was removed. The cells were incubated at 37°C with 2 ml of Ham's F-10 medium containing 200 μg of ^{125}I-lipoproteins for 24 hr. The medium was then analyzed for thiobarbituric acid reactive substance (TBARS) after the method of Patton and Kurtz (15). An aliquot containing 5 μg of the ^{125}I-lipoproteins that had been incubated with the cells or copper ions was tested for degradation using a fresh culture of resident MPM or isolated foam cells, as described above.

Extraction of Lipoproteins from Lesions

Aortas and plasma samples were obtained from four NZW rabbits that had been fed a 2% cholesterol–containing diet for 6 months. The aortic tissue was minced with a McIlwain tissue chopper. Both the minced tissue and whole plasma were incubated overnight at 4°C under nitrogen in a saline extraction buffer containing antioxidants and protease inhibitors, as previously described (29). Lipoproteins within the extract were isolated using density gradient ultracentrifugation. The LDL fraction was further analyzed for the presence of oxidation-specific epitopes using SDS-PAGE and Western blot techniques (29). Antisera Mal-2 and YE-1 (generated against WHHL LDL and recognizing rabbit apoB) were utilized for the Western blots.

RESULTS

Previous studies by Parthasarathy et al. (14) have demonstrated that β-VLDL can be oxidized following incubation with copper ions or endothelial cells. Oxidized β-VLDL is in turn taken up and degraded approximately twofold more than native β-VLDL and leads to significantly more incorporation of labeled oleate into cellular cholesteryl-esters in mouse peritoneal macrophages. β-VLDL isolated from probucol-treated rabbits was resistant to oxidation *in vitro;* it was not degraded any more avidly by the cultured macrophages than was the corresponding β-VLDL that was not exposed to oxidizing conditions (Table 2).

The above *in vitro* data suggest that β-VLDL may undergo oxidation *in vivo* in an fashion analogous to LDL. However, to date there is no evidence for the presence of oxidized β-VLDL or LDL *in vivo* in the cholesterol-fed rabbit. Figure 1 shows the results of the immunocytochemical analysis of atherosclerotic lesions

TABLE 2. *Oxidative modification of β-VLDL from cholesterol-fed rabbits*

β-VLDL	TBARS (nmol/mg)	Mac degr. (μg/5 hr/mg)	^{14}C-chol oleate (nmol/mg protein)
From untreated rabbits			
Nonincubated control	12.81	1.86	66.2
After incubation with			
endothelial cells	78.56	4.32	147.9
After incubation with			
copper ions	116.68	4.56	N.D.
From probucol-treated rabbits			
Nonincubated control	11.92	1.65	46.2
After incubation with			
endothelial cells	17.63	1.55	33.5
After incubation with			
copper ions	23.56	1.38	N.D.

N.D., not determined; TBARS, thiobarbituric acid reactive substances; Mac degr., macrophage degradation; ^{14}C-chol oleate, incorporation of labeled oleate into macrophage cholesteryl-esters.

β-VLDL from control or probucol-treated rabbits were incubated with cultured rabbit aortic endothelial cells or copper acetate (5 μM) in 2 ml of Ham's F-10 medium at 100 μg/ml for 24 hr. TBARS, macrophage degradation, and oleate incorporation were determined as described previously (14). Values shown are the averages of four determinations from duplicates of two separate experiments. (Data are reproduced from *Arteriosclerosis,* 1989; 9:398–404, by copyright permission of the American Heart Association.)

in the abdominal aorta of NZW rabbits that had undergone balloon denudation of the endothelium and had been fed a high cholesterol diet for 12 weeks. The tissue was stained with a guinea pig antiserum generated against malondialdehyde-conjugated LDL (MDA-LDL) and shows specific localization to areas of the lesion rich in immunoreactive macrophages. Thus, the data demonstrate the presence of oxidation-specific lipid-protein adducts potentially derived from β-VLDL or LDL in a distribution identical to that observed in macrophage-rich lesions of the WHHL rabbit.

Figure 2 further demonstrates that the foam cells isolated from lesions identical to that shown in Fig. 1 retain the oxidation-specific lipid-protein adducts. In this case, the isolated cells were immunostained with a monoclonal antibody that also specifically recognizes MDA-LDL. This figure also demonstrates that the isolated cells are macrophages, because they are immunoreactive with the rabbit macrophage-specific monoclonal antibody RAM-11.

We also performed Western blot analyses of plasma LDL and lesion LDL isolated from cholesterol-fed rabbits (data not shown). The silver-stained SDS-PAGE showed a large number of bands from the lesion LDL indicative of the oxidative breakdown of apoB. A similar degree of degradation was not apparent with plasma LDL. The Western blot using the antiserum YE-1 (generated against LDL from WHHL rabbits and recognizing rabbit apoB) also showed multiple bands of immunoreactive apoB fragments. Again, the plasma LDL apoB was largely intact. Finally, the Western blot using antiserum Mal-2 showed several immunoreactive bands in the lesion LDL but no MDA containing adducts in the plasma fraction. In addition, agarose gel electrophoresis of the isolated lesion LDL showed a marked increase in electrophoretic mobility consistent with oxidative modification of the LDL.

One of the advantages to studying isolated foam cells in comparison to *in vitro* models of macrophages loaded with acetyl-LDL etc., is their massive content of cholesterol. The isolated foam cells contain, on average, 600 μg of cholesterol per mg of cell protein with greater than 80% of the cholesterol stored in the esterified form [(data not shown), (19)]. This level of lipid loading and distribution is difficult to achieve in *in vitro* systems.

By studying the properties of the cells within 24 hr of removal from the artery wall, a time during which there is no apparent loss of foam cell phenotype, we have concluded that the observed activities closely reflect the capacities of these cells *in vivo*. We used the freshly isolated foam cells to study the capacity of these cells to bind and degrade modified lipoproteins. Figure 3 shows that the isolated foam cells can bind and degrade LDL, acetyl-LDL, oxidized LDL, and β-VLDL comparably to mouse peritoneal macrophages.

The isolated foam cells are also capable of oxidizing lipoproteins. Table 3 shows the capacity of the isolated foam cells to oxidize LDL in comparison to rabbit aortic endothelial cells and mouse peritoneal macrophages. Despite plating the foam cells at a much lower density, the foam cells generate equivalent amounts of malondialdehyde per mg of LDL protein, as do the other cell types. In addition,

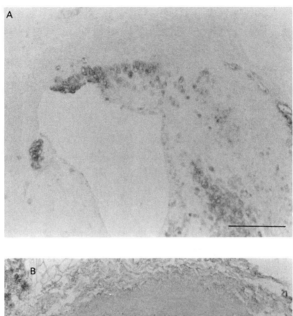

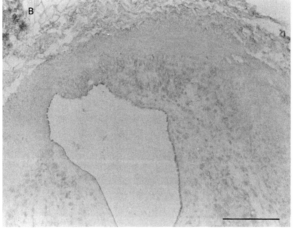

FIG. 1. Macrophages within atherosclerotic lesions from ballooned, cholesterol-fed rabbits contain oxidation specific lipid-protein adducts. Immunocytochemical staining of sections of the abdominal aorta containing atherosclerotic lesions, with antibodies generated against malondialdehyde conjugated LDL (Mal-2) and macrophages (RAM-11). **(A)** RAM-11; **(B)** and **(C)** guinea pig polyserum Mal-2, **(D)** nonspecific serum (goat), phase contrast. The final magnification of panels A, B, and D = ×220, bars = 100 μ. Panel C = ×2,200, bars = 10 μ. All staining utilized an avidin-biotin-alkaline phosphatase procedure, as described previously (19).

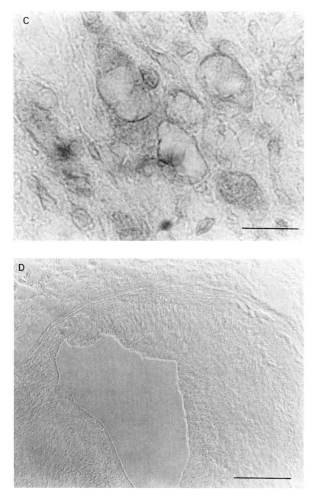

FIG. 1. *Continued.*

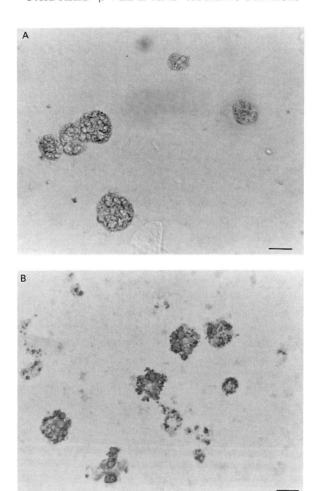

FIG. 2. Isolated foam cells contain oxidation-specific lipid-protein adducts. Immunocytochemical staining of the isolated foam cells with monoclonal antibodies generated against malondialdehyde-conjugated LDL and rabbit macrophages. **(A)** mouse monoclonal antibody MDA-2; **(B)** mouse monoclonal antibody RAM-11. The final magnification of panels A and B = ×890, bars = 10 μ. All staining utilized an avidin-biotin-alkaline phosphatase procedure as described previously (19).

→

FIG. 3. Comparison of the capacity of isolated rabbit arterial foam cells and mouse peritoneal macrophages to degrade LDL, modified forms of LDL, and β-VLDL. Monolayers of cells were incubated with 10 μg protein/ml of LDL, acetyl-LDL (Ac-LDL), Cu^{++} oxidized LDL (Ox-LDL) and β-VLDL in the absence and presence of 25-fold unlabeled lipoproteins for 5 hr at 37°C. Degradation products were determined in the media as described previously (6). n = number of separate experiments. Values shown are the means of n experiments where each experiment yielded an average of duplicate wells. (Data reproduced from ref. 19 by copyright permission of the American Society of Clinical Investigation.)

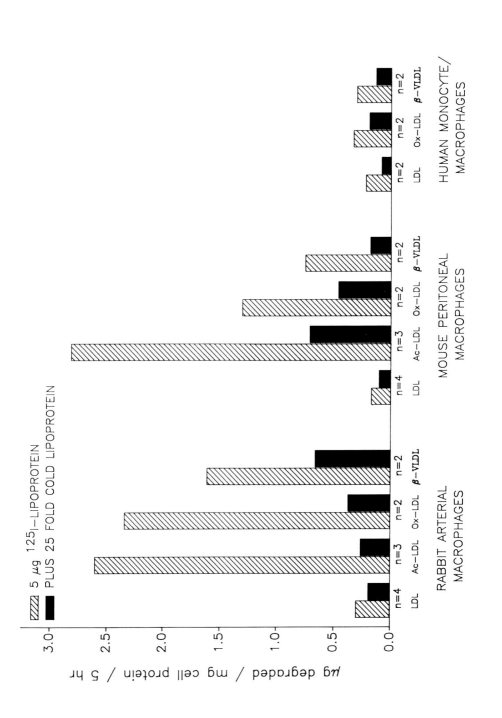

TABLE 3. *Comparison of the capacity of different cell types to oxidize LDL and the degradation of the oxidized LDL by mouse peritoneal macrophages*

	Oxidation (nmol MDA/mg LDL protein)		Degradation (μg/mg cell protein)	
Cell type	Exp. 1	Exp. 2	Exp. 1	Exp. 2
Native LDL (cell-free)	0.3	2.7	0.4	0.3
Rabbit endothelial cells	44	45	5.4	7.3
Mouse peritoneal Mφ	56	53	5.9	5.8
Isolated foam cells	42	38	6.6	3.5

Monolayers of cells were incubated with 200 μg/ml of human ^{125}I-LDL in Ham's F-10 medium for 24 hr at 37°C. The medium was then analyzed for TBARS activity, as described previously (15); 5 μg of the ^{125}I-LDL that had been incubated with the cells was added to fresh MPM. Degradation products were measured as described previously (6). Values shown are the average of triplicate wells, except for isolated foam cells where values are the average of duplicate wells. All cell types were plated at 2.5×10^6 cells/well, except for isolated foam cells, where cells were plated at 5×10^5 cells/well. (This data is reproduced from ref. 19 by copyright permission of the American Society of Clinical Investigation.)

the isolated foam cells are also capable of oxidizing β-VLDL, as demonstrated by the capacity of mouse peritoneal macrophages to degrade the altered β-VLDL (Table 4).

DISCUSSION

We have previously shown that oxidized LDL is a prominent component of atherosclerotic lesions in WHHL rabbits (12,20,29). Furthermore, chronic probucol administration is effective in inhibiting atherosclerosis in the aorta of WHHL rabbits (4,8). Those data strongly support the hypothesis that oxidative modification of LDL is an important event in mediating the atherogenicity of LDL in the WHHL rabbit. Based on the observations presented in this article

TABLE 4. *Isolated foam cells oxidize β-VLDL*

	Mouse peritoneal macrophage degradation (μg/mg cell protein)		
	Total	TCA-soluble	Cell-associated
Incubation			
Native β-VLDL	1.4	1.0	0.4
Foam cells (Exp. 1)	9.2	7.3	1.9
Foam cells (Exp. 2)	8.4	5.3	3.1
No cell control	1.7	0.3	1.4

Monolayers of cells were incubated with 200 μg/ml of rabbit ^{125}I-β-VLDL in Hams F-10 medium for 24 hr at 37°C; 5 μg of the ^{125}I-β-VLDL that had been incubated with the cells was added to fresh cultures of mouse peritoneal macrophages. Degradation products were measured as described previously (6). Values shown are the average of triplicate wells. The foam cells were plated at 2.5×10^6 cells/well for the oxidation phase and the mouse cells were plated at 1×10^6 cells/well for the degradation phase.

as well as additional previous data, we believe that oxidized lipoproteins also occur in the cholesterol-fed rabbit. This model should be an appropriate model for studying antioxidant effects on atherosclerosis.

Comparative morphologic studies of the WHHL and comparably hypercholesterolemic cholesterol-fed rabbits (18,27) showed that there were no differences in the sequence of cellular events that occur in the initiation and progression of lesions in the aorta. In addition, over a 12-month period, comparable amounts of cholesterol were deposited in the arteries of these two different rabbit models. Thus, although there are differences in the predominant lipoprotein (LDL versus β-VLDL), the arteries of these animals appear to respond in a fashion similar to a hypercholesterolemic insult.

Our current observations concerning the presence of oxidation-specific lipid protein adducts are consistent with the earlier comparative studies showing marked similarities in these two animal models. In both the WHHL and cholesterol-fed rabbits, we demonstrated the presence of the lipid-protein adducts primarily associated with macrophage-derived foam cells (12,13,20). Furthermore, we have demonstrated that oxidized LDL can be extracted from the same WHHL rabbit lesions that contain the oxidation specific lipid-protein adducts; and we now report that the LDL that is immunoreactive for the oxidation-specific epitopes can be extracted from lesions of cholesterol-fed rabbits as well. However, to date we have not yet isolated β-VLDL–like particles from the arteries of cholesterol-fed rabbits to determine if they too have evidence of oxidative modification.

Our studies of the isolated foam cells demonstrate that despite the fact that they contain on average 600 μg cholesterol per milligram protein and are immunoreactive for the oxidation specific lipid-protein adducts, these cells are still capable of binding and degrading oxidized lipoproteins. Moreover, they are also capable of oxidizing LDL and β-VLDL comparably to other cell types previously studied *in vitro.* The data suggest that macrophage-derived foam cells oxidize and take up LDL and β-VLDL *in vivo,* because the activity of the isolated foam cells studied within 24 hr of isolation likely reflects their behavior *in vivo.*

Finally, it should be noted that oxidized lipoproteins within the artery wall may not only contribute to the atherogenic process by stimulating foam cell formation. Recent studies suggest that oxidized LDL may itself be chemotactic for monocytes (16) and may activate other cells within the artery to produce chemotactic factors and cytokines as well as express specific adherence molecules (3,17). Thus, future studies of the effects of antioxidants on atherogenesis in the cholesterol-fed rabbit should be designed to include assessment of the multiple roles that oxidized lipoproteins may play in this disease process.

ACKNOWLEDGMENT

This work was supported in part by NIH grants HL-42617, HL-14197, and HL-34724. The authors thank Michael Burson, Paula Sicurello, and Elizabeth

Miller for their excellent technical contributions and Drs. Daniel Steinberg and Joseph Witztum for helpful discussions.

REFERENCES

1. Basu, S. K., Goldstein, J. L., Anderson, R. G. W., and Brown, M. S. (1976): Degradation of cationized low density lipoprotein and regulation of cholesterol metabolism in homozygous familial hypercholesterolemia fibroblasts. *Proc. Natl. Acad. Sci. USA*, 73:3178–3182.
2. Berberian, P. A., Jenison, M. W., and Roddick, V. (1985): Arterial prostaglandins and lysosomal function during atherogenesis II. Isolated cells of diet-induced atherosclerotic aortas of rabbit. *Exp. Molec. Pathol.*, 43:36–55.
3. Berliner, J. A., Territo, M. C., and Sevanian, A., et al. (1990): Minimally modified low density lipoprotein stimulates monocyte endothelial interactions. *J. Clin. Invest.*, 85:1260–1266.
4. Carew, T. E., Schwenke, D. C., and Steinberg, D. (1987): Antiatherogenic effect of probucol unrelated to its hypercholesterolemic effect: evidence that antioxidants in-vivo can selectively inhibit low density lipoprotein degradation in macrophage-rich fatty streaks and slow the progression of atherosclerosis in the Watanabe heritable hyperlipidemic rabbit. *Proc. Natl. Acad. Sci. USA*, 84:7725–7729.
5. Daugherty, A., Zweifel, B. S., and Schonfeld, G. (1989): Probucol attenuates the development of aortic atherosclerosis in cholesterol-fed rabbits. *Br. J. Pharmacol.*, 98:612–618.
6. Goldstein, J. L., Basu, S. K., and Brown, M. S. (1983): Receptor-mediated endocytosis of low density lipoprotein in cultured cells. *Methods Enzymol.*, 98:241–260.
7. Havel, R. J., Kita, T., and Kotite, L., et al. (1982): Concentration and composition of lipoproteins in blood plasma of the WHHL rabbit: an animal model of human familial hypercholesterolemia. *Arteriosclerosis*, 2:467–474.
8. Kita, T., Nagano, Y., and Yokode, M., et al. (1987): Probucol prevents the progression of atherosclerosis in Watanabe heritable hyperlipidemic rabbit, an animal model for familial hypercholesterolemia. *Proc. Natl. Acad. Sci. USA*, 84:5928–5931.
9. Kritchevsky, D., Kim, H. H., and Tepper, S. A. (1971): Influence of 4,4'-(Isopropylidenedithio)bis(2,6-di-t-butylphenol) (DH-581) on experimental atherosclerosis in rabbits. *Proc. Soc. Exp. Biol. Med.*, 136:1216–1221.
10. Niendorf, A., Brasen, J. H., Peters, S., Finckh, B., Niendorf, D. S., and Beisiegal, U. (1990): Reduced atherosclerosis in probucol-treated WHHL rabbits is due to a low foam cell and necrosis formation. *Arteriosclerosis*, 10:843a.
11. O'Brien, K. D., Chait, A., Gown, A. M., Nagano, Y., and Kita, T. (1989): Probucol treatment decreases macrophage content of atherosclerotic plaques in Watanabe heritable hyperlipidemic rabbits [Abstract]. *Circulation*, 80:II-331; no. 1321.
12. Palinski, W., Rosenfeld, M. E., and Ylä-Herttuala, S., et al. (1989): Low density lipoprotein undergoes oxidative modification in vivo. *Proc. Natl. Acad. Sci. USA*, 86:1372–1376.
13. Palinski, W., Ylä-Herttuala, S., and Rosenfeld, M. E., et al. (1990): Antisera and monoclonal antibodies specific for epitopes generated during the oxidative modification of low density lipoprotein. *Arteriosclerosis*, 10:325–335.
14. Parthasarathy, S., Quinn, M. T., Schwenke, D. C., Carew, T. E., and Steinberg, D. (1989): Oxidative modification of beta-very low density lipoprotein: potential role in monocyte recruitment and foam cell formation. *Arteriosclerosis*, 9:398–404.
15. Patton, S., and Kurtz, G. W. (1951): 2-Thiobarbituric acid as a reagent for detecting milk fat oxidation. *J. Dairy Sci.*, 34:669–674.
16. Quinn, M. T., Parthasarathy, S., Fong, L. G., and Steinberg, S. (1987): Oxidatively modified low density lipoproteins: a potential role in recruitment and retention of monocyte/macrophages during atherogenesis. *Proc. Natl. Acad. Sci. USA*, 84:2995–2998.
17. Rajavashisth, T. B., Andalibi, A., and Territo, M. C., et al. (1990): Induction of endothelial cell expression of granulocyte and macrophage colony-stimulating factors by modified low-density lipoproteins. *Nature*, 344:254–257.
18. Rosenfeld, M. E., Tsukada, T., Gown, A. M., and Ross, R. (1987): Fatty streak initiation in Watanabe Heritable Hyperlipemic and comparably hypercholesterolemic fat-fed rabbits. *Arteriosclerosis*, 7:9–23.

19. Rosenfeld, M. E., Khoo, J. C., Miller, E., Parthasarathy, S., Palinski, W., and Witztum, J. L. (1991): Macrophage-derived foam cells freshly isolated from rabbit atherosclerotic lesions degrade modified lipoproteins, promote oxidation of low-density lipoproteins, and contain oxidation-specific lipid-protein adducts. *J. Clin. Invest.,* 87 (in press).
20. Rosenfeld, M. E., Palinski, W., Ylä-Herttuala, S., Butler, S. W., and Witztum, J. L. (1990): Distribution of oxidation specific lipid-protein adducts and apolipoprotein B in atherosclerotic lesions of varying severity from WHHL rabbits. *Arteriosclerosis,* 10:336–349.
21. Salacinski, P. R. P., McLean, C., Sykes, J. E. C., Clement-Jones, V. V., and Lowry, P. J. (1981): Iodination of proteins, glycoproteins, and peptides using a solid-phase oxidizing agent, 1,3,4,6-tetrachloro-3,6-diphenyl glycouril (Iodogen). *Anal. Biochem.,* 117:136–146.
22. Shore, V. G., Shore, B., and Hart, R. G. (1974): Changes in apolipoproteins and properties of rabbit very low density lipoproteins on induction of cholesterolemia. *Biochemistry,* 13:1579–1585.
23. Stein, Y., Stein, O., Delplanque, B., Fesmire, J. D., Lee, D. M., and Alaupovic, P. (1989): Lack of effect of probucol on atheroma formation in cholesterol-fed rabbits kept at comparable plasma cholesterol levels. *Atherosclerosis,* 75:145–155.
24. Steinberg, D., Parthasarathy, S., Carew, T. E., Khoo, C., and Witztum, J. L. (1989): Beyond cholesterol: modifications of low-density lipoprotein that increase its atherogenicity. *N. Engl. J. Med.,* 320:915–924.
25. Steinbrecher, U. P., Parthasarathy, S., Leake, D. S., Witztum, J. L., and Steinberg, D. (1984): Modification of low density lipoprotein by endothelial cells involves lipid peroxidation and degradation of low density lipoprotein phospholipids. *Proc. Natl. Acad. Sci. USA,* 83:3883–3887.
26. Tanzawa, K., Shimada, Y., Kuroda, M., Tsujita, Y., Arai, M., and Watanabe, H. (1980): WHHL-rabbit: a low density lipoprotein receptor deficient animal model for familial hypercholesterolemia. *FEBS Lett.,* 118:81–84.
27. Tsukada, T., Rosenfeld, M. E., Ross, R., and Gown, A. M. (1986): Immunocytochemical analysis of cellular components in atherosclerotic lesions. Use of monoclonal antibodies with the Watanabe and fat-fed rabbits. *Arteriosclerosis,* 6:601–613.
28. Tsukada, T., Tippens, T., Gordon, D., Ross, R., and Gown, A. M. (1987): HHF-35, a muscle-actin–specific monoclonal antibody. *Am. J. Pathol.,* 126:51–60.
29. Ylä-Herttuala, S., Palinski, W., and Rosenfeld, M. E., et al. (1989): Evidence for the presence of oxidatively modified low density lipoprotein in atherosclerotic lesions of rabbit and man. *J. Clin. Invest.,* 84:1086–1095.

Atherosclerosis Reviews, Volume 23,
edited by P. C. Weber and A. Leaf.
Raven Press, Ltd., New York © 1991.

Significance of Risk Factors in the Prediction of Atherosclerosis

D. Seidel, P. Cremer and Dorothea Nagel

Institute for Clinical Chemistry, Klinikum Großhadern, Ludwig Maximilians University, Marchioninistraße 15, D-8000 Munich 70, Germany

There is ample evidence that diseases resulting from premature atherosclerosis—the leading event is myocardial infarction (MI)—have great impact on health care in industrialized countries (11,13). These illnesses are the most common cause not only of death but also of early retirement. No doubt this has contributed to the fact that atherosclerosis, together with cancer, is a primary consideration in experimental, clinical, and preventive medicine. The results of many studies have shown that there are a large number of factors involved in atherogenesis. The following factors seem to be the most important: disturbances in lipid metabolism, familial history of MI, hypertension, smoking, elevated blood glucose, overweight, male sex, and age. Most recently, Lp(a) (10) and fibrinogen (8) have been added to the list.

It is important that the translation of experimental and statistical data into advice for clinical practice is done with caution, with a good sense of proportion, a realistic approach, and consideration of a risk:benefit:cost relationship for the individual and society in general. It is necessary to be simple without oversimplification and to differentiate clearly between the goals of primary prevention and the goals of secondary prevention. It is important to realize that there is no such disease as hypertension or hypercholesterolemia by itself, but only a sick person who is suffering from such a disturbance or is at risk because of the disturbance. Finally, it is very important to focus on the risk factors that have been proven to be causal for the disease. All this is particularly true for coronary artery disease (CAD) in humans.

The evidence for the role of blood lipids, lipoprotein families, or apolipoproteins in the etiology of atherosclerosis and coronary heart disease comes from a number of sources, including studies of cell biology, experimental pathology, clinical biochemistry, prospective and case control studies, as well as intervention trials. This chapter reports on the apparent discrepancy between the established causal relationship of low-density lipoprotein (LDL) cholesterol and CAD and its relatively weak predictive power as seen in most epidemiological studies.

There are very few clinical or epidemiological studies in which LDL cholesterol ranks as the number one risk factor. The reason for this may be that in the past, little attempt has been made to directly measure LDL cholesterol. However, it is obvious and logical that the predictive power of a risk factor not only depends on the factor as such but also on the methods used to measure the factor.

The Göttingen Risk, Incidence, and Prevalence Study (GRIPS) (4,7) is the first prospective cohort study in which LDL cholesterol was measured directly and its predictive power compared with that of lipids, high-density lipoprotein (HDL) cholesterol, apolipoproteins, etc. In the GRIPS study, over 6,500 industrial workers were examined in early 1982. Since then, this group has been regularly checked by follow-up examinations, with special attention to the incidence of coronary and other diseases. The observation time of the study will last 15 years. The basic analysis in 1982 included recording of the family status, family history for atherosclerotic disease, school education, social position, professional stress, physical activity, dietary habits, alcohol consumption, smoking, present health status, and present medication. Special emphasis was placed on the precision and accuracy of the biochemical methods for quantification of the separate lipoproteins and apoproteins. LDL cholesterol was measured directly by three different methods, each of which showed a coefficient of variance of less than 2%. These included quantitative lipoprotein electrophoresis (12), dextrane sulfate precipitation (1), and acid heparin precipitation (2). Because of their low precision (CV, 5%–10%), such indirect methods as the Lipid Research Clinic (LRC) technique or the Friedewald formula were not used to quantify LDL.

Of the total group examined in GRIPS during 1982, 5,738 were men of German origin who were free of atherosclerosis and other diseases. This report presents

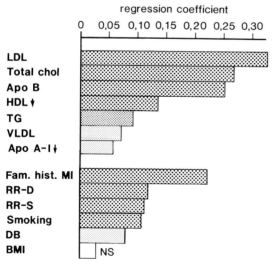

FIG. 1. Grading of variables reveals LDL as predominant factor for myocardial infarction risk within a 5-year interval according to univariate regression analysis.

TABLE 1. *GRIPS (B): grading of variables according to their predictive power by multivariate logistic regression analysis*

Pos	Variable	χ^2	p	OR	CI
1	LDL chol (4 Cat)[a]	95	***	2.32 (12)[b]	1.9–2.8
2	Family history of MI	31	***	4.07	2.6–6.4
3	HDL chol ($</\geq$35 mg/dl)	17	***	2.70	1.7–4.3
4	Age ($</\geq$50 yr)	16	***	2.29	1.5–3.3
5	Hypertension	6	*	1.36	1.1–1.8
6	Cigarette smoking	5	*	1.63	1.1–2.4
7	Glucose ($</\geq$120 mg/dl)	4	*	1.72	1.1–2.8

OR, odds ratio, CI, confidence interval for odds ratio, χ^2, 2 log likelihood ratio, ***$p < 0.001$, *$p < 0.05$.
[a] <150, 150–169, 170–189, ≥190 mg/dl.
[b] High-risk group versus low-risk group.

the first 5-year follow-up data of GRIPS. The responder rate was 95.2%. Of our subjects, 5,132 remained free of atherosclerotic disease (reference group), whereas 107 developed a first MI, and 148 developed another cardiovascular disease between 1982 and 1987. This report will focus on the MI subjects (incidence group) and compare them with the reference group.

Univariate analyses, indicate that LDL cholesterol was the strongest predictor of MI risk, followed by total cholesterol, apoB, HDL cholesterol (inversely related), etc. (Fig. 1). Among the nonlipid parameters, family history for MI was the strongest predictor, followed by high blood pressure, cigarette smoking, di-

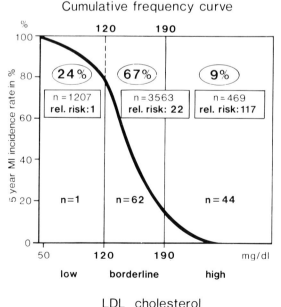

FIG. 2. Cumulative frequency of LDL cholesterol showing the relative risk in three different concentration groups.

abetes, and body mass index. This ranking is substantiated on the basis of a multivariate logistic regression analysis (Table 1). LDL cholesterol ranks first, followed by familial MI history, etc.

The cumulative frequency curve of LDL cholesterol (Fig. 2) reveals three subgroups with impressing differences in their relative risk for MI. The low-risk group (LDL cholesterol < 120 mg/dl) represents 24% of the cohort, with only one event in 5 years. If this is counted as risk 1, the relative MI risk for the high-risk group (LDL cholesterol ≥ 190 mg/dl) counts 117. Nine percent of the cohort belongs to the high-risk group; they have a 10% chance to suffer an MI event within 5 years. Two-thirds of the total cohort show LDL cholesterol concentrations between 120 mg/dl and 189 mg/dl. This subgroup reveals a relative MI risk of 22, i.e., six times lower than that of the high-risk group. The influences of other factors on MI risk were important in the high and intermediate LDL groups. However, their impact was negligible in the low-LDL group. These findings are not in full agreement with most epidemiological studies. For example, a recent report of the Framingham Study (3) claims the strongest predictive power for the HDL cholesterol/total cholesterol ratio. The most likely explanation for this misleading discrepancy is the frequent use of inadequate biochemical methodology.

The multivariate model confirms (Figs. 3 and 4) that only if LDL cholesterol exceeds a critical threshold concentration of approximately 120 mg/dl, other risk factors influence the MI risk considerably (Figs. 3 and 4).

In regard to the question of primary and secondary prevention, it is most interesting to compare the relationship between LDL cholesterol concentrations and MI risk in subjects free of atherosclerosic diseases at the beginning of the study (1982) and in those who had suffered at least one event of MI before 1982 (Fig. 5). During the first 5 years of our study, 9% of the high-risk, (LDL cholesterol ≥ 190 mg/dl), initially MI-negative group developed a first MI, whereas 100% of the high-risk, initially MI-positive group developed additional MI events. Analogous differences concerning the MI incidence were found in lower-risk groups (LDL cholesterol < 150 mg/dl: 0.6% versus 31%; LDL cholesterol 150–

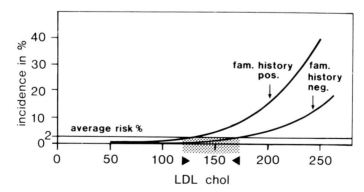

FIG. 3. Potentiation of LDL risk by family history of myocardial infarction.

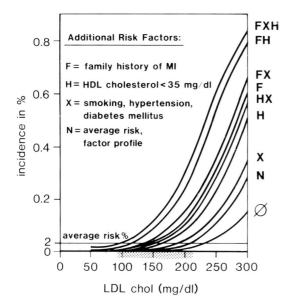

FIG. 4. Potentiation of LDL risk for myocardial infarction (MI) by other risk factors.

189 mg/dl: 2.6% versus 50%). Pekkanen et al. reported similar results in their analysis of a subgroup of the Lipid Research Clinics Program Prevalence study (6). These data clearly indicate the clinical need to carefully differentiate the goals of primary and secondary prevention.

To date, the conclusion of the GRIPS study and our recommendations for a strategy to classify subjects according to their MI risk are as follows (Fig. 6): A

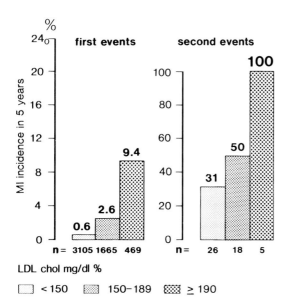

FIG. 5. Five-year myocardial infarction incidence of subjects with and without previous events in three different LDL concentration groups.

physical examination, and a record of other risk factors including family history of cardiovascular events are used to classify a subject into one of three groups: (group 1) patients with coronary artery disease; (group 2) patients without signs of coronary artery disease but with other risk factors (familial history of CHD, hypertension, cigarette smoking); and (group 3) patients without signs of coronary artery disease and without risk factors.

Whereas measurement of lipoproteins is always recommended for group 1, screening for total cholesterol and triglycerides is initially sufficient for groups 2 and 3. The following cutoff points are recommended: triglycerides 200 mg/dl for both groups; total cholesterol 200 mg/dl for group 2, and 240 mg/dl for group 3. If one of these threshold concentrations is exceeded, lipoprotein analysis is obligatory.

The recommended therapeutic goals for LDL cholesterol are <110 mg/dl for group 1, <150 mg/dl for group 2, and for those group 3 subjects with HDL cholesterol <35 mg/dl; <190 mg/dl for the remaining group 3 subjects. These therapeutic goals differ from those of the U.S. National Cholesterol Education Program Expert Panel (5), which are 130 mg/dl (groups 1 and 2) or 160 mg/dl (group 3), respectively (5). Analogous therapeutic goals of the European Consensus Conference are 135 and 155 mg/dl, respectively (9). Due to the small difference between these two threshold values, the latter recommendations (9) neither allow a reliable classification of subjects according to their MI risk nor are they a valid basis for strategies in the treatment of hypercholesterolemia. Undoubtedly, LDL cholesterol is not the only risk indicator for coronary heart disease; however, it seems to be the most important and so far the only one with a convincingly documented causal relationship.

If we want to do something against the current epidemic of coronary heart disease, we must attempt to focus on what is important. It is time to realize that LDL cholesterol can be measured directly and precisely. If the risk of a person

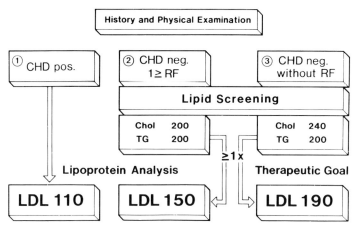

FIG. 6. Strategy to estimate coronary heart disease risk.

is to be estimated, LDL cholesterol deserves first priority. For the definition of therapeutic goals in the primary and secondary prevention of coronary heart disease one should also focus on LDL cholesterol. However, the decision for therapy should never be based on a plasma lipid or plasma lipoprotein concentration value alone. The entire person (additional risk factors, coronary status) must always be taken into consideration.

ACKNOWLEDGMENT

This work was supported by Bundesministerium für Forschung und Technologie (BMFT), Förderkennzeichen 07063216.

REFERENCES

1. Armstrong, V. W., and Seidel, D. (1985): Evaluation of a commercial kit for the determination of LDL cholesterol in serum based on precipitation of LDL with dextran sulfate. *Ärztl. Lab.,* 31:325–330.
2. Armstrong, V. W., Wieland, H., and Seidel, D. (1983): A new sensitive method for measuring low-density lipoproteins and its application to the screening for hyperlipoproteinemia. In: Benson, F., ed. *Screening and management of potentially treatable genetic metabolic disorders.* MTP Press, 115–125.
3. Castelli, W. P., Wilson, P. W. F., Levy, D., and Anderson, K. (1990): Serum lipids and risk of coronary artery disease. In: Leaf, A., and Weber, P. C., eds. *Atherosclerosis reviews,* vol. 21. New York: Raven, pp. 7–19.
4. Cremer, P., and Muche R. (1990): Göttinger Risiko-, Inzidenz- und Prävalenzstudie (GRIPS). Empfehlungen zur Prävention der koronaren Herzkrankheit. *Ther. Umsch.,* 6:482–491.
5. National Cholesterol Education Program Expert Panel. (1988): Report of the National Cholesterol Education Program Expert Panel on detection, evaluation and treatment of high blood cholesterol in adults. *Arch. Intern. Med.,* 148:36–69.
6. Pekkanen, X., Linn, S., Heiss, G., et al. (1990): 10 year mortality from cardiovascular disease in relation to cholesterol level among men with and without preexisting cardiovascular disease. *N. Engl. J. Med.,* 322:1700–1707.
7. Seidel, D., and Cremer, P. (1986): Guidelines for the clinical evaluation of risk factors: first report from the Göttingen Risk, Incidence, and Prevalence Study. In: Gotto, A. M., and Paoletti, R., eds. *Atherosclerosis reviews,* vol. 14. New York: Raven Press, pp. 61–89.
8. Smith, E. B. (1990): Transport, interactions and retention of plasma proteins in the intima: the barrier function of the internal elastic lamina. *Eur. Heart J.,* 11(suppl. E):72–81.
9. Study Group, European Atherosclerosis Society. (1988): The recognition and management of hyperlipidaemia in adults: a policy statement of the European Atherosclerosis Society. *Eur. Heart J.,* 9:571–600.
10. Utermann, G. (1989): The mysteries of lipoprotein(a). *Science,* 246:904–910.
11. WHO Expert Committee. (1982): Prevention of coronary heart disease. *WHO Techn. Rep. Series.* Geneva: WHO: 678.
12. Wieland, H., and Seidel, D. Quantitative lipoprotein-electrophoresis. In: Lewis, L. A., ed. *CRC handbook of electrophoresis,* vol. 3. Boca Raton, Fla.: CRC Press, pp. 83–102.
13. Witels, E. H., Hay, J. W., and Gotto, A. M. Jr. (1990): Medical costs of coronary artery disease in the United States. *Am. J. Cardiol.,* 15:432–440.

Atherosclerosis Reviews, Volume 23,
edited by P. C. Weber and A. Leaf.
Raven Press, Ltd., New York © 1991.

N-3 and N-6 Fatty Acids, Cholesterol, and Coronary Heart Disease

Michael L. Burr

*MRC Epidemiology Unit (South Wales), Llandough Hospital,
Penarth, South Glamorgan CF6 1XX, Wales*

This chapter reviews the role of n-3 and n-6 fatty acids in relation to coronary heart disease (CHD), with special reference to evidence from intervention studies in human subjects. Observational evidence is certainly important because it draws attention to associations which can then be investigated experimentally. But observed associations are not necessarily causal. People who choose one kind of diet differ in various ways from people who choose another kind of diet, and the nondietary differences may represent more important factors in the development of CHD than the dietary patterns associated with them. The experimental approach allows diet to be altered while other factors are kept constant. Animal models are useful because they allow experiments that are impractical or unethical in human subjects. But there will always be reservations concerning the relevance to human disease of conditions induced in other species, particularly if the diets are quite unlike anything the animal would normally eat.

N-3 FATTY ACIDS AND CHD

The fatty acids of the n-3 series are mostly derived from seafood. The main n-3 fatty acids relevant to human nutrition are eicosapentaenoic acid (EPA) (20:5n-3) and docosahexaenoic acid (DHA) (22:6n-3). They are synthesized by algae and phytoplankton at the bottom of the marine food chain and incorporated into all forms of seafood, and are especially abundant in fish with a high content of oil.

Attention was first drawn to n-3 fatty acids as potentially protective against CHD by observations in Greenland Eskimos (2,3). The rarity of CHD in these people was linked with their low plasma concentrations of cholesterol and (especially) triglycerides (TG), which were attributed to the high levels of polyunsaturated fatty acids (principally of the n-3 series) in their diet. The possibility of a protective effect was reinforced by evidence from cohort studies, which showed a lower CHD mortality in subjects who eat a moderate amount of fish than in subjects who ate little or no fish (16,27).

TABLE 1. *Outcome of the diet and reinfarction trial (5)*

	Fish advice group		No fish advice group
Total no. subjects	1,015		1,018
No. deaths	94 (9.3%)	*	130 (12.8%)
No. CHD deaths	78 (7.7%)	**	116 (11.4%)
No. nonfatal MI	49 (4.8%)		33 (3.2%)
No. CHD events	127 (12.5%)		149 (14.6%)

$* p < 0.05, ** p < .001.$

These and other observations have led to intervention studies designed to investigate the possibility that n-3 fatty acids confer some protection against CHD. The Diet and Reinfarction Trial (DART) examined the effect of fatty fish on survival after myocardial infarction (MI) (5). In this trial, 2,033 men under the age of 70 years were recruited during their recovery from acute MI and randomly allocated to receive (or not to receive) advice to eat fatty fish at least twice a week. Those who could not tolerate fatty fish were supplied with fish oil capsules. The 2-year mortality of men given advice to eat fish was significantly lower than that of the men not given this advice; the difference was attributable to a reduction in CHD deaths. Nonfatal reinfarction occurred somewhat more frequently in the group advised to eat fish (although the difference was not statistically significant), so that the incidence of CHD events (deaths attributed to CHD plus nonfatal reinfarctions) did not differ significantly between the two groups (Table 1).

These results suggest that some protection against CHD is given by a modest intake of oily fish (about 300 g weekly, corresponding to a daily dose of approximately 0.6 g n-3 fatty acids). There must inevitably be some reservations as to whether the results of a single study should be regarded as conclusive; other confirmatory trials are undoubtedly needed. It is even questionable whether the benefit was attributable to the increased intake of n-3 fatty acids in the intervention group or to the concomitant decrease in other foods replaced by fatty fish. However, this is a very unlikely explanation. The reductions in other foods (meat, cheese, and eggs) were very small and markedly less than the reductions in these foods occurring as a consequence of independently randomized advice that had no effect on mortality.

N-3 FATTY ACIDS AND RESTENOSIS

Percutaneous transluminal coronary angioplasty is increasingly being used to dilate stenosed coronary arteries. A major problem of this technique is that restenosis frequently occurs in the dilated vessels, usually within the first 6 months. Several controlled trials have been conducted in which fish oil has been investigated as a possible means of preventing restenosis. Table 2 summarizes the results of some of these trials; dosages are expressed in terms of total n-3 fatty acids for purposes of comparison.

TABLE 2. *Randomized trials of fish oil in preventing restenosis after coronary angioplasty*

Reference	n-3 fatty acids (g/day)	Numbers of subjects[a]		Duration	Assessment	Evidence of benefit
		Fish oil group	Control group			
Slack (28)	1.8–2.7	67	71	6 mo.	Stress test	Yes
Ilsley (15)	3.6	36	37	6 mo.	Symptoms, angiography	Yes
Milner (19)	4.5	71	78	6 mo.	Symptoms, stress, angiography	? Yes
Dehmer (8)	5.4	43	39	6 mo.	Angiography	Yes
Grigg (12)	3.0	43	49	4 mo.	Angiography	No
Reis (22)	6.0	124	62	6 mo.	Symptoms, angiography	No
Franzen (11)	3.15	67	62	4 mo.	Angiography	No

[a] Numbers relate to subjects for whom results were obtained.

It is not clear why some trials have shown a favorable effect of fish oil whereas others have not. In each study, various other types of treatment were given to all patients, and it is possible that the efficacy of fish oil is related to the fact that other medication was given. The three negative trials all employed olive oil as a placebo, and it is conceivable that this oil has some antistenotic action. The duration of fish oil administration prior to angioplasty may well be important, since the trials varied considerably in this regard. They also differed in numbers of subjects, doses of fish oil, and criteria of outcome. Therefore, further trials should require that fish oil be given for several weeks prior to angioplasty and that blind clinical and angiographic assessment be performed subsequently.

Nevertheless, we must acknowledge that the prevention of restenosis after angioplasty is a special activity. We cannot assume that the process of restenosis in these highly artificial circumstances necessarily resembles the formation of primary stenotic lesions, nor that the determinants will be the same.

POSSIBLE MODE OF ACTION OF N-3 FATTY ACIDS

Assuming that the n-3 fatty acids confer some protection against CHD, we still need to determine the likely mechanism. The DART study suggested that moderate amounts of oily fish affect CHD mortality within a few months (5). Similar conclusions were drawn from a "natural experiment" at the start of World War II, when a change in the Norwegian diet from meat to fish was followed within a year by a substantial fall in CHD mortality (1). Such an immediate reaction to dietary change can hardly be mediated by an effect on the atheromatous process, which presumably operates over years or decades. Some other mechanism must therefore be involved.

One possible mode of action is an effect on the blood platelets and other aspects of the clotting process. Several randomized controlled trials have demonstrated that fish oil reduces platelet aggregation and the production of thromboxane B_2 (4,18), prolonging the bleeding time (20) or the heparin thrombin clotting time (24). However, these studies all employed doses of n-3 fatty acids much greater than would normally be supplied by dietary sources; it remains to be demonstrated whether clinically important changes in clotting mechanisms can be obtained by means of smaller amounts.

N-3, N-6 AND CHOLESTEROL

There have been numerous studies investigating the effects of n-3 fatty acids on serum lipids. It seems that a reduction in serum cholesterol occurs only if very large doses (4.5–6 g EPA or 6.5–10 g n-3 fatty acids per day) are given (6). Smaller amounts of n-3 fatty acids appear to have no effect, or even to cause a slight increase (5,26). The blood concentration of very-low-density lipoproteins is reduced (20,26), and TG levels are also reduced even when the amount of fish oil is quite small (9). It seems therefore that a reduction in serum cholesterol *per se* is not an important part of the protective action of oily fish, although other effects on the serum lipids may be.

Of the fatty acids in the n-6 series, linoleic acid (18:2n-6) has been investigated in particular detail. Its principal nutritional sources are vegetables, nuts, and seeds. Unlike EPA and DHA, it has a well-documented cholesterol-lowering effect; for this reason, it has long been regarded as an important agent in preventing CHD.

N-6 FATTY ACIDS AND CHD

Numerous studies have investigated the possible role of n-6 fatty acids—particularly linoleic acid—in preventing CHD. These studies have usually involved reducing total fat and replacing saturated with polyunsaturated fatty acids in the diet, or else supplementing the diet with vegetable oils rich in linoleic acid. They can be conveniently classified as primary and secondary prevention trials, according to whether or not the subjects had already suffered from MI. It must be recognized that these trials have not investigated the effect of linoleic acid (or any other fatty acid) in isolation. In each case, the intention was primarily to reduce the serum cholesterol concentration. The linoleic acid intake was increased to varying degrees for this purpose. It is seldom possible to determine the amounts of linoleic acid that were taken by the subjects. More attention was usually given to the ratio of polyunsaturated to saturated fatty acids in the subjects' diets (in the published accounts of these studies, "polyunsaturated" largely denotes linoleic acid).

Table 3 summarizes the primary prevention trials in which the allocation was randomized; only the Minnesota Coronary Survey (10) included women. The WHO trial (32) differed from the others in that paired factories rather than

TABLE 3. *Randomized controlled trials involving linoleic acid in primary CHD prevention*

Reference	Total no. of subjects	Other factors	Duration	Serum cholesterol change		Outcome
				Intervention	Controls	
Dayton (7)	846	—	≤100 mo.	−11% (at 2 yr)	+2%	Reduction in athero- sclerotic but not total mortality
Hjermann (13)	1,232	Smoking	5 yr	−20%	+4%	MI incidence reduced
MRFIT (21)	12,866	BP, smoking	7 yr (mean)	−4% (at 2 yr)	−1%	No significant differences
WHO (32)	60,881	BP, smoking, exercise, obesity	5–6 yr	−2.2%[a] (at 4 yr)	—	No overall differences
Wilhelmsen (29)	30,022	BP, smoking	12 yr (mean)	−0.6% (at 4 yr)	+0.6%	No significant differences
Frantz (10)	9,057	—	$4\frac{1}{2}$ yr	−15%	−2%	No significant differences

[a] Net change after subtracting change in control group.

individual subjects were randomized. The subjects in the Oslo trial (13) and Multiple Risk Factor Intervention Trial (MRFIT) (21) were selected as being at high risk (smoking, blood pressure, or serum cholesterol); in those subjects and in the WHO trial subjects, the intervention "package" included nondietary components. In the Göteborg trial (29), the group randomized to intervention was then screened for hypertension, hypercholesterolemia, and smoking; dietary advice was given to subjects whose serum cholesterol exceeded 6.8 mmol/liter, and intensive attention was paid to those whose serum cholesterol exceeded 7.8 mmol/liter. The changes in serum cholesterol in these trials were not all calculated in the same way, but they give some idea of the relative effects of the diets.

The Veterans Study showed some reduction in atherosclerotic mortality in the intervention group (7). This was, however, balanced by a small excess of deaths from other causes (trauma and cancer), so that overall mortality was similar in the two groups. The Oslo Study (13) showed a reduction in MI incidence, but it is difficult to know how much was attributable to smoking cessation and how much to dietary change. The MRFIT results (21) showed no reduction in mortality or CHD incidence, but the differential reduction in risk factors was less than expected, due partly to spontaneous changes in the control group. Thus, the differences between plasma cholesterol concentrations were small, and by 6 years a reduction of 3% in the control group had occurred in comparison with a reduction of 5% in the intervention group. The WHO trial (32) involved centers in seven countries, with substantial differences in compliance. The Belgian component of the trial had good compliance and showed a significant reduction in both CHD incidence and total mortality (31).

The Göteborg trial (29) was similarly disappointing; after 10 years, the serum cholesterol had fallen to virtually the same extent in the intervention and control groups (6.5% and 6.4%, respectively), and there were no significant differences in mortality or CHD incidence.

The Minnesota Coronary Survey (10) had roughly equal numbers of men and women, all of whom lived in institutions. The intervention diet included 15% polyunsaturated fatty acids, compared with 5% in the control diet, but no reduction in total fat. No significant differences occurred in mortality or CHD incidence.

Other intervention studies have been conducted in which the allocation was not randomized. Several of them have claimed to show a beneficial effect of a diet high in polyunsaturated fat (i.e., linoleic acid), but considerable reservations must attach to nonrandomized studies in view of the possibility of bias.

Randomized secondary prevention trials are shown in Table 4. The trial by Rose et al. (25) included some women; in the other trials, all the subjects were men. The WHO trial (33) differed from the others in that dietary advice was given only to subjects considered to have a high serum cholesterol level. None of these trials showed any reduction in overall mortality—in fact, one trial (30) showed a significant increase. As in the primary prevention trials, the differential reduction in serum cholesterol attributable to the diet was disappointing in some cases, and the trials that achieved the largest reductions in serum cholesterol were probably insufficient in size.

Overall, it seems that the results of increasing the consumption of n-6 fatty acids have been disappointing so far. It is possible that larger studies would show an effect, or that a longer period of time is necessary. It is difficult to devise a study in which a random half of the subjects can be induced to achieve and maintain profound dietary changes while the others are insulated from the background health education that tends to cause similar changes to a lesser degree.

POSSIBLE MODE OF ACTION OF N-6 FATTY ACIDS

It has generally been assumed that linoleic acid has a favorable effect on CHD risk by means of a reduction in cholesterol concentrations in serum or plasma.

TABLE 4. *Randomized controlled trials involving linoleic acid in secondary CHD prevention*

| Reference | Total no. of subjects | Duration | Serum cholesterol change | | Outcome |
			Intervention	Controls	
Rose (25)	80	2 yr	−20%	−3%	No difference
Research Committee (23)	393	2–7 yr	−22%	−6%	No difference
Leren (17)	412	10–12 yr	−18%	−4%	"Fatal MI" reduced; total mortality unaffected
Woodhill (30)	458	2–5 yr	−11%	−7%	Total mortality increased
WHO (33)	3,184	3 yr	—	—	No difference
Burr (5)	2,033	2 yr	−2%	+1%	No difference

The known relationship between serum cholesterol and the atheromatous process suggests that any beneficial effect of linoleic acid might be expected to operate over several years, by opposing or conceivably reversing the formation of atheromatous plaques.

It has been suggested, however, that other n-6 fatty acids—metabolites of linoleic acid such as dihomogammalinolenic acid (20:3n-6) and arachidonic acid (20:4n-6)—may be responsible for the cholesterol-lowering action of linoleic acid and may have certain additional protective effects, including a reduction in platelet aggregability (14). Some arachidonic acid is obtained from the diet, especially from meat and eggs; dihomogammalinolenic acid is absent from the diet (apart from human milk). Clinical studies are needed to investigate the relevance of these fatty acids in the control of CHD.

CONCLUSIONS

Fatty acids in the n-3 series are mainly derived from seafood; they are currently attracting great interest because of the likelihood that they protect against CHD. Their mode of action is uncertain but may well involve clotting mechanisms; it is unlikely that an effect on serum cholesterol is relevant. The n-6 fatty acids, by contrast, have a cholesterol-lowering effect that is probably clinically important. Only linoleic acid has been investigated in any detail in this connection. Randomized dietary trials have been rather disappointing, possibly because they have been too small and too short. Given the high incidence of CHD and the wide public interest in its prevention, it should not be impossible to conduct trials of secondary (if not primary) prevention of CHD that would demonstrate more clearly the benefits of increasing the intake of these fatty acids.

REFERENCES

1. Bang, H. O., and Dyerberg, J. (1981): *Acta Med. Scand.,* 210:245–248.
2. Bang, H. O., Dyerberg, J., and Hjorne, N. (1976): *Am. J. Clin. Nutr.,* 33:2657–2661.
3. Bang, H. O., Dyerberg, J., and Nielsen, A. B. (1971): *Lancet,* 1:1143–1146.
4. Brox, J. H., Killie, J.-E., Gunnes, S., and Nordoy, A. (1981): *Thromb. Haemost.,* 46:604–611.
5. Burr, M. L., Fehily, A. M., Gilbert, J. F., et al. (1989): *Lancet,* 2:757–761.
6. Davidson, M. H., McKenna, R., Sullivan, D. P., Liebson, P. R., Schoenberger, J. A., and Messer, J. V. (1987): *J. Am. Coll. Cardiol.,* 9:185A.
7. Dayton, S., Pearce, M. L., Goldman, H., et al. (1968): *Lancet,* 2:1060–1062.
8. Dehmer, G. J., Popma, J. J., van den Berg, E. K., et al. (1988): *N. Engl. J. Med.,* 319:733–740.
9. Fehily, A. M., Burr, M. L., Phillips, K. M., and Deadman, N. M. (1983): *Am. J. Clin. Nutr.,* 38: 349–351.
10. Frantz, I. D., Dawson, E. A., Ashman, P. L., et al. (1989): *Arteriosclerosis,* 9:129–135.
11. Franzen, D., Höpp, H. W., Günther, H., Schannwell, M., Oette, K., and Hilger, H. (1990): *Eur. Heart J.,* 11(suppl.):367.
12. Grigg, L. E., Kay, T. W. H., Valentine, P. A., et al. (1989): *J. Am. Coll. Cardiol.,* 13:665–672.
13. Hjermann, I., Byre, K. V., Holme, I., and Leren, P. (1981): *Lancet,* 2:1303–1310.
14. Horrobin, D. F., and Yuang, Y.-S. (1987): *Int. J. Cardiol.,* 17:241–255.
15. Ilsley, C. D. J., Nye, E. R., Sutherland, W., Ram, J., and Ablett, M. B. (1987): *Aust. N. Z. J. Med.,* 17:559.

16. Kromhout, D., Bosschieter, E. B., and Coulander, C de L. (1985): *N. Engl. J. Med.*, 312:1205–1209.
17. Leren, P. (1970): *Circulation*, 42:935–942.
18. Mehta, J. L., Lopez, L. M., Lawson, D., Wargovich, T. J., and Williams, L. L. (1988): *Am. J. Med.*, 84:45–52.
19. Milner, M. R., Gallino, R. A., Leffingwell, A., Pickard, A. D., Rosenberg, J., and Lindsay, J. (1988): *Circulation*, 78(Suppl. II):634.
20. Mortensen, J. Z., Schmidt, E. B., Nielsen, A. H., and Dyerberg, J. (1983): *Thromb. Haemost.*, 50:543–546.
21. Multiple Risk Factor Intervention Trial Research Group. (1982): *J. Am. Med. Assoc.*, 248:1465–1477.
22. Reis, G. J., Boucher, T. M., Sipperly, M. E., et al. (1989): *Lancet*, 2:177–181.
23. Research Committee. (1968): *Lancet*, 2:693–700.
24. Rogers, S., James, K. S., Butland, B. K., Etherington, M. D., O'Brien, J. R., and Jones, J. G. (1987): *Atherosclerosis*, 63:137–143.
25. Rose, G. A., Thomson, W. B., and Williams, R. T. (1965): *Br. Med. J.*, 1:1531–1533.
26. Schmidt, E. B., Kristensen, S. D., and Dyerberg, J. (1988): *Artery*, 15:316–329.
27. Shekelle, R. B., Missell, L., Paul, O., Shryock, A. M. and Stamler, J. (1985): *N. Engl. J. Med.*, 313:820.
28. Slack, J. D., Pinkerton, C. A., Van Tassel, J., et al. (1987): *J. Am. Coll. Cardiol.*, 9:64A.
29. Wilhelmsen, L., Berglund, G., Elmfeldt, D., et al. (1986): *Eur. Heart J.*, 7:279–288.
30. Woodhill, J. M., Palmer, A. J., Leelarthaepin, B., McGilchrist, C., and Blacket, R. B. (1978): *Adv. Exp. Med. Biol.*, 109:317–330.
31. World Health Organization Collaborative Group. (1983): *Eur. Heart J.*, 4:141–147.
32. World Health Organization Collaborative Group. (1986): *Lancet*, 1:869–872.
33. World Health Organization Regional Office for Europe. (1983): *Euro Reports and Studies 84.* Copenhagen: WHO, pp. 1–99.

Atherosclerosis Reviews, Volume 23,
edited by P. C. Weber and A. Leaf.
Raven Press, Ltd., New York © 1991.

Pharmacological Prevention of Myocardial Infarction and Stroke

Carlo Patrono

University of Chieti, G. D'Annunzio School of Medicine, Chieti, Italy

Thrombotic occlusion of a major coronary or cerebral artery is an unpredictable complication of atherosclerotic lesions. Several pharmacological strategies have been used to reduce the risk of potentially fatal outcomes, i.e., myocardial infarction (MI) and stroke. These strategies include lowering of blood lipids (14) and high blood pressure (4), blockade of β-adrenergic receptors (21) or calcium channels (11), and inhibition of various hemostatic functions (19). Suppression of some forms of platelet activation (e.g., thromboxane-dependent platelet activation) is perhaps the most widely investigated pharmacological intervention during the last 20 years, both in secondary and primary prevention studies (12). Moreover, within the class of inhibitors of platelet aggregation, a single drug— aspirin—provides approximately 70% of all the available information, thus allowing some comparison of the efficacy of this pharmacological intervention in different types of patients.

Aspirin has been studied in over 20 randomized, placebo-controlled clinical trials involving more than 60,000 subjects (12). The evidence supporting its antithrombotic efficacy can be considered conclusive for the prevention of MI, stroke, and vascular death in secondary prevention studies (1,12). Nevertheless, the evidence is limited to prevention of MI in primary prevention trials (12). Doubts remain about the potential impact of aspirin therapy on the incidence of stroke (possibly enhanced) and vascular death (possibly unchanged), because of the small number of such events in primary prevention studies.

ANTIPLATELET DRUGS CAN PREVENT MYOCARDIAL INFARCTION AND STROKE

Clinical efficacy—a statistically significant reduction in "hard" end points— has been demonstrated in patients with previous (occurring weeks or months before starting therapy) or acute (within 24 hr after the onset of symptoms) MI, unstable angina, transient ischemic attacks, and stroke as well as in apparently healthy male physicians.

Interestingly, patients entering these studies because of coronary heart disease

(CHD) were protected by aspirin against both coronary (i.e., MI or reinfarction) and cerebral (stroke) thrombotic complications. The converse is also true; patients with cerebrovascular disease treated with aspirin had a reduced incidence of both stroke and MI. These observations might be taken to suggest that a common underlying cause (e.g., a fissured atherosclerotic plaque) may be present in either vascular district and that such an acute vascular lesion is transduced, at least in part, by a common mechanism (i.e., thromboxane-dependent platelet aggregation) into sudden occlusive events. Measurement of urinary thromboxane metabolites supports this notion by showing episodic increases in metabolite excretion in patients with unstable coronary syndromes (7,9,20) as well as in patients with transient ischemic attacks (Ciabattoni, Koudstaal, and Patrono, unpublished observations).

The remarkable clinical efficacy of a short-term (4 weeks) treatment with aspirin initiated within 24 hr of the onset of symptoms of suspected acute MI (13) is not surprising if one accepts the idea that a dynamic thrombotic process (i.e., episodic thrombus formation and fragmentation) is present in the early phase of coronary thrombosis (as discussed elsewhere in this volume) and that such a process can be equally hampered in its further progression by either slowing platelet aggregation or accelerating fibrinolysis.

If we take vascular death as the primary end-point for the analysis of clinical efficacy, aspirin is the only antiplatelet agent for which a statistically significant reduction has been clearly demonstrated in a single large trial (ISIS-2) (13) as well in an overview of several smaller studies (1). Variable reductions in the incidence of MI and stroke have also been reported with sulfinpyrazone (1) or ticlopidine (2,8,10) in secondary prevention trials. It is unknown whether aspirin and ticlopidine prevent the same type of vascular occlusive events. Because of their different mechanism of action in inhibiting platelet function, the possibility of obtaining additive effects is currently being explored.

SIZE OF THE EFFECT

Because there was no obvious large difference among the effects of antiplatelet therapy in the different types of trials reviewed by the Antiplatelet Trialists' Collaboration (1), information from all trials was combined regardless of the type of prior vascular disease at entry into therapy. The following reductions in risk were found: nonfatal MI, $32 \pm 5\%$; nonfatal stroke, $27 \pm 6\%$; total vascular death, $15 \pm 4\%$; any major vascular event (i.e., the three combined), $25 \pm 3\%$. Thus, treatment of 100 such patients for 2 years would on average avoid one vascular death and two nonfatal events.

Table 1 compares the ISIS-2 results on short-term antiplatelet treatment of suspected acute MI with the overview of the results on long-term antiplatelet treatment of patients with a history of MI. The general pattern is quite similar, with very definite reductions in each of the three types of vascular events from

TABLE 1. *Suspected evolving myocardial infarction (MI) and survivors of myocardial infarction: reductions in risk (% ± SD) in vascular events among those assigned antiplatelet therapy*

Endpoint	Suspected evolving MI (ISIS-2)[a]	Survivors of MI (antiplatelet overview)[b]
Nonfatal reinfarction	49 ± 9	31 ± 5
Nonfatal stroke	46 ± 17	42 ± 11
Total vascular death	23 ± 4	15 ± 5
Any vascular event	28 ± 4	25 ± 5

[a] One month of daily aspirin (13).
[b] Longer-term months or years of daily treatment (1).

both short-term (4 weeks) and long-term (1–2 years) therapy. Treatment of 100 patients with acute MI with aspirin for 1 month can preclude approximately two vascular deaths and one nonfatal event (12). Continuation of this therapy for 1 or 2 years could probably preclude another two deaths and three nonfatal events, making the total avoided by early and late treatment equal to four fatal and four nonfatal events.

Based on the results of published trials, there is no convincing evidence that any of the newer antiplatelet agents is distinctly superior to aspirin in the secondary prevention of major vascular events, although ticlopidine has been found somewhat more effective than aspirin in reducing the risk of nonfatal stroke or death in high-risk patients (8).

In terms of primary prevention trials, a recently published overview of the U.S. Physicians' Health Study and British Doctors' Trial yields a highly significant ($p < 0.0001$) 32 ± 8% reduction in the risk of nonfatal MI, a nonsignificant 18 ± 13% increase in the risk of nonfatal stroke, and a nonsignificant 5 ± 10% reduction in total cardiovascular death, thus resulting in a statistically significant ($p < 0.05$) 13 ± 6% reduction in any vascular event (12). Although the percentage risk reduction for MI in apparently healthy male subjects is very similar to that obtained in secondary prevention trials, it is important to realize the markedly different size of the population exposed to treatment and the duration of such exposure. Thus, in the U.S. Physicians' Health Study, approximately 110 subjects had to be treated for 5 years in order to prevent one MI.

ANY RELATIONSHIP WITH THE DOSE?

A wide range of doses have been employed in the published clinical trials of aspirin, ranging from as low as 75 mg (18) to as high as 1,500 mg (1). In terms of clinical efficacy, no obvious dose-response relationship has been found over this 20-fold range of daily dosage, although a direct comparison of different doses within the same trial is limited to the UK-TIA trial (17). This is not surprising, inasmuch as a maximal suppression of platelet TXA_2 biosynthesis is obtained with a daily administration of 30 to 50 mg, and no additional effects on platelet biochemistry or function can be demonstrated with 324 mg/day in patients with unstable angina (5) or MI (6).

Several trials of low-dose (30–50 mg/day) aspirin are currently underway, but the results are not yet available. Thus, there is no clear indication today that one needs to use more than 75 to 100 mg (the content of a baby aspirin, in most countries) and, more importantly, the available evidence fails to justify repeated (e.g., three or four times daily) dosing to achieve the desired antithrombotic effect.

Only the U.S. Physicians' Health Study has used alternate-day dosing (325 mg every other day). However, no compelling argument exists to suggest that this might be the ideal dosing regimen. In fact, this particular regimen is not devoid of gastrointestinal toxicity (see below), and it impairs vascular prostacyclin production to a greater extent than the daily administration of lower doses (3).

LONG-TERM SAFETY OF ANTIPLATELET AGENTS

The mechanism of action of aspirin and the markedly different renewal rates of prostaglandin G/H synthase in platelets (over days, as a function of platelet turnover) and other cell types (over hours, as a function of *de novo* enzyme synthesis) theoretically should allow us to dissociate the desired antiplatelet effects from the unwanted vascular, gastric, and renal effects (16). In fact, evidence derived from large-scale clinical trials indicates that the incidence of side effects is dose-related in the range of doses tested so far (75–1,500 mg), whereas antithrombotic efficacy is not. Safety comparisons of different aspirin regimens in different clinical trials are difficult because of heterogeneity with respect to dosing interval, length of treatment, and aspirin formulation (e.g., regular versus enteric-coated). The only direct comparison is provided by the UK-TIA trial, as detailed in Table 2.

TABLE 2. *UK-TIA trial: percentage of patients ever reporting gastrointestinal side effects (mean, 4-year follow-up)*

	Allocated treatment			Statistical significance of difference (2p)	
	Placebo (n = 814)	Aspirin 300 mg/day (n = 806)	Aspirin 1,200 mg/day (n = 815)	Placebo vs. both aspirin	300 mg vs. 1,200 mg aspirin
Constipation	2.3	5.6	6.0	<0.001	NS
Indigestion, nausea, heartburn, etc.	24.0	29.0	39.0	<0.001	<0.001
Any gastrointestinal bleed	1.6	2.6	4.7	<0.01	<0.05
Serious gastrointestinal bleed (requiring hospital admission)	0.9	1.5	2.3	<0.05	NS

Data from ref. 17.
NS, not significant.

This clinical observation is consistent with the demonstration that a single daily administration of 300 to 325 mg will inhibit extraplatelet (e.g., gastric mucosa) cyclooxygenase activity substantially less (i.e., for only 4 hr–6 hr after dosing) than a twice, three-, or four-times daily regimen. However, it should be noted that even 325 mg every other day was associated with increased risk of upper gastrointestinal ulcers when given to apparently healthy male physicians for approximately 5 years (12).

Aspirin is unlikely to affect prostaglandin-dependent renal function when administered at 75 to 325 mg daily, because of the different dose-dependence of the inhibition of renal cyclooxygenase activity (15). The long-term safety of doses lower than 75 mg is not known; however, it can reasonably be assumed to be consistent with improved biochemical selectivity. It should be emphasized, however, that hemorrhagic complications (including the potential for excess cerebral bleeding) are inherently associated with the desired pharmacological effect and unlikely to be reduced by a further reduction in dosage.

Considerably less information is available on the long-term safety of newer antiplatelet agents. In the case of ticlopidine, both the possible occurrence of severe neutropenia and a significant increase in total cholesterol level (8) may be a source of concern. The safety of combining different antiplatelet agents is largely unknown, with the exception of aspirin plus dipyridamole or aspirin plus sulfinpyrazone combinations. Because none of these combinations has been shown to be superior to aspirin alone (1), the risk of additional toxicity does not appear to be justified.

ACKNOWLEDGMENT

I thank Maria Luisa Bonanomi and Pinuccia Protasoni for expert editorial assistance.

REFERENCES

1. Antiplatelet Trialists' Collaboration. (1988): *Br. Med. J.,* 296:320–331.
2. Balsano, F., Rizzoni, P., Violi, F., et al. (1990): *Circulation,* 82:17–26.
3. Clarke, R., Mayo, G., Price, P., and FitzGerald, G. A. (1990): *Circulation,* 82:III–602[Abstract].
4. Collins, R., Peto, R., MacMahon, S., et al. (1990): *Lancet,* 335:827–838.
5. De Caterina, R., Boem, A., Gazzetti, P., et al. (1991): *Thromb. Res.* (in press).
6. De Caterina, R., Giannessi, D., Boem, A., et al. (1985): *Thromb. Haemost.,* 54:528–532.
7. Fitzgerald, D. J., Roy, L., Catella, F., and FitzGerald, G. A. (1986): *N. Engl. J. Med.,* 315:983–989.
8. Gent, M., Blakely, J. A., Easton, J. D., et al. (1989): *Lancet,* 1:1215–1220.
9. Hamm, C. W., Lorenz, R. L., Bleifeld, W., Kupper, W., Wober, W., and Weber, P. C. (1987): *J. Am. Coll. Cardiol.,* 10:998–1004.
10. Hass, W. K., Easton, D., Adams, H. P., et al. (1989): *N. Engl. J. Med.,* 321:501–507.
11. Held, P. H., Yusuf, S., and Furberg, C. D. (1989): *Br. Med. J.,* 299:1187–1192.
12. Hennekens, C. H., Buring, J. E., Sandercock, P., Collins, R., and Peto, R. (1989): *Circulation,* 80:749–756.
13. ISIS-2. (1988): *Lancet,* 2:349–360.

14. O'Connor, P., Feely, J., and Shepherd, J. (1990): *Br. Med. J.,* 300:667–672.
15. Patrignani, P., Filabozzi, P., and Patrono, C. (1982): *J. Clin. Invest.,* 69:1366–1372.
16. Patrono, C. (1989): *TIPS,* 10:453–458.
17. Peto, R., Warlow, C., and the UK-TIA Study Group. (1988): *Br. Med. J.,* 296:316–320.
18. RISC Group. (1990): *Lancet,* 336:827–830.
19. Stein, B., Fuster, V., Halperin, J. L., and Chesebro, J. H. (1989): *Circulation,* 80:1501–1513.
20. Vejar, M., Fragasso, G., Hackett, D., et al. (1990): *Thromb. Haemost.,* 63:163–168.
21. Yusuf, S., Peto, R., Lewis, J., Collins, R., and Sleight, P. (1985): *Prog. Cardiovasc. Dis.,* 27:335–371.

Atherosclerosis Reviews, Volume 23,
edited by P. C. Weber and A. Leaf.
Raven Press, Ltd., New York © 1991.

Intervention Studies in Peripheral Vascular Disease

Hubert Stiegler and Eberhard Standl

*Department of Metabolic and Vascular Disease, City Hospital Schwabing,
Munich 40, D-8000 Germany*

Atherosclerosis of the lower limb results in peripheral vascular disease (PVD) and may lead to intermittent claudication, rest pain, gangrene, and finally amputation (7). Although major progress has been achieved during recent years in efficient lumen reconstructive procedures applicable to the arteries of the legs (7,26,30), in terms of intervention studies, peripheral vascular disease, as compared to coronary heart disease (CHD), has been largely neglected. Perhaps the need for such studies appeared to be less striking because of the successful development of the more invasive treatment options, e.g., percutaneous angioplasty with and without local thrombolysis, which also often represents the first step for an effective treatment approach of coronary artery disease (CAD) (7). In addition, there are also obvious difficulties with intervention studies in PVD, in particular with the appropriate assessment techniques (7). This review, therefore, deals mainly with the state of intervention studies in PVD and the imminent difficulties.

MORBIDITY AND PROGRESSION RATES

Apparent morbidity and progression rates of PVD depend largely on the method of assessment used. Considering only intermittent claudication or amputation—as in studies including the Framingham Study (15)—leads to a gross underestimation of significant disease. With more appropriate oscillometric techniques, a threefold higher prevalence and incidence rate was found in the Basle Artery Project, close to the figures for CHD (34). Amputation nowadays is rarely necessary, provided the patient is not a diabetic. On the other hand, the symptomatology of claudication and the need for amputation may be heavily influenced by factors other than peripheral vascular disease (7,26). Palpating pulses represent a subjective, investigator-dependent method and lead to insufficiently accurate and reproducible results. A minimal prerequisite for objective assessment also useful for epidemiological studies are additional ultrasound Doppler pressure readings and flow curve recordings (14). No anatomical imaging, however, is obtained by this approach. In terms of intervention studies, until recently, repeated high resolution angiograms and a sophisticated scoring system seemed to be warranted to yield at least a semiquantitative rating (4). Patients had to be subjected to the burden and potential risks of several angiograms for the purpose of scientific evaluation. Only a few intervention studies with a limited number of patients have been performed on that basis.

SPECIFIC RISK PREDICTORS AND PATHOGENETIC FACTORS

Any intervention has to be controlled for all other variables affecting the outcome of the disease. Although atherosclerotic disease of the lower limb is certainly within the framework of atherosclerosis as a generalized disease and its pathogenesis, little is known about specific risk predictors and pathogenetic factors of this distinct disease subentity. Several prospective population-based studies have emphasized cigarette smoking, diabetes, hypertension, and hyperlipidemias as independent risk predictors of peripheral vascular disease, with an overall predictive power of about 70% (7,13–15,25,32,34). None of these risk parameters, however, has been established as a true risk factor proven by intervention. The evaluation by multivariate analytical methods suggests a considerable contribution of parameters other than the above-mentioned ones to the risk of promoting PVD. Other likely candidates are hemostasiological abnormalities, which often are thought to be rather secondary than primary pathogenic events (7,24). Recently, microalbuminurea has been shown to be a highly significant marker of PVD, but the common denominator for this finding might be hypertension or a constitutional alteration in the extracellular vessel matrix (31).

A very important confounding factor in many studies seems to be age, which is a powerful risk marker and predictor in its own right and interacts intensively with a number of the other risk parameters (7,13–15,25,32,34). Accounting for age (and sex) is an apparent need for all PVD intervention studies. Moreover, the strong interdependence among most risk markers or predictors might be another pitfall when attempts are made to single out one particular risk factor by means of multivariate statistical analysis. In the light of recent observations in relation to syndrome X, this might be indeed misleading. The cluster of abnormalities characterizing the hyperinsulemia/insulin resistance syndrome includes:

Insulin resistance
Hyperinsulinemia
Central obesity
Hypertension
Glucose intolerance
Increased serum VLDL triglyceride
Decreased serum HDL cholesterol
Hyperuricemia
Increased risk of macrovascular disease

Insulin resistance appears to be genetically determined and may be present in predisposed individuals without obesity or evidence of impaired glucose tolerance (9,35). Those hyperinsulinemic subjects, however, compared to control subjects, exhibit relatively higher systolic and diastolic mean blood pressure values and serum triglyceride concentrations in addition to relatively lower HDL cholesterol levels in the absence of—and many years before—overt hypertension, dyslipo-proteinemias, and diabetes mellitus (35). Thus, it seems to be the long-term clustering of risk potential that precedes atherosclerotic disease without necessarily expressing all the manifest risk conditions later on. In fact, hyperinsulinemia and insulin resistance have been incriminated as risk factors for atherosclerotic complications as a result of a whole series of independent, large-scale, prospective studies (25,28). Interestingly enough, higher endogenous insulinemia and higher daily doses of insulin treatment have been found to be associated with and also predict PVD in a large group of diabetic patients.

In all, it seems difficult to control intervention studies in PVD for all risk parameters at the present time, not to mention the problem of a differential impact of risk conditions for different localizations—e.g., peripheral versus more proximal localization—of "peripheral" vascular disease.

INTERVENTION STUDIES

Although most textbooks list elimination of risk factors as first-line therapy of PVD, no clear-cut evidence is available to validate this recommendation on the basis of large-scale intervention studies. There are one open trial, one controlled trial, and one unpublished controlled trial in which repeated femoral angiograms have been rated in a limited number of hyperlipidemic and hypertensive patients secondary to intervention (1,8,16). Lipid-lowering was attempted according to the type of hyperlipidemia and compounds used, including cholestyramine, niacin, colestipol, clofibrate, neomycin, and lovastatin. The reported results were striking. After 13 months and $2\frac{1}{2}$ years, respectively, regression or slower progression of PVD was found in response to a significant lowering of blood lipids, but the "responder" or treatment groups consisted of a little more than 10 patients in each trial, and no (or only partial) effort was made to control for all the other risk variables.

Much larger series of patients have been recruited for secondary prevention trials evaluating antiplatelet agents, such as acetylsalicylic acid, dipyridamol, or ticlopidine. Hess et al. have reported a double-blind, placebo-controlled, prospective study in which 240 patients with PVD were randomly assigned to one of three treatment groups: aspirin 330 mg, dipyridamole 75 mg plus aspirin 330 mg, or placebo (12). An angiogram scoring system at entrance and at 2-year follow-up indicated that progression of the disease was most pronounced in the placebo-treated group and significantly less in the active treatment groups, in particular with regard to newly occurring occlusions (Fig. 1). But even in this larger series, it was difficult to control for all the other risk variables; in fact,

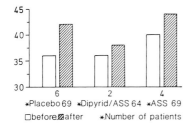

45 ⌐
40 -
35 -
30 ⌐
      6   2   4
*Placebo 69   *Dipyrid/ASS 64   *ASS 69
☐before.▨after   *Number of patients

FIG. 1. Angiographic sum score.

serum cholesterol, blood glucose, fibrinogen, systolic and diastolic blood pressure, and smoking habits changed—i.e., improved—during the course of the study in all three groups. When subgroups were considered, evidence was found that smokers and hypertensive subjects may benefit from antiplatelet drugs, in contrast to diabetics or hyperlipidemics. On the basis of smaller numbers, however, these effects were not significant. Of course, side effects such as gastrointestinal bleeding have to be measured against those "benefits." That aspirin, either alone or in combination with dipyridamole, might retard the progression of femoral artery stenosis to complete occlusion has also been suggested by Schoop et al. (21).

In another double-blind, randomized trial with a similar study protocol, the effect of ticlopidine was assessed (29). After a 1-year follow-up, 21 patients on ticlopidine—which, unlike aspirin, acts through mechanisms other than cyclooxygenase inhibition—showed a significantly reduced angiographic progression of PVD compared to 22 controls. Risk factors were said not to have been different between the two study groups.

Divergent effects have been observed with coumadine versus acetylsalicylic acid in large prospective trials subsequently to femoropopliteal endarterectomy or bypass (5,17,20). Whereas aspirin significantly decreased the rate of reocclusion after endarterectomy compared to anticoagulation with coumadine over 2 years (84 versus 58% patency; $p < 0.02$), coumadine was superior to aspirin in cases of femoropopliteal bypass operation (87 versus 65% patency after 2 years; $p < 0.05$). After transfemoral catheter angioplasty, the beneficial effects of aspirin in terms of decreased early and late reocclusion rate have been substantiated by several studies indicating that platelet aggregation and thrombus formation play an important role secondary to injuries of the intimal vessel layer, e.g., by angioplasty and endarterectomy (3,21,36).

There is only one double-blind, placebo-controlled aspirin trial, but it had a 7-year follow-up, subsequent to leg amputation due to gangrene (6). No favorable effect, however, could be proven in patients with severely advanced PVD who in addition were all diabetic. Hence, early stenosing PVD and secondary prevention of (re-)occlusion after intima lesions in the context of therapeutical procedures seem to be the best evaluated indications for the use of aspirin and related compounds in PVD.

Still, the situation in terms of so called vasoactive agents is particularly complex (3,27). Although numerous compounds have been developed since the 1930s

TABLE 1. Evaluation of "vasoactive" compounds in relation to severity of peripheral vascular disease (Fontaine grades II–IV)

"Vasoactive" compound	Suggested action	Efficacy tested in Fontaine stage		
		II	III	IV
(1) Buflomedil	Improved hemorheology. Effect on metabolic and cellular factors.	+	+	
(2) Naftidrofuryl	As for (1) + aggregation inhibition.	+	+	+
(3) Pentoxifylline	Improved hemorheology; aggregation inhibition.	+		+
(4) Prostaglandin E_1	As for (1) and (2) + vasodilatation and activation of fibrinolysis.	+	+	+

and countless studies have been performed, only recently have complaints been raised again about the unsatisfactory nature of our notions. Rarely, those intervention studies were performed based on sequential ratings of angiograms rather than on clinical grounds such as pain-free walking or disappearance of rest pain. This approach, however, may be severely hampered by the fact that any newly occurring obliteration of a main artery will induce collateral circulation, which

TABLE 2. "Vasoactive" agents: double-blind, placebo-controlled, prospective studies with significant improvement of intermittent claudication

Studies (ref.)	Agent	Length of treatment	Total patients (on "vasoactive" compound)	% Gain of pain-free walking distance
Becker et al. (1979)	N i.v.	14 days	210 (106)	183
Trübestein et al. (1982)	B	12 wk	93 (47)	97
Porter et al. (1982)	P	24 wk	128 (61)	56
Maas et al. (1984)	N	12 wk	104 (54)	68
Adhoute et al. (1986)	N	24 wk	118 (54)	94
Kiesewetter et al. (1987)	P[a]	4 wk	30 (15)	23
Rudofsky et al. (1988)	P i.v.	14 days	154 (75)	70
Kriessmann et al. (1988)	N[a]	12 wk	136 (71)	77
Rudofsky et al. (1988)	PE$_1$[a] i.v.	28 days	50 (25)	73
Diehm et al. (1989)[b]	PE$_1$[a] i.v. N[a]	21 days	(24) (24)	99 97
Lindgärde et al. (1989)	P	24 wk	150 (75)	80

N = Naftidrofuryl; B = Buflomedil; P = Pentoxifylline; PE$_1$ = Prostaglandin E$_1$.
[a] Trial following long-term exercise program.
[b] Randomized prospective trial.

will in turn improve, e.g., the ability to walk spontaneously, for up to 1 year. Furthermore, regular exercise has been shown to improve the walking ability of patients with intermittent claudication as much as 200% to 300%, depending on the localization of occlusion. The reported beneficial effects attributed to drug intervention have often not been better than the potential exercise effect.

With these limitations in mind, several scientific angiologic committees or associations have issued guidelines for the evaluation of "vasoactive" agents (2,33). In the meantime, a few longer-term double-blind, placebo-controlled trials with well-defined protocols and agents without "steel effects" have been completed. Table 1 lists those compounds, their suggested mechanisms of action, and the stage of PVD according to Fontaine in which they have been tested. In addition, Table 2 gives detailed data on trials in relation to claudicating patients, the numbers enrolled, the duration of the prospective double-blind study, and the effect on walking ability (27). In patients with early gangrene, prostaglandin E_1 seems to be superior to other compounds. Continuing controversies, however, should not be denied; negative results have also been obtained with the compounds just mentioned.

FUTURE PERSPECTIVES

New hopes have been raised for appropriate assessment and quantification of PVD without the need of sequential angiografies. Noninvasive Duplex sonography with high-resolution B mode imaging and color-coded Doppler devices allows high-precision measurement of the intima-media thickness of peripheral arteries and also shows more advanced arterial lesions with excellent quality in a three-dimensional way (10,11,22) (Fig. 2). Using this approach, a significant impact of serum cholesterol concentrations on extracranial carotid artery disease in young patients with familial hypercholesterolemia was established (23). Likewise, a marked reduction of intima-media thickness was observed during the first days after carotid endarterectomy when aspirin was administered (19).

In addition, new compounds are now on the horizon or already available for a better-targeted intervention. Increased glycosylation of the extracellular matrix of the vessel wall might become preventable and with it, advanced glycosylation end-products specific attacks of macrophages. Syndrome X and hyperinsulinemia

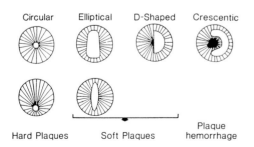

Circular   Elliptical   D-Shaped   Crescentic

Hard Plaques   Soft Plaques   Plaque hemorrhage

FIG. 2. Schematic diagram of atherosclerotic plaques from ultrasound cross sections.

can be approached by α-glucosidase inhibition and reduced postprandial blood glucose (18). Finally, powerful antihypertensive drugs (including ACE inhibitors and Ca-channel blockers and cholesterol-lowering agents such as HMG-CoA reductase-inhibitors) can now be safely administered in large-scale, long-term trials. It is now time for new intervention studies in PVD early in life, with new concepts, promising compounds, and noninvasive imaging.

REFERENCES

1. Barndt, R., Blankenhorn, D. H., and Crawford, D. W. (1977): Regression and progression of early femoral atherosclerosis in treated hyperlipoproteinemic patients. *Ann. Intern. Med.,* 86: 139–146.
2. Böhme, H., and Heidrich, H. (1988): Naftidrofuryl. *Vasa,* suppl 24:1–75.
3. Bollinger, A. (1988): Medikamentöse Therapie bei peripherer arterieller Verschlußkrankheit. *Schweiz Med. Wochenschr.,* 118:1283–1289.
4. Bollinger, A., Breddin, K., Hess, H., et al. (1981): Semiquantitative assessment of lower limb atherosclerosis from routine angiographic images. *Atherosclerosis,* 38:339–346.
5. Bollinger, A., and Brunner, U. (1985): Antiplatelet drugs improve the long term patency rates after femoro-popliteal endarterectomy. *Vasa,* 14:272–279.
6. Colwell, J. A., Bingham, S. F., Abraira, C., et al. (1986): Veterans Administration cooperative study on antiplatelet agents in diabetic patients after amputation for gangrene: II. Effects of aspirin and dipyridamol on atherosclerotic vascular disease rates. *Diabetes Care,* 9:140–148.
7. Dormandy, J., Stock, G., eds. (1990): *Critical leg ischaemia—its pathophysiology and management.* Berlin: Springer, pp. 1–172.
8. Duffield, R. G., Lewis, B., Miller, N. E., et al. (1983): Treatment of hyperlipidaemia retards progression of symptomatic femoral atherosclerosis. A randomized controlled trial. *Lancet,* 2: 639–642.
9. Eriksson, J., Franssila-Kallunki, A., Ekstrand, A., et al. (1989): Early metabolic defects in persons at increased risk for non–insulin-dependent diabetes mellitus. *N. Engl. J. Med.,* 321:337–343.
10. Gostonzyk, J. G., Heller, W. D., Gerhard, P., et al. (1988): B-scan ultrasound examination of the carotid arteries within a representative population (Monica Project Augsburg). *Klin. Wochenschr.,* 66(suppl):58–65.
11. Hennerici, M., and Steinke, W. (1988): Three-dimensional ultrasound imaging for the evaluation of progression and regression of carotid atherosclerosis. In: Hennerici, M., Sitzer, G., and Weger, H.-D., eds. *Carotid artery plaques.* Basel: Karger, pp. 115–132.
12. Hess, H., Mietaschk, A., and Deichsel, G. (1985): Drug induced inhibition of platelet function delays progression of peripheral occlusive arterial disease. *Lancet,* 2:415–419.
13. Janka, H. U. (1985): Five year incidence of major macrovascular complications in diabetes mellitus. *Horm. Metabol. Res.* suppl 15:15–19.
14. Janka, H. U., Standl, E., and Mehnert, H. (1980): Peripheral vascular disease in diabetes mellitus and its relationship to cardiovascular risk factors: screening with the Doppler-ultrasound technique. *Diabetes Care,* 3:207–213.
15. Kannel, W. B., and McGee, D. L. (1979): Diabetes and glucose tolerance as risk factor for cardiovascular disease: the Framingham Study. *Diabetes Care,* 2:120–126.
16. Kramsch, D. M., Blankenhorn, D. H., Azen, S. D., and Hemphill, L. C. (1990): Regression of atherosclerosis. Presented at the Symposium on treatment of severe dyslipoproteinemia in the prevention of coronary heart disease. Munich, Germany.
17. Kretschmer, G., Wenzl, E., Piza, F., et al. (1987): The influence of anticoagulant treatment on the probability of function in femoropopliteal vein by pass surgery: analysis of a clinical series (1978–1985) and interim evaluation of a controlled clinical trial. *Surgery,* 102:453–459.
18. Lebovitz, H. (1990): Treatment principles of reducing insulin resistance in NIDDM and pre-NIDDM (incl. a-glucosidase inhibition). In: Standl, E., ed. *Perspectives of the hyperinsulinemia/ insulin resistance syndrome in NIDDM.* München: MMV Medizin, pp. 82–95.
19. Rudofsky, G., Hirche, H., Meyer, P., and Altenhoff, B. (1986): Die Erfassung und Verlaufsbeo-

bachtung präklinischer Arteriosklerose mit dem Ultraschall-real-time-scan. *Klin. Wochenschr.,* 64(suppl 5:235–236.

20. Schneider, E., Brunner, U., and Bollinger, A. (1979): Medikamentöse Rezidivprophylaxe nach femoro-poplitealer Arterienrekonstruktion. *Angio* 2:73–77.

21. Schoop, W., Levy, H., Schoop, B., and Gaentzsch, A. (1983): Experimentelle und klinische Studien zu der sekundären Prävention der peripheren Arteriosklerose. In: Bollinger, A., and Rhyner, K., eds. *Thrombozytenfunktionshemmer, Wirkungsmechanismen, Dosierung und praktische Anwendung,* Stuttgart: Thieme, pp. 49–58.

22. Seifert, H., Jäger, K., Jöhl, H., and Bollinger, A. (1988): Stellenwert der Duplex-Sonographie in der Diagnose peripherer arterieller Durchblutungsstörungen. *Schweiz. Med. Wochenschr.,* 118: 554–557.

23. Spengel, F. A., Kaess, B., Keller, Ch., et al. (1988): Atherosclerosis of the carotid arteries in young patients with familial hypercholesterolemia. *Klin. Wochenschr.,* 66:65–68.

24. Standl, E., Janka, H. U., and Mehnert, H. (1984): Plasma-β-thromboglobulin and platelet aggregation in peripheral vascular disease. In: Balas, P., ed. *Angiology: new developments.* New York: Plenum, pp. 245–248.

25. Standl, E., Stiegler, H., Janka, H. U., et al. (1988): Risk profile of macrovascular disease in diabetes mellitus. *Diab. Metab.,* 14:505–511.

26. Standl, E., Stiegler, H., Janka, H. U., et al. (1989): Cerebral and peripheral vascular disease. In: Mogensen, C. E., and Standl, E., eds. *Prevention and treatment of diabetic late complications.* Berlin: De Gruyter, pp. 169–198.

27. Standl, E., Stiegler, H., Mathies, R., et al. (1991): Pharmacologic prevention and treatment of diabetic foot problems. In: Mogensen, C. E., and Standl, E., eds. *Pharmacology of diabetes.* Berlin, New York: De Gruyter, pp. 221–238.

28. Standl, E., and Vague, P. (1987): Hyperinsulinemia as a possible risk factor of macrovascular disease in diabetes mellitus. *Diabetes Metab. Rev.,* 13:277–394.

29. Stiegler, H., Hess, H., Mietaschk, A., et al. (1984): Einfluß von Ticlopidin auf die periphere obliterierende Arteriopathie. *Dtsch. Med. Wochenschr.,* 109:1240–1243.

30. Stiegler, H., Hufen, U., Weichenhain, B., et al. (1990): Ergebnisse der lokalen Thrombolyse unter Berücksichtigung einer diabetischen Stoffwechsellage. *Med. Klinik.,* 85:171–175.

31. Stiegler, H., Standl, E., Standl, R., et al. (1990): Risk profile and macroangiopathy of patients with type II-diabetes mellitus in general practice. *Vasa,* 19:119–128.

32. Uusitupa, M. I. J., Niskanen, L. K., Siitonen, O., Voutilainen, E., and Pyörälä, K. (1990): 5-Year incidence of atherosclerotic vascular disease in relation to general risk factors, insulin levels, and abnormalities in lipoprotein composition in non–insulin-dependent diabetic and nondiabetic subjects. *Circulation,* 82:27–36.

33. Widmer, L. K. (1981): Provisorische Richtlinien zur Prüfung der therapeutischen Wirksamkeit peripherer vasoaktiver Medikamente bei arterieller Durchblutungsstörung. *Vasa,* 4:337–341.

34. Widmer, L. K., Biland, L., and Delley, A. (1986): Risikoprofil bzw. Morbidität bei peripherer arterieller Verschlußkrankheit. In: Trübestein, G., ed. *Conservative therapy of arterial occlusive disease.* Stuttgart: Thieme, pp. 513–518.

35. Zavaroni, I., Bonora, E., Pagliara, M., et al. (1989): Risk factors for coronary artery disease in healthy persons with hyperinsulinemia and normal glucose tolerance. *N. Engl. J. Med.,* 320: 702–706.

36. Zeitler, E., Reichold, J., Schoop, W., and Loew, G. (1973): Einfluß von Acetylsalicylsäure nach perkutanter Rekanalisation arterieller Obliterationen nach Dotter. *Dtsch. Med. Wochenschr.,* 98:1285–1288.

Atherosclerosis Reviews, Volume 23,
edited by P. C. Weber and A. Leaf.
Raven Press, Ltd., New York © 1991.

The Cholesterol Story

More Questions Than Answers

A. Weizel

Heinrich-Lanz-Krankenhaus, Mannheim, Germany

Cholesterol has been under discussion worldwide during the last few years. Several programs have been initiated to inform the public and practicing physicians of the latest developments in the scientific field. Practical consequences with regard to prophylaxis and therapy have been put forward by panels of scientists and medical associations. Among these programs are The National Cholesterol Education Program in the U.S. and The German Cholesterol Initiative (3,8).

The basis of our therapeutic approach is the belief that elevated plasma cholesterol is a risk factor for coronary heart disease (CHD), and that lowering of cholesterol by whatever means possible can help to prevent CHD.

There is not much doubt about the statistical association of elevated cholesterol with CHD. However, the recommendations that have been given, as far as treatment of elevated cholesterol is concerned, have not been acclaimed universally. Criticism has come not only from outside sources but also from within the medical community. One example of this criticism was an article published in 1989 by Brett in the *New England Journal of Medicine* which was titled "How should practicing physicians interpret the published data for patients?" (2).

The problem for the practicing physician is indeed to decide the degree to which scientific results can be applied in daily practice. A scientist can recommend a therapy on the basis of statistically significant results accepting the fact that an "insignificant" number of patients will not profit from this therapy. However, a practicing physician wants a therapy that will benefit every single patient. In my opinion, recent developments have made the decision to treat individual patients even more difficult for the practicing physician.

Our goal as practicing physicians is to prevent CHD and in particular fatal myocardial infarction, which is one of the leading causes of death in Western countries. This general and often cited objective should be examined more closely. Unfortunately there are not much data on the incidence of coronary events in the general population, other than fatal myocardial infarction.

If we look at this data, however, there are two distinct trends: (a) fatal myocardial infarction is decreasing in incidence within the male population (Table

TABLE 1. *Mortality from myocardial infarction in West Germany*

	1985	1986	1987
Male (no.)	48,056	46,515	45,986
Female (no.)	33,970	33,771	33,768

1) and (b) fatal myocardial infarction is an event that occurs predominantly in the age group older than 65 years. In West Germany only 30% of fatal myocardial infarctions were found in the age group younger than 65 years (Table 2).

It seems that, at least in West Germany, fatal myocardial infarction is predominantly a disease in old and very old people and therefore a consequence of medical progress and increased life span. It is an almost philosophical question as to whether we should try to prevent myocardial infarction in this age group, and I think we should be very reluctant with regard to therapy of these persons. There is, however, no doubt that we should undertake every effort to define persons who are candidates for early myocardial infarction.

CHD has two clinical aspects which do not necessarily occur in the same patients—myocardial infarction and other coronary events, e.g., angina pectoris. Whereas data on fatal myocardial infarctions is registered in most countries, data on the prevalence of nonfatal myocardial infarction and other coronary events is not so easy to find. Recent studies have given some insight into the prevalence of these cardiovascular events.

The Lipid Research Clinics Study (LRC) and the Helsinki Heart Study (HHS) have produced pertinent data (5,7). Both studies were studies of primary prevention in persons without clinical signs of CHD at the beginning of the study. Intervention was performed by administration of cholestyramine in the LRC study and by administration of gemfibrocil in the HHS study. The effect of either drug was compared with placebo.

In both studies, only men who were considered to belong to the high-risk group were included. At the end of the studies there was no significant difference in mortality between the treated and the placebo group but there were marked differences in the frequency of nonfatal coronary events. The interesting aspect of these results was the fact that the incidence of these coronary events was rather low. The incidence in the untreated control group was 9.8% in the LRC study and 4.1% in the HHS. The incidence in the treated group was lower, as was

TABLE 2. *Age adjusted mortality from myocardial infarction in West Germany, 1987*

Age (years)	Number	Percentage
25–45	941	2
45–65	13,237	29
65–75	13,308	29
75+	18,490	40

expected, but not very much lower. The incidence dropped from 9.8% to 8.1% in the LRC study and from 4.1% to 2.7% in the HHS. These data have given rise to discussions of interpretation. Brett (2) has pointed out that these data are misleading, if these small, absolute differences are expressed as rather large relative differences.

The manufacturers of the drugs that were used in these studies claim that there was a reduction of coronary events by 20% to 30%. Although this is perfectly correct, these impressive relative numbers are based on rather small absolute numbers. These results might entail therapeutic consequences. If coronary events occur at a relatively low incidence even in high-risk groups, one must conclude that a large number of patients (especially those at low risk) will undergo treatment without justification. Unfortunately, I believe that we are undoubtedly treating large numbers of persons who will never suffer from coronary sclerosis at all. In other words, we seem unable to identify correctly the persons at risk, if we take total cholesterol as a criterion for therapy.

Bearing this in mind, it is interesting to see that there are two approaches to CHD. There are somewhat confusing because they seem to be pointing in diametrically opposite directions: identification of high-risk persons with refined biochemical markers vs. population-wide screening with total cholesterol determinations. On the one hand, we have the much publicized campaign aimed at screening complete populations to identify people at risk, based solely on determinations of cholesterol, in special cases supported by high-density lipoprotein (HDL)- and low-density lipoprotein (LDL)-cholesterol determinations. On the other hand, there are numerous scientists in many laboratories worldwide trying to identify biological markers that will better characterize patients at risk.

I believe this is a thoroughly necessary task because recent findings have shown that not even elevated cholesterol levels in familial hypercholesterolemia are true indicators of coronary risk. Wiklund et al. (12) and Seed et al. (13) have shown that even this group is not homogenous. There are patients with familial hypercholesterolemia who develop premature CHD and others who do not follow that pattern. The difference that seems to distinguish these two groups is the level of Lp(a). Patients with elevated cholesterol and elevated Lp(a) seem to be the persons at risk (Table 3). If there are such enormous differences of morbidity in a group that has been one of the solid bases of our decisions to treatment, how can we deal with "normal" hypercholesterolemic patients?

However, it is not only the Lp(a) that is confounding the picture. There are

TABLE 3. *Familial hypercholesterolemia: coronary heart disease (CHD), total cholesterol (TC), and LP(a) levels*

	No CHD	CHD
TC mmol/L	10.0 (9.9)	9.6 (10.1)
Lp(a) mg/L	144 (180)	283 (250)

Data from refs. 12 and 13.

other factors as well that have not been completely elucidated with regard to their connection with CHD. These include (a) apoproteins and subfractions, (b) coagulation factors, e.g., plasminogen activator inhibitor (PAI-I), and possibly (c) triglycerides (TGs).

Some apoproteins seem to have good predictive values. It has been shown that some lipoprotein subfractions may be better indicators than total lipoprotein fractions. It has also been claimed that lipoproteins need oxidation to be truly pathogenic. The blood clotting system may be more involved than we thought, e.g. fibrinogen and PAI-I.

One extremely obscure area in my opinion is the question of the atherogenicity of TGs, complicated even more by the fact that recent developments seem to indicate that not only fasting TGs but also postprandial TGs should be considered (11).

Here again, as a clinician, I wonder how to proceed. All therapeutic studies have been performed on patients with "pure" hypercholesterolemia. This disorder is infrequent in daily practice. The majority of patients with dyslipidemia fall into the categories of mixed hyperlipemia with elevated TG levels in addition to elevated cholesterol levels. To my knowledge, there are no convincing studies that have shown that treatment of mixed hyperlipidemia gives the same encourging results as does the therapy of pure hypercholesterolemia. The same uncertainties prevail, if one considers treatment of hypercholesterolemia in women and elderly people. To date, there are no data to justify therapy in these groups.

If one bears all these uncertainties of diagnostic procedures and unconvincing indications in mind, one wonders if we are not putting the "cart before the horse" if we initiate population-wide screening programs and recommend therapeutic interventions based on determinations of total cholesterol, HDL cholesterol and LDL cholesterol.

The situation does not get much easier if we turn our attention to the official therapeutic recommendations. It is generally agreed that dietary and drug therapy can be used to lower plasma cholesterol. Both therapies are controversial.

As far as diet is concerned, there is no doubt, that a statistical association exists between the intake of cholesterol and the amount of saturated fatty acids, and the incidence of CHD. Therefore, it seems logical to change the plasma cholesterol levels by modification of the diet. However, dietary intervention studies are rare and subject to many technical problems. It is impossible to conduct a double-blind dietary study and it is exceedingly difficult to monitor dietary adherence.

Dietary therapy as such has come under criticism. The principles of a lipid-lowering diet are low cholesterol intake, partial replacement of saturated fatty acids with unsaturated fatty acids, and reduction of total fat calories. This recommendation is not without problems. As far as dietary cholesterol is concerned, it is known that great interindividual variations exist in response to dietary cholesterol. The level of 300 mg of dietary cholesterol/day that is recommended is an arbitrary level that is not supported by experimental evidence. If we do not find suitable tests that distinguish dietary responders from nonresponders a large number of persons will undergo dietary modifications with no effect on their cholesterol levels.

The situation is clearer if we look at saturated fatty acids. We have fairly good evidence that these fatty acids influence cholesterol in an undesirable fashion. Therefore, there are not too many objections to reducing saturated fatty acids in the diet.

There is more disagreement as far as the *unsaturated fatty acids* are concerned. For many years, we have recommended that persons with elevated cholesterol levels consume a certain percentage of polyunsaturated fatty acids. Safflower oil and corn oil have been some of the favored oils in the hypolipidemic diets. However it has been shown that these fatty acids lower LDL cholesterol but have no positive influence on HDL cholesterol. A recent article showed that HDL cholesterol was higher on a diet with polyunsaturated fatty acids compared to a diet rich in monounsaturated fatty acids (4).

For many years *monounsaturated fatty acids* were considered to be neutral with respect to plasma cholesterol levels. Here again, there has been a gradual change in thinking. Nutritionally interested lipidologists now recommend monounsaturated fatty acids, for example, in the form of olive oil. Olive oil is a product that has been consumed in many countries for long periods without adverse effects, and recent studies have shown that adequate doses of oleic acid can lower LDL cholesterol without adverse effects on HDL cholesterol (6,9).

There is a new group of fatty acids that so far have not played any part in the discussion—the *trans-fatty acids*. Trans-fatty acids are found in milk (4 g/100 g of milk fat), certain margarines, and shortenings and fats used for frying. The trans-fatty acids are formed during hydrogenation of polyunsaturated fatty acids. Roughly 6% to 8% of total fat is consumed as trans-fatty acids. In a report by Mensink and Katan (10) that was recently published, the authors showed that trans-fatty acids raised LDL cholesterol and lowered HDL cholesterol. It is not clear whether these new developments will change our dietary approach again.

ω-3 *Fatty acids* have been under discussion for much longer periods, and here again, it is not certain how much they influence our dietary approach.

If one looks at the results of studies (that is, the LRC study and HHS) in which diet was a part of the therapy, it is obvious that the effect of the dietary intervention was not very convincing. Even in these studies in which there was a large degree of medical presence, the average lowering of cholesterol was about 5%. Therefore, I am very skeptical about the effect of dietary advice on a large community- or population-wide scale.

One of the drawbacks of dietary therapy is the fact that most physicians (at least in Germany) have no formal training in dietary therapy; therefore, many of them are simply not qualified to give sound dietary advice. As a consequence, we find in hyperlipidemia, as in many other metabolic diseases, that failure of dietary therapy or the lack of dietary advice often leads to drug therapy.

Our concept of drug therapy as far as CHD is concerned is largely based on the results of large-scale drug trials, e.g., the LRC Study and the HHS (5,7). For a practicing physician, it is interesting to look at the drugs that were used in these studies and to establish whether the results can be reproduced in daily practice. Four lipid-lowering drugs and their controversial aspects are discussed below.

(a) Cholestyramine was used in the LRC Study. It is a very effective lipid-lowering drug and it is most effective in higher doses—it is also a very unpleasant drug. The LRC Study has shown that only about one-half of the participants were able to take the prescribed dose of 24 g/day and this is the common experience of most physicians who have worked with this drug. In addition, we do know that cholestyramine has no effect on HDL cholesterol, which makes this drug less desirable. (b) Nicotinic acid could be an alternative drug. But here again we find the problem of compliance. It is an effective drug but many patients will not take it because they cannot tolerate the side effects. (c) What about the fibrates? In Europe, these drugs have been the most widely used drugs in the treatment of hyperlipidemia. The side effects with these drugs are fewer than with other drugs, although the lithogenic effect of some fibrates is troublesome in long-term therapy. Unfortunately, however, these drugs exert their main effect on the very-low-density lipoprotein (VLDL) fraction and to a lesser degree on the LDL fraction. In some instances, there is even a completely undesirable rise of LDL concentration when the VLDL concentration falls. Taking all the facts together, most people with high cholesterol who need cholesterol lowering usually do not profit very much from fibrate therapy. (d) For some time now, the group of HMG CoA-reductase inhibitors has been available. This group of drugs fulfills the requirements for cholesterol lowering by lowering the LDL cholesterol fraction and raising the HDL cholesterol fraction at the same time. It seems to be the ideal solution to our problems provided long-term toxicity does not prevent the application of these drugs. What makes these drugs so attractive is the fact that they usually lead to a marked reduction of plasma cholesterol of up to 30%. Recent studies in patients with coronary bypass surgery have shown that a lowering of plasma cholesterol of this order of magnitude can lead to regression of atherosclerotic plaques (1).

It is my impression that this is the first realistic approach to treatment of patients with elevated cholesterol in daily practice. The other regimens—cholestyramine and nicotinic acids—are difficult to maintain outside of clinical studies and specialized lipid clinics. It has been shown that a lowering of cholesterol of 20% to 30% is necessary to halt progression or even induce regression in secondary prevention and I would not be surprised if a similar degree of cholesterol lowering was necessary to prevent effectively development or progression of lesions in primary prevention.

To date, this class of drugs seem to be the drugs of choice for persons with cholesterol levels above 300 mg/dl, and fibrates or statins for persons who have cholesterol values in the range between 240 and 300 mg/dl, elevated LDL cholesterol levels and/or associated risk factors. Between 30% and 40% of the normal

TABLE 4. Distribution of cholesterol in a normal population

Age (years)	Cholesterol levels		
	200–249 mg/dl	250–299 mg/dl	300 mg/dl
25–29	39%	10%	1%
30–39	43%	20%	5%
40–49	44%	29%	9%
50–59	44%	31%	9%
60–69	39%	30%	12%

population have been shown to have cholesterol levels between 200 and 250 mg/dl (Table 4). These people are often worried about our statement that the ideal level is below 200 mg/dl. What approach should be taken when dealing with these patients? In my opinion, therapeutic interventions should be exercised with caution. If these people are of normal weight, normal LDL-cholesterol values and no other risk factors intervention is not indicated at all. If risk factors are present, it is to be decided on an individual basis if treatment is justified.

SUMMARY AND CONCLUSION

Elevated cholesterol plasma levels are established risk factors for CHD. HDL cholesterol and LDL cholesterol determinations are additional discriminators to define persons at risk. Other biochemical parameters such as (apoproteins, LP(a), and others will help physicians to focus on patients with high risk. Population-wide programs encounter tremendous difficulties because present diagnostic instruments are not able to define clearly persons at risk. There are no data to justify prophylactic measures in women and elderly people. Dietary therapy suffers from a lack of information concerning the effects of different dietary constituents on lipid parameters. Drug therapy shows significant and reproducible effects. However, some of the drugs lead to problems of compliance, and other drugs influence the VLDL fraction rather than the LDL fraction. Long-term toxicity may be a problem with some of the newer drugs. The ideal situation for intervention is achieved when a dedicated physician works together with a cooperative patient who fulfills the criteria, according to our present knowledge, of a high-risk patient.

REFERENCES

1. Blankenhorn, D. H., Neslm, S. A., Johnson, R. L., Sammarco, M. E., Azen, S. P., and Cashin-Hemphill, L. (1987): Beneficial effects of combined Colestipol-Niacin therapy on coronary atherosclerosis and coronary venous bypass grafts. *JAMA,* 257:3233–3240.
2. Brett, A. S. (1989): Treating hypercholesterolemle. How should practicing physicians interpret the published data for patients? *N Engl J Med,* 321:676–679.
3. Deutsche Cholesterin Initiative. (1990): *Deutsches Ärzteblatt,* 87:1358–1362.
4. Dreon, D. M., Vranizan, K. M., Krauss, R. M., Austin, M. A., and Wood, P. D. (1990): The

effects of polyunsaturated fat vs monounsaturated fat on plasma lipoproteins. *JAMA,* 263:2462–2466.

5. Frick, M. H., Elo, O., Haapa, K., et al. (1987): Helsinki Heart Study: primary-prevention trial with gemfibrozil in middle-aged men with dyslipidemia: safety of treatment, changes in risk factors, and incidence of coronary heart disease. *N Engl J Med,* 317:1237–1245.

6. Grundy, S. M. (1989): Monounsaturated fatty acid and cholesterol metabolism: implication for dietary modification. *J Nutr,* 119:529–533.

7. Lipid Research Clinics Program. The Lipid Research Clinics Primary Preventions Trial results. Reduction in incidence of coronary heart disease. (1984): *JAMA,* 251:351–364.

8. Report of the National Cholesterol Education Program. Expert Panel on detection, evaluation and treatment of high cholesterol in adults. (1988): *Arch Intern Med,* 148:36–69.

9. Mensink, R. P., de Groot, M. J., van den Broeke, C. T., Severijnen-Nobel, A. P., Denacke, P. N., and Katan, M. B. (1989): Effect of monounsaturated fatty acids versus complex carbohydrates on serum lipoproteins and apoproteins in healthy men and women. *Metabolism,* 38: 172–178.

10. Mensink, R. P., and Katan, M. B. (1990): Effect of dietary trans fatty acids on high-density and low-density lipoprotein cholesterol levels in healthy subjects. *N Engl J Med,* 323:439–445.

11. Schettler, G., and Klör, H. U., eds. (1990): Postprandialer Lipoproteinstoffwechsel und Atherosklerose. *Klin Wschr,* 68(suppl XXII) III-V.

12. Seed, M., Hoppichler, F., et al. (1990): Relation of serum lipoprotein (a) concentration and apolipoprotein (a) phenotype to coronary heart disease in patients with familial hypercholesterolemia. *N Engl J Med,* 322:1494–1499.

13. Wiklund, O., Angelin, B., et al. (1990): Apolipoprotein (a) and ischaemic heart disease in familial hypercholesterolemia. *Lancet,* 335:1360–1363.

Atherosclerosis Reviews, Volume 23,
edited by P. C. Weber and A. Leaf.
Raven Press, Ltd., New York © 1991.

Subject Index